The Natural Approach To Essential Oils

2nd Edition

Jane Lawson

DISCLAIMER

The information in this book is not a substitute to medical advice. You the reader should never delay seeking medical advice, disregard or replace medical advice or discontinue medical treatment based on the information in this book. To the extent that you rely on any information in this book, you assume all risks involved in such reliance.

CONTENTS

1   Introduction   1

2   Come Into the Garden   6

3   What Are Essential Oils?   13

4   Contraindications Of Essential Oils   18

5   The Citrus Garden - Emotions   28

6   The Mental Garden - Mental   53

7   The Arbour - Relationships   83

8   The Herb Garden - Physical   112

9   Exotics & Grasses – Dreams & Aspirations   157

10   Safety and Blending   193

ACKNOWLEDGMENTS

This book was conceived in Aberdeen some 25 years ago. During its gestation it has travelled to Anglesey, Devon, Cheshire and finally to Gloucestershire.
In 2022 I decided it was time to review and revise the original, the results of which you hold in your hand now.

First and foremost, I want to thank my teacher Irene Latter who set me on this path of lifelong learning and discovery.
To my friends Sandy, Glen and Nerys in Anglesey who encouraged and supported me during the early years.
My steadfast friend Lorna, who ironically hails from Aberdeen, who has been my support and mentor and unfailing friend through the following years. I could never have done this without my Personal Angel.
Merlin, my astrologer friend, for his spiritual guidance and un-wavering support.
Sam Neffendorf, for 'tapping' me over the last hurdle for the first edition.
But most of all my pendulum, (Teach) and my clients and students over the decades. With gratitude to them, I have learnt more about Essential Oils than I have from any lecture, book or chemistry.

INTRODUCTION

It's my birthday. With a mug of tea in my hand, I look through the dining room window and see that my garden is a mess. It has lain dormant and neglected for the past seven to eight years. I am not sure, and cannot recall exactly when I stopped paying attention to what had been my sanctuary. I do remember various events, which began to pull my attention away and distract me. These events culminated in an explosion of negative emotions, which drained me of any energy I had to tend my garden. With a lack of energy, no enthusiasm, and a very distrustful and cynical heart, I became a hedgehog. Armed for protection with my prickly spikes I curled myself up into a little ball and hibernated.

But my hibernation was fitful. Every time I uncurled to take a peek at my garden, I was attacked again and again. The onslaught was so relentless that the day came where I could no longer curl up into the safety of my prickly orb, and the only escape route left to me was to make a run through a small door which was left ajar in the wall surrounding my garden.

My garden had been perfect for me. It was almost totally enclosed by a red brick wall. It was not square like a box, but more egg shaped. The wall had fallen down a little at the narrow end, where the sun rose in the morning. Where the sun set at the wider end the bricks formed seven archways. The seventh, in the middle, was the door through which I escaped.

I would get up of a morning and enter my garden to be greeted by the sun rising through the tumbledown part of the wall. I spent my days, weeding, pruning, planting, harvesting and pottering in the glorious sunshine. I soaked up the wonderful aromas the herbs and flowers released during the day. I would listen to the grasses and leaves of the trees as they whispered to me in the gentle breeze. I had my own daily, living rainbow in the foray of colours my plants showed me. My taste buds were periodically tickled as I nibbled at chives here, an apple there. My hands became sensitive to the array of botanical requests each individual plant required. Some needed a gentle, loving touch; others preferred a firmer, steady hand. I talked, whispered and sometimes sang ceaselessly through the day. Daily, my senses were overwhelmingly intoxicated. I was content and full of joy as my heart was filled with love for my garden. Tranquility and peace enveloped me as my garden returned love and bliss to me.

Just before sunset I would sit in what I called my 'meditation spot', and gaze through the seventh archway, to contemplate and reflect on the day's events. I would bask myself in the gratitude I felt to the 'powers that be' for having given me yet another wonderful day.

Each night I would retire to bed knowing that as long as I tended to my garden with love, honesty and diligence, all would be well in my world. So, I fell into a peaceful slumber each night, trusting that everything was as it should be in my universe.

What began this steady, almost systematic destruction of my sanctuary garden?

I awoke one morning feeling off balance, my instincts knew that something was not right. I got out of my bed and went to my garden, only to find that the sun was not shining brightly as it usually did. I surveyed my garden, section-by-section, part-by-part, looking for a sign of where the disruption had happened. A cloud came over the sun. My whole garden was plummeted into dark shadows. The aromas withdrew themselves. The breeze stopped; there was an eerie silence. Colours became hidden in the shadows. The sweet taste in my mouth had turned bitter. My once steady, strong yet gentle hands shook uncontrollably. My throat became dry and felt strangled. No gentle words of love came out, but a desperate, heart-rending cry from the depths of my soul, which brought me to my knees. My father had been diagnosed with cancer.

My father's diagnosis was like the first tumbleweed to invade my garden. Just like cancer, it twists and turns itself around healthy plants. Just like cancer, you don't notice it at first, until you discover one of your plants; shrubs or bush is dying or already dead. Just like cancer this weed is pervasive, arrogant, stubborn and destroys everything in its path as it sucks the life force out of other living organisms. This horrible, most terrible and spiteful weed, just like the cancer, had started its attack on the focal point of my garden, my world. My beautiful oak tree which had always stood tall and firm and strong, giving shade and coolness in the heat of the day, shelter from the rain and wind, was slowly being eaten away. My oak, that had lived, and therefore seen and experienced much more of this world than I had, or could ever hope to. My oak, which had taught me so much from its wisdom of the ages through its whisperings, as I rested my weary back against its trunk. From this central point in my garden, I could walk around its massive trunk and look at each aspect of my universe. If there were a part of my garden that was not as well as it should be and I could not see what needed to be done to love it better, my oak would always whisper a solution for me. But now my oak was dying, my father was dying, their whisperings were becoming fewer and fewer.

While I grieved an all-consuming living grief over my dying oak, while I battled to save my dying friend through memories at least, this relentless tumbleweed continued its onslaught of total annihilation of my garden. I was so blind to its attack that I never noticed it was going on in the rest of my world. Until one morning, on entering my garden, to love my oak some more, to ease its pain in its final death throws; a blanket of large, white, trumpet shaped flowers confronted me. The tumbleweed had taken over, and won. My father had passed over. My beautiful oak was dead. My garden, my world was in ruin, no longer recognisable. Utterly disfigured by this cancerous weed that I had allowed to eat away at everything I held like a precious gift, which I called my life. That was over twenty-five years ago.

Twenty years ago, discarding my prickly orb I escaped with my children through the seventh archway. We headed south towards the sun armed with nothing more than our love for each other that bonded the four of us together like super glue and our individual determinations to re-build our gardens, our lives.

We all at some stage in our lives experience unavoidable personal emotional heartache. These experiences teach us something about our own strengths and weaknesses.   They leave us with a plethora of feelings that we do our best to evaluate and learn from. Sometimes though, we cannot deal with or handle the responses we have to these emotions and it becomes easier to just bury them deep within our subconscious, rather than face them head on. Sometimes we just don't like our responses, and what deep hidden depths of our personalities suddenly come to the surface, so it's easier to 'just don't go there'. But whom are we kidding? Avoidance of the issues just puts things off for another day. We keep avoiding, running away or burying those parts of our personalities we would just rather not face - thank you very much! It's not because it's too much like hard work, or a fatalistic sense of 'that's just life'. The reality and truth of the matter is that it's the pain we would have to go through to resolve these issues. Yep, that's the REAL issue, the pain. Pain and hurt will only go away, and if you can only take this one thought away from this book, if you LOVE IT BETTER.

Sometimes it's just mundane things that get to us. One off little thing that can aggravate us, to a greater or lesser extent. Other times there are ongoing niggles which don't seem to go away, until the day comes when we wake up and realise that it is down to ourselves to reach a resolution. Many a time, by this stage only what seems to be drastic action is the only course left for us to take.

Wouldn't it be just wonderful if we could not only pre-empt any given horrid situation, but even better, know that whatever life chooses to throw at us we can handle and deal with it in a calm, cool, collected, rational and most importantly a wise way? A way which is a win / win situation for all rather than confrontational? Of course, it would! Take this a step further, and one of the basic laws of physics teaches us this - like attracts like! So, the more you can deal with your life from this calm, cool and collected place, I will call this a 'centered' space, the more of the same you will attract! Wonderful!

But how do you start to turn your perspective of life around? How quickly can you come from this place of centeredness? How much of your time do you have to invest to achieve this peaceful pace to your life? How much emotional pain will you have to go through to achieve this? You have already started to turn your perspective on life around by choosing to read this book. The speed by which this can be achieved is totally individual to your circumstances and how committed you are to improving your life. You don't have to invest very much time at all! That's right, the processes I will show you in this book can be done in tandem with your everyday life routines. The emotional pain ah, that old chestnut. Well, do you want to improve your life? Do you want to attract to you only that which serves your highest good? Isn't crossing a small bridge of emotional pain to reach the opposite bank where the sun shines, you have a smile on your face and most importantly you feel empowered, worth it? Of course, it is! I would like to introduce you to a model that you can use to help you with unresolved issues, past, present and even the ones that might be looming on the horizon for you in the future. Tools that will help you cross that little bridge to a better way of life. This tool is all around you, it's Mother Nature's gift to us, and it's the plant kingdom. But before I do that, let's have a look at a few other aspects in a little more detail. We are going to do this so that you can get your own starting point, find the right key to unlock your door to a more loving, peaceful, joyful future, your garden of serenity.

2.

COME INTO THE GARDEN

How about your garden? How is it looking? No, don't imagine your actual garden if you have one. Not even what you would like your back yard to look like, perfect urban chic. Stretch your imagination. Let your imagination run free, run wild, get right into nature. Your garden has no limits, if you want, let it be so large, that no matter where you are, whatever part of your garden you are in, nobody can see you. A visitor would need to call your name to find out where you are.

Close your eyes. Begin with a blank canvas. There are many ingredients to your garden. A small arbour of trees, an herb garden, a flowerbed or two, or three! Grasses, citrus trees, what else? You know. You can see the colours. You can hear the breeze rustle the leaves and grasses. You can smell all the different scents as you begin to wander through your sanctuary, your life. You can taste the orange you have gently plucked from your tree. You can feel the different textures of the leaves and petals. This is your garden, your fantasy. Can you see it? Can you create your garden with each of these ingredients? Add an ornament here; a beautiful bench seat there, a pond or a pool to surprise you as you round a corner. What about a child's garden toy? Or an abandoned walking stick? A book left open on a grassy patch? Whatever aspect of your life you look at, it always has an emotional response, be it either a good or bad reaction. Our emotional response to a situation will govern how we deal and handle that situation.

If you start with emotional peace, mentally you will think more clearly. You are then in a better position to deal with your relationships. As these upward spiral progresses, your physical wellbeing improves and your immune system is fighting fit as it becomes less compromised. With all these elements in place, you are more open and prepared for your spiritual journey. This could be interpreted to mean achieving your dreams and aspirations, or discovering what really makes you tick. Whatever path your spiritual journey takes it will bring you full circle back to your emotional self. The constant circle of life is now working in a positive upward motion, and not fighting against the tide in a negative, downward spiral.

Everything we do in life, everything we experience, has its root in our emotional attitude and reaction.

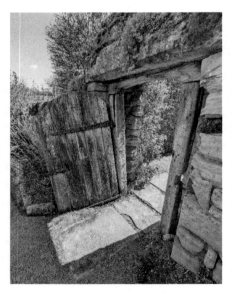

Photo reproduced by kind permission of Paula-Marie Turner in Felley Priory Gardens, Nottinghamshire, UK

In the following two diagrams I have used work as an example to demonstrate the positive and negative life cycles we have. You can substitute work with the emotions you have perhaps towards your partner or children. Play around with the two cycles substituting whatever you like from your life, but always start at the emotional point.

Dreams & Aspirations – Grasses and Exotic Garden

Here comes that promotion! Or you might want to try something new. You have the energy, support, positive mental attitude, and feel totally confident to try it!

Emotional – The Citrus Garden

Imagine your work situation, which is your dream job, you are completely happy and satisfied with it. You look forward to the next day at work with a smile on your face.

Physical – The Herb Garden

Physically you can't remember the last time you popped a painkiller, let alone visited the doctor!

Mental – The Flower Garden

You make decisions with clarity and optimism.

Relationships The Tree Garden

Your boss is happy; you go home your partner is glad to see you because you don't bring your work home, your children are happy because you still have bags of energy for them!

Negative Cycle Starts here

Dreams and Aspirations – Grasses and Exotic Garden

Life seems a constant struggle, and all those dreams and aspirations you have for you and those you love seem a million light years away.

Emotional – The Citrus Garden

Emotionally, you are not happy with your job. You are constantly thinking about a better one and how you can get out of this one.

Physical – The Herb Garden

As this negative situation persists, you begin to develop physical symptoms e.g., migraines, sore back, allergies, sinus problems, lack of interest in sex etc.

Mental – The Flower Garden

Eventually you are not thinking straight!

Relationships – The Tree Garden

These problems begin to affect your relationships be it either with time off work, impatient with your children, or less attention to your partner.

I am not telling you anything new here. You are well aware of upward and downward cycles, and how different aspects of our lives can affect others. But what I am hopefully going to be able to do, is show you a game plan, pointing you in the direction of that seventh arch, the doorway to the staring post, which once you commit to the game, **your** game, and begin to weed and prune all the negatives out, become inspired to plant new seeds and encourage new seedlings as you work your way round your garden - your life.

I want you to take a notebook and on a separate page for each ingredient of your garden, I want you to write the following: Citrus, Flower, Trees, Herb, and finally Grasses and Exotics. Let's look at the ingredients of your garden in a little more depth and apply different aspects of you and your life to each of these ingredients.

These aspects of you and your garden are:

a) Citrus/Fruit represents your **emotional** wellbeing, your feelings and 'heart' self.

b) Flowers represent your **mental** wellbeing, your logical, cognitive mind.

c) Trees represent your **relationships** with your children, family, friends, colleagues and even yourself.

d) Herbs represent your **physical** wellbeing.

e) Exotics, resins and the grasses represent your **spiritual** wellbeing - your **dreams and aspirations**, your work and life purpose.

Each of these ingredients and their aspects - the citrus, flowers, trees, herbs, exotics and grasses, will be explained through each of their individual essences, their life force, or what is commonly known today as their Essential Oil properties.

Each part or aspect of your garden will contain an encyclopedia of the relevant Essential Oil and their healing properties in the following chapters.

Now I want you to split the individual pages into two columns. Shut your eyes, quiet your mind, and let your breathing relax. Take your time don't rush. Take days if necessary to revisit different aspects of your garden. Visit each ingredient one at a time in whichever order is comfortable for you. In your first column make notes of what you see. Some of the things I have already mentioned at the beginning of this chapter perhaps? Maybe some other things? Do they remind you of people, places, events, and situations in your life? Don't worry if you don't know the names of the plants or trees, this is not important at this stage. Don't **construct** your garden; **let your garden come to you**. Allow your imagination to give you surprises. It is through your free-flowing imagination that your soul self, will whisper little insights to you. The little ornaments you might come across or physical things like the walking stick or open book or children's toy I mentioned will be clues for you, and you alone. These clues are very important. They are symbolic of things that are either positive or negative in your life. Positive because maybe you haven't accepted or realise something's significance in your life, or negative because they symbolise what needs attention. They could even be regarded as some sort of symbolic message, which at the moment does not make sense.

 Maybe there won't be anything other than the plants or trees. Maybe there will be an ingredient, a part of the garden that is just missing, may be the flower garden for example. This is all right too. If an aspect is missing, question it, in the sense of why is it missing? Is it an area of your life then that you have totally shut out or an area which is perfectly ok with you? I would suggest that if you think it is alright then it should appear in your quiet moments and appear perfect. So go back to that area and be honest with yourself! Just relax, imagine the warm summer sun on your face as you wander and make notes.

Now, re-visit each ingredient and in your second column write down the 'jobs' that you can see that need doing. Each of these jobs reflects you and your life.

What do you need to prune or cut back on, do less of? For example, perhaps drink less caffeine? What do you need to dead head, or stop doing so that stronger plants can grow? Is it time to re-evaluate your finances? What do you need to weed, or cut out of your life altogether? How about cutting out a habit like smoking?

What do you need to sow, or put into motion an idea you have always wanted to start or try? How about making a commitment to that new hobby? What do you need to plant? Is there something or somebody new who has just come into your life and does it really fit into that part of your garden? Where do you need to plant it for its best potential and yours to grow? What about the rubbish? It sounds easy to get rid of rubbish, but this is usually the hardest part of 'gardening'. We know the rubbish has to go but our 'rubbish' usually has strong emotional links and ties, which make it very difficult to put these things in the bin. Try to think of your rubbish going to a compost heap. This way it is easier, knowing that whatever goes there will be changed into something more useful and positive, if not something more positive to you but maybe somebody else. Some of us will visit the compost bin of life more often than others!

So whether you have Mother Nature's healing gifts to use in your garden, local park or woodland, or their essence captured in a little bottle, you can begin to weed-out, prune and cultivate a healthier, more complete, serene you. You will have as a result more time to *being* you, as opposed to *doing*. Any *problems* will become just *situations*. You will start coming from *within,* your soul self, as opposed to *out with* yourself, what you think everybody else expects of you. Ultimately this is being true to you, which means you will be true to others and you will attract the same from them. You will begin to *love yourself better.*

So let's begin with what Essential Oils are.

3.

WHAT ARE ESSENTIAL OILS?

To state the obvious, all plants, shrubs and trees have their own life support system, and this is what we extract to give us essential oils. They are capable of adapting to their environment. Take for example Lavender, the higher the altitude this plant is grown at, the more healing properties it is reputedly supposed to have. Rosemary grown in Spain is going to be very different to the Rosemary grown in Tunisia. When harvested in Spain to make an essential oil, it is done before the Rosemary flowers. In Tunisia, it is harvested when it comes into flower. Using your imagination alone would tell you that something, which contains flowers, would smell different to the plant harvested before flowering. Therefore, logic tells us that the essence extracted from the life support system of that plant will be very different in both cases. In the case of essential oils, the country of origin can play an important part as to which would work best for an individual. Over the years I have found that some people just don't like the smell of Geranium. The most common Geranium oil available comes from Egypt. But when I ask a client to smell Geranium oil, which has come from China, their reaction is quite the opposite. It also works the other way round. Those who like the smell of the common Geranium do not like the Chinese Geranium. For the gardeners amongst you, there are of course many, many Geraniums available for you to select your favourite.

The life force of the plant is extracted in many different ways. The extraction process is determined by the plant or tree. Citrus will give its life force quite easily through distillation or pressure. Some flowers life force requires to be extracted by a process known as enfleurage, not often used today, sadly. This process involves plates of glass thinly coated with odourless fat and flowers such as Jasmine, which don't give up their life force that easily, and would be pressed between the glasses. The flowers would be replaced frequently until the 'chassis', as the fat is called, would become saturated with the essence of the plant. Once saturated the chassis is known as a 'pomade'; the pomade is then treated by an extraction process involving alcohol to separate the oil from the fat, this then gives us the plants essential oil. Some trees give off a resin or sap, and this is their life force. If you want to learn more about how essential oils are obtained from the plants, there are many books available explaining the various processes in detail.

The Orange Blossom, or more correctly tree, gives us three very different essential oils. When we harvest the blossoms, we get oil called Neroli. This oil like Jasmine requires tons of blossoms before we can acquire any respectable volume of oil, hence the reason why it is very expensive. From the leaves, bark and twigs we obtain Petitgrain. This has a woody odour with an underlying hint of the perfume of the blossoms, and a subtle citrus overtone. Finally, we obtain Sweet Orange from the fruit.

As individual we are as human beings, so too are each of the plants, shrubs and trees. The enthusiastic and avid gardeners amongst you would testify I am sure that no two plants grown from the same parent plant are the same either.

So, why are we so naturally attracted to the plant kingdom? Who hasn't bought a bunch of flowers to cheer themselves or a friend up? Or taken a walk in the local woods for some peace and exercise? Or lazed, with a cool drink at the end of a day's gardening? Or spent an afternoon strolling around the local garden center? Who hasn't been to their local chemist or health food shop to look for Echinacea, or St. John's Wort? No? What about a homoeopathic remedy? An essential oil perhaps? Bet you've tried one of those herbal extract shampoos or bubble baths! What about trying an organic produce from your local market?

You see, Mother Nature is calling us all the time, even in subliminal ways that we just haven't stopped long enough to ask why? What is the telepathic link we have with her which calls us and we respond to at different times for different reasons?

This is your 'little voice', your inner self, your soul self, which is responding and reacting to help the physical you maintain a healthy mind, body, spirit and soul. But what exactly does your soul self and Mother Nature know that we physically have no idea **why** we always turn to her, or at the very least 'give her a go' to help us?

I will tell you. The DNA of plants is almost identical to the DNA of us humans. The DNA of a plant is a closer match to ours than any other living animal on this planet. Now, go make yourself a cup of tea or coffee and think about that in all its implications before you continue reading!

So why are the plants DNA the closest match to our own? I am going to put this simply, not scientifically! The first living things on this planet were algae's, lichens and mosses. These gradually evolved to grasses, which eventually gave us shrubs, which then evolved to trees. I said this would be put simply! This was a very slow and gradual process over millions of years. Whilst this process was going on, the oxygen level in our atmosphere was increasing, along with many other changes due to the increase and diversity of 'plants'. Eventually 'something' happened, to begin the creation of other life forms. That 'something' still eludes our scientists today. There are many theories and possibilities. Any one, or even a little bit of each, could be the right answer as to how the animal kingdom, which includes us, came into being. Whichever way you look at it, whatever you believe, how we came into being is a little bit like making a cake! There are basic ingredients - the plant kingdom, the increase in oxygen, the various other gasses in our atmosphere, the new chemicals created from the mingling and combining of these gasses, the water, which, when combined with possibly the 'x' factor that the scientists cannot pin point, created the first animal or creature on earth. So, somewhere down our ancient ancestral past a part of us came from plants. This makes me think of Eve eating the apple!

So, how do you feel now? Quite a thought, isn't it? If you are still doubting this little bit of 'illumination', consider this, why are over 80% of modern allopathic medicines derived from plants? Why are pharmaceutical corporations spending up to 75% of their profits, sending teams of chemists and biochemists back into the forests and grasslands of Africa, India and South America, for instance? Why are they sending teams of anthropologists to learn from indigenous peoples in these areas of their medicinal cures? Because this little bit of information is the very bit of information, they don't want you to know! Why? Because, they cannot patent Mother Nature's gifts to us to make more money from you. They also know and realise that as new diseases appear over the horizon to affect us humans, the plant kingdom is already adapting and adjusting its own life force, its own DNA for its survival. The plant kingdom is far ahead of us. Right, I am stepping down off my political 'soap box'.

However, as I have already mentioned, most individual plants in their essential oil format, will cover almost all the different aspects of your garden. But each plant has its own particular strength, which will put it much more in one category rather than another.

An excellent example of this paradox, and one, which is probably familiar to most of you is Tea-Tree oil. As its name suggests, it is indeed a tree, and as such will come into that aspect of your garden, which we have equated with our relationships for example with our children, family, friends and colleagues etc. We all know and recognise Tea-Tree as being immensely anti-viral, anti-bacterial and antiseptic. These properties we would think, would put it in the part of our garden which deals with our physical wellbeing, which are the herbs - which Tea-Tree is not! So why am I going to tell you that Tea-Tree will stay firmly in the arbour, dealing with our children, family and friends, and not come into the herb garden to deal with our colds and flu's? This is why ….

Think of a situation with your child, a family member or a friend, who is causing you (or has caused you) worry or anguish to the point you are **exhausted** and **tired** with it all, exhaustion being the key word here. Have you thought of one? Good. Now, what is the one word you would use to describe this exhaustion or tiredness that you feel when you think of this person and situation? May I suggest the word might be stress? What does stress do? It compromises our immune system, leaving you wide open to the 'Invasion of the Viruses'! How does Tea-Tree actually combat viruses and bacteria? Because of its chemical compounds it kills the virus or bacteria, and supports your immune system as it is also a pro-biotic. So, in these situations, using Tea-Tree gives our physical wellbeing a helping hand by boosting our immune system, and at the same time 'killing-off' any viruses that come near, just waiting to attack our weakened state. Tea-Tree can be used like smelling salts when somebody is light headed or has fainted. When you are **exhausted** and **tired** of an ongoing situation, reaching for Tea-Tree revives you emotionally and mentally and thus equips your immune system to fight off infection.

OK, this child, family, friend situation is continuing, no abatement. You are dealing with the situation the best you can, but not thinking once about how this is affecting your immune system, and therefore not making use of Tea-Tree oil until one day wham! You wake up with the first signs of a virus, a sore throat. By now the streptococci or staphylococci virus has got you. Tea-Tree would help to some degree - remember it has anti-viral properties. But look to the herbs, because now you have a physical situation. Within the herbs, your physical remedies, you have for example Thyme oil. Thyme (if it is a safe oil for you to use) will kill off a strep or staph bug in about 20 minutes! Tea-Tree cannot do that. But if you had used Tea-Tree the minute you started feeling **exhausted** and **tired** and the situation was elevating your stress levels, it would have given you and your immune system the helping hand you needed before the child/family/friend/colleague situation snowballed and compromised your immune system to become a physical problem.

This is *being* and responding from a place of awareness. Not *doing* and responding 'after the event'. In turn, what you will do for yourself from this place of awareness and **being**, using Tea-Tree oil as in the above example at a time of stress, you might suggest its use to your child, family member or friend to help them. So begins the upward spiral to wellness, as Tea-Tree also brings with it a mental cleansing and clarity to a situation.

All right, so we know essential oils can help and heal us on many different levels. But, by the same token, they can also exacerbate other physical problems you might have, for example high blood pressure. Some oils, Thyme is one example, will raise blood pressure. This is all right if you have low blood pressure, but obviously not if your blood pressure is already above the normal range. So, before we go any further, let's do one more quick exercise, and sort out which oils you need to avoid. This does not apply to plants, so don't go digging up the Thyme plant from your garden if you have some!

4.

CONTRAINDICATIONS OF ESSENTIAL OILS

Before you begin to read about the aspects of your garden, and the essential oils there in, you must first check if there are any of the oils that you cannot use. I have done this as simply as possible for you. Below you will find some questions, after each question there is a list of oils. If you can answer any of the questions with a "yes", then you MUST NOT use any of the oils listed pertaining to that question.

As you work your way through the questions, cross off the oils that you cannot use, so that you are left with a personal list of essential oils. After all, this is a workbook! I want to see your book well used, dog eared with notes in the margins and post-it notes sticking out from your pages!

Please remember though, that **ANY** oil can cause a skin reaction. This is usually similar to a heat rash and will clear up in under an hour. This is called irritation in Aromatherapy. If you have such a reaction, cross that essential oil off too. To err on the side of caution, if you have sensitive skin, do a patch test first. Also please remember NEVER use ANY essential oil within at least 24 hours of using a sunbed or even sunbathing. The most important oils to avoid in this circumstance are the citrus oils. Some oils on the other hand, such as Chamomile, Immortelle, Lavender and Patchouli can be very soothing to the skin after sunbathing.

1. Are you pregnant, or intending to get pregnant or breast feeding?

Please do not use: Angelica (root and seed), Basil, Benzoin, Black Pepper, Cedarwood, Chamomile, Clary-Sage, Cypress, Dill, Eucalyptus, Fennel, Geranium, Ginger, Hyacinth, Jasmine, Juniper, Lavender, Marjoram, Melissa, Myrrh, Peppermint, Rose, Rosemary, Sage, Spikenard, Thyme and Yarrow.

2. Are you undergoing treatment for cancer, or still in remission from cancer?

*HC = Hormonal Cancer/ oestrogen-related cancers.

Please do not use: Angelica (root or seed), Basil (HC), Benzoin (HC), Black Pepper, Cedarwood (any), Chamomile (HC), Clary-Sage (HC), Cypress (HC), Dill (HC), Eucalyptus (any), Fennel, Geranium, Hyacinth (HC), Jasmine (HC), Juniper, Lavender (any), Lemon, Lime, Marjoram (HC), Melissa in prostatic hyperplasia, Myrrh (HC), Neroli, Peppermint (HC), Rose, Sage (HC), Spikenard (HC), Thyme (all and HC), Yarrow (HC).

3. Do you suffer from epilepsy, petit mal, grand mal or convulsions?

Please do not use: Eucalyptus, Fennel, Peppermint, Rosemary, Sage, Thyme, Yarrow.

4. Do you have stomach ulcers?

Please do not use: Cardamon and Ginger.

5. Do you have hemophilia, or taking blood–thinning drugs such as Warfarin?

Please do not use: Fennel, Geranium or Immortelle.

6. Do you have Hypertension (high blood pressure)?

Please do not use: Angelica (root and seed), Eucalyptus, Rosemary, Sage, Thyme.

7. Do you have Hypotension (low blood pressure)?

Please do not use: Clary-Sage, Lavender, Lemon, Marjoram, Melissa, Tagetes, Ylang-Ylang.

8. Are you taking Iron or iodine supplements?

Please do not use: Clary-Sage or Lavender.

9. Do you have any kind of kidney problem?

Please do not use: Angelica, Benzoin, Black Pepper, Cedarwood, Chamomile, Cypress, Eucalyptus, Fennel, Geranium, Guaiacwood, Juniper, Lavender, Patchouli, Rose, Rosemary, Sage, Sandalwood, Yarrow.

10. Do you have Diabetes?

Please do not use: Angelica and Rosemary are established as interfering with diabetic medication. However, research is still scant and depending what you read, the following essential oils have also been cited: Dill, Fennel, Geranium, Lemon, May Chang, Melissa, Peppermint, and Sage. I could not find any scientific research papers about the afore mentioned essential oils except an article by one Dr Sharon Baisil MD who is the founder of an Android app called Beat Diabetes. Other than avoiding Angelica or Rosemary if you are on diabetic medication, I would suggest erring on the side of caution with the others until we know more.

11. Do you have Endometriosis?

Please do not use: Fennel.

12. Do you have a Thyroid imbalance?

Please do not use: Thyme (over active thyroid).

13. Do you have Glaucoma?

Please do not use: Melissa.

14. Have you been diagnosed as clinically depressed and/or on antidepressant medication?

Please do not use: Patients on bupropion antidepressants should not use May Chang, Melissa, Palmarosa, Sandalwood, Yarrow. Neither should Sandalwood be used if you have been diagnosed with clinical depression but not on medication.

15. Are you taking any Homoeopathic Remedies?

Please do not use: Eucalyptus, Peppermint, Rosemary, Spearmint.

16. Are you taking statins, medication for malaria, lupus or Sjogren's Syndrome?

Please do not use: Grapefruit: The 'jury is still out' in the case of the medication as the essential oil comes from the skin, not the fruit we eat. I would suggest it depends on the individual and proceed with caution if you must use the essential oil.

These are just the basic questions, please read through 'Contraindications and Advisories in More Detail', starting with the Essential Oils you already have.

Contraindications and Advisories in More Detail

Angelica Root (Angelica sinensis): Not to be used in pregnancy or whilst breast feeding. This also implies that the root should not be used on children or babies. People with diabetes, high blood pressure, cysts, tumours, undergoing treatment for or still in remission from cancer should not use it. Avoid if on blood thinning medication. There is scientific research showing Angelica Root being an anti-coagulant.
Advisory: It may cause insomnia in some people. The root is highly phototoxic, as such should not be applied to the skin for 24-48 hours before or after being exposed to sunlight or sunbed.

Angelica Seed (Angelica archangelica): No known contraindications, some say same contraindications as the root. HOWEVER, I would err on the side of caution and avoid in pregnancy, breast feeding, using on babies and children and undergoing treatment for cancer. It is however far less phototoxic than the root.

Basil (Sweet & Linalool) (Ocimum basilicum): Not to be used if pregnant, breast feeding or on babies and children. Not to be used if undergoing treatment for a hormonal/oestrogen cancer.
Advisory: Possible skin irritant to a few.

Benzoin (Styrax benzoin): Not to be used if pregnant, breast feeding or on babies and children. Not to be used if undergoing treatment for a hormonal/oestrogen cancer.
Advisory: Possible skin irritant to a few.

Bergamot (Citrus bergamia): Phototoxic as such should not be applied to the skin for 24-48 hours before or after being exposed to sunlight or sunbed. Bergamot FCF (FCF Has the Bergaptens/Furanocoumarins removed, thus making it unlikely to react in sunlight).

Black Pepper (Piper nigrum): Not to be used if pregnant, breast feeding or on babies and children. Not to be used if undergoing treatment for cancer.

Advisory: Possible skin irritant.

Cardamon (Elettaria cardamomum): Do not use if you have stomach ulcers.

Advisory: Possible skin irritant.

Cedarwood (Himalayan): Currently it is best to follow the same contraindications of the more popular Cedarwood Atlas, until we know more if it is a safer alternative. Not to be used if pregnant, breast feeding or on babies and children. Not to be used if undergoing treatment for cancer. Can cause severe thirst therefore not suitable for those with kidney disorders.

Advisory: Possible skin irritant.

Chamomile Roman (Chamaemelum nobile): Not at any stage of pregnancy if there has been a history of miscarriage or breakthrough bleeding, otherwise not during first trimester of pregnancy.

Advisory: It can trigger underlying allergies in some.

Clary-Sage (Salvia sclarea): Not to be used if pregnant, breast feeding or on babies and children. It can lower blood pressure, so take care if you have low blood pressure as it could lower it further. Do not use within 24 hours of consuming alcohol, it can result in night terrors. Do not use if taking iron supplements. Not to be used if undergoing treatment for cancer or oestrogen-related cancers.

Cypress (Cupressus semperivens): Not to be used if pregnant, breast feeding or on babies and children. Not to be used if undergoing treatment for oestrogen-related cancers

Dill (Anethum gravolens): Not to be used if pregnant, breast feeding or on babies and children, but can ease childbirth. Phototoxic as such should not be applied to the skin for 24-48 hours before or after being exposed to sunlight or sunbed. Not to be used if undergoing treatment for oestrogen-related cancers

Advisory: Possible skin irritant.

Elemi (Canarium luzonicum):

Advisory: Possible irritant to sensitive skins.

Eucalyptus (Eucalyptus globulus): Not to be used during the first trimester of pregnancy. Personally, I would use other safer alternatives such as Niaouli. Not to be used if undergoing treatment for cancer. Not to be used if you have high blood pressure, or have epilepsy. Avoid using if you are also taking homeopathic remedies. Not to be used on children under the age of 6 years. Personally, I prefer not to use it on pre-pubescent children.
Advisory: Possible skin irritant.

Fennel (Foeniculum vulgare): Not to be used if pregnant, breast feeding or on babies and children. Not to be used if undergoing treatment for cancer. Not to be used if you have endometriosis, epilepsy or taking warfarin or other blood thinning drugs.
Advisory: Possible skin irritant.

Frankincense (Boswellia carterii): No known contra-indications, although I would urge caution during pregnancy and not use it until the 3rd trimester.

Galangal (Alpina officinarum): No known contraindications.

Geranium (Pelargonium graveolens): Not to be used if pregnant, breast feeding or on babies and children. Not to be used by people on blood thinning medication such as warfarin, Not to be used if undergoing treatment for cancer.
Advisory: Possible skin irritant.

Ginger (Zingiber officinale): Not to be used if pregnant, breast feeding or on babies and children. Do not use if you have stomach ulcers. Some people are allergic to Ginger, so the essential oil must be avoided as well.
Advisory: Very possible skin irritant. I would suggest localised treatment only, as it will raise temperature.

Grapefruit (Citrus x paradisi): Not to be used if on statins, on medication for malaria, lupus or Sjogren's syndrome. The 'jury is still out' in the case of the medication as the essential oil comes from the skin, not the fruit we eat. I would suggest it depends on the individual and proceed with caution if you must use the essential oil.
Advisory: Possible skin irritant.

Guaiacwood (Bulnesia sarmienti): No known contra-indications.

Hyacinth (Hyacinthus orientalis): Not to be used if pregnant, breast feeding or on babies and children. Classified as a narcotic and hypnotic, use in tiniest amounts and with care. Not to be used if undergoing treatment for oestrogen-related cancers

Immortelle (Also known as Helichrysum from its botanical name Helichrysum angustifolium): Not to be used if on blood thinning medication such as warfarin.

Jasmine (Jasminum officianalis): Not to be used if pregnant, breast feeding or on babies and children.

Juniper (Juniperus communis): Not to be used if pregnant, breast feeding or on babies and children. Not to be used if there are kidney problems, or have been on long-term steroids in past seven years. Not to be used if undergoing treatment for cancer.

Lavender (Lavendula angustifolia): Not at any stage of pregnancy if there has been a history of miscarriage or breakthrough bleeding, otherwise not during first trimester of pregnancy. It can lower blood pressure, take care if you have low blood pressure. Not to be used if undergoing treatment for cancer. Do not use if taking preparations containing Iodine or Iron is being taken.

English Lavender has higher Linalool content.

Advisory: It can trigger underlying allergies in some.

Lemon (Citrus limon): Not to be used if undergoing treatment for cancer. Phototoxic as such should not be applied to the skin for 24-48 hours before or after being exposed to sunlight or sunbed, unless you are certain the essential oil has been steam distilled.

Advisory: Possible skin irritant.

Lime (Citrus aurantifolia): Not to be used if undergoing treatment for cancer. Phototoxic as such should not be applied to the skin for 24-48 hours before or after being exposed to sunlight or sunbed, unless you are certain the essential oil has been steam distilled.

Advisory: Possible skin irritant.

Mandarin (Citrus reticulata):

Advisory: Possible skin irritant.

Marjoram (Origanum majorana): Not to be used if pregnant, breast feeding or on babies and children.
Advisory: Possible skin irritant.

May Chang (Also known by its botanical name Litsea cubeba): Patients on bupropion antidepressants should avoid it.
Advisory: Possible skin irritant. I would be extremely careful when applying to the skin.

Melissa (Melissa officinalis): Not to be used if pregnant, breast feeding or on babies and children. Not to be used if you have glaucoma, or diagnosed with prostatic hyperplasia. Patients on bupropion antidepressants should avoid it. People who are diabetic must be extremely careful when using this oil.
Advisory: Possible skin irritant.

Myrrh Commiphora myrrha): Not to be used if pregnant, breast feeding or on babies and children. Not to be used if undergoing treatment for oestrogen-related cancers.

Myrtle (Myrtus communis):
Advisory: Over-use may cause damage to mucus membrane/tissues.

Neroli (Citrus aurantium var. amara): Not to be used if undergoing treatment for cancer.

Niaouli (Melaleuca viridiflora): No known contra-indications.

Palmarosa (Cymbopogon martini): Patients on bupropion antidepressants should proceed with caution.

Patchouli (Pogostemon cablin):
Advisory: May cause loss/decrease in appetite in some people.

Peppermint (Mentha piperata): Not to be used if pregnant, breast feeding or on babies and children. Not to be used if you have epilepsy, Petit Mal, heart disease or cardiac fibrillation. Do not use if you have a fever as it will raise temperature even further. It is a neurotoxic if over used. Not to be used if undergoing treatment for oestrogen-related cancers.
Advisory: Possible skin irritant. Not to be used if you are taking homeopathic remedies.

Petitgrain (Citrus aurantium): No known contra-indications.

Rose (Absolute, Rosa damascena): Not to be used if pregnant, breast feeding or on babies and children. Not to be used if undergoing treatment for cancer.

Rosemary (Rosmarinus officianalis): Not to be used if pregnant, breast feeding or on babies and children. Not to be used if you have epilepsy, Petit Mal or have high blood pressure. People who are diabetic must be extremely careful when using this oil.
Advisory: Possible skin irritant. Not to be used if you are taking homeopathic remedies.

Rosewood (Aniba rosaeaodora): No known contra-indications.

Sage (Salvia lavendulaefolia): Not to be used if pregnant, breast feeding or on babies and children. Not to be used if you have epilepsy, Petit Mal or high blood pressure. Not to be used if undergoing treatment for oestrogen-related cancers.
Advisory: Possible skin irritant. Excessive inhalation can cause vertigo.

Sandalwood Santalum album): Avoid in cases of diagnosed clinical depression, as it may lower your mood further particularly if you are on antidepressant medication.

Spearmint (Mentha spicata):
Advisory: Not to be used if you are taking homeopathic remedies.

Spikenard (Nardostachys jatamansi): Not to be used if pregnant or on babies and children or by nursing mothers. Not to be used if undergoing treatment for oestrogen-related cancers

Sweet Orange (Citrus sinensis):
Advisory: Possible skin irritant. Will improve the absorption of Vitamin C supplements. Be aware as it could trigger a bout of diarrhea.

Tangerine:
Advisory: Possible skin irritant.

Tagetes (Tagetes minuta):
Advisory: possible skin irritant.

Tea-Tree Melaleuca alternifolia):
Advisory: Possible skin irritant to small percentage of people.

Thyme (Thymus vulgaris, also known as White Thyme): Not to be used if pregnant, breast feeding or on babies and children. Nor is it to be used if you have high blood pressure, epilepsy or hypothyroidism.

Advisory: Possible skin irritant.

Thyme (Linalool higher in linalool than White Thyme): Same as above until more research is done, although it is regarded as a safer alternative.

Advisory: Possible skin irritant.

Vetiver (Vetiveria zizanioides): No known contra-indications.

Yarrow (Achillea millefolium): Not to be used if pregnant, breast feeding or on babies and children. Not to be used if you have epilepsy, Petit Mal or running a fever. Not to be used if undergoing treatment for cancer. Patients on bupropion antidepressants should proceed with caution.

Advisory: Possible skin irritant. Prolonged use may cause headaches.

Ylang-Ylang (Cananga odorata): Lowers blood pressure, care should be taken if you have low blood pressure. It reduces tachycardia and can stabilize arrythmia, so would be advisable not to use if you are on heart regulating medications.

Advisory: Possible skin irritant. May cause nausea or headaches in high concentrations or prolonged use.

Start here

The Exotic & Grasses Garden – Dreams and Aspirations

Myrrh, Spikenard, Frankincense, Elemi, Guaiacwood, Benzoin, Palmarosa, Vetiver, Galangal, Patchouli

Citrus Garden – Emotional

Bergamot, Mandarin, Sweet Orange, Tangerine, Lime, Lemon, Black Pepper, Grapefruit, May Chang

The Herb Garden – Physical

Angelica, Basil, Cardamon, Clary-Sage, Dill, Fennel, Ginger, Lavender, Marjoram, Rosemary, Peppermint, Sage,

Flower Garden – Mental

Chamomile, Geranium, Hyacinth, Immortelle, Jasmine, Lavender, Melissa, Neroli, Rose, Tagetes, Ylang-Ylang

The Arbour – Relationships

Cedarwood, Cypress, Eucalyptus, Juniper, Myrtle, Niaouli, Petitgrain, Rosewood, Sandalwood, Tea-Tree

5.

THE CITRUS GARDEN – EMOTIONS

Emotions are our subconscious feeling and reaction to a situation. Mental processing of a situation is our conscious reaction to a situation, and can often be confused with our emotional reaction. We often, if not almost always forget that our emotions are our first reaction to any given situation, and because we forget, that is when we can make mistakes, errors of judgments, and even dismiss our emotional response simply because it does not *seem* like the *logical* way to deal with the situation. Whereas in fact we should be far more aware of our initial emotional response as that is the closest to the truth of the situation. It is our gut instinct or as I have already mentioned our soul self, sending you the REAL signal, so that if you recognised and accepted this soul self-message, (your emotions) you would be *being you* rather than *doing*.

How are you feeling emotionally?

I am not even going to begin the never-ending list of negative emotions, suffice to say that if you are not feeling comfortable, contented, at peace or happy, then you are emotionally stressed and wish that you felt someway or something else. This 'something else' is diametrically opposite to the way you are feeling right now. Ever the optimist, I have elected to show you what and where these oils can take you emotionally by describing situations to you, situations that should evoke positive feelings. Only you will know where and how you **want to be** other than where you are at right now.

Our emotions can be governed or can be likened to the seasons and the elements. Let's face it, don't most of us start feeling happier when spring starts to poke its head out of the winters cold and gloom? There are others of us who feel a lot happier when we are hibernating like a bear and thoroughly relish the idea of being tucked up and cosy during the winter months.

Do you feel you have more of an affinity with spring, summer, autumn or winter? Do you feel that if you were more airy, fiery, earthy or going with the flow like water, your life would be more contented? Maybe you could do with a season and a dash of the elements added perhaps?

As already mentioned in Chapter 3, all the plants although botanically speaking fall into specific groups, do have properties, which overlap them into other aspects of your garden. For example, if you feel down or even depressed, the following description of Bergamot might describe exactly how you would *like* to feel, you might also find that the cause of your 'down' state is cystitis, depression or feeling down being a symptom of cystitis, for which Bergamot is a first-rate remedy.

The Season's
Bergamot – Spring

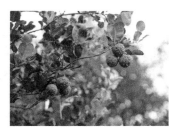

Botanical Name: Citrus bergamia
Plant Part: Peel
Country of origin: SE Asia, 80% now comes from Italy
Note: Top
Extraction method: Cold pressed and steam distilled

Contraindications: Phototoxic as such should not be applied to the skin for 24-48 hours before or after being exposed to sunlight or sunbed. Bergamot FCF (FCF Has the Bergaptens/Furanocoumarins removed, thus making it unlikely to react in sunlight).

Emotional: Bergamot can be relaxing and calming by balancing and uplifting our emotions. It encourages confidence and joy and helps emotional anxiety and inner nervousness.

Mental: A gentle oil for mental depression. It is also refreshing without being too stimulating to the mind. This is in turn brings a positive outlook, raises self-esteem, motivation and enthusiasm. It also helps where a little more concentration and focus is required. Can be useful for insomnia, depending on the 'trigger'.

Relationships: Ah, peace and contentment over a cup of Earl Grey tea on the back lawn. Whether you have the style and eloquence of a favourite Great Uncle; or the grace, panache and chic of a Great Aunt. You feel at peace with yourself and the world. You have seen it, done it and nothing fazes you. You know you have the wisdom of experience to deal with anything life throws at you in a calm, centred, even humorous way. You have brushed off your winter wrappings and trappings, got dressed in your best and now exude an air of calm quite confidence, ready for anything. You become that calm port amidst a spring storm both for yourself and everyone else.

It brings empathy, companionship, harmony, kind consideration and caring to any relationship.

Physical:

Muscular/Skeletal System: Not the best, but can ease general muscular tension.

Circulatory System:

Lymphatic/Immune System: Helps to reduce fever (febrifuge). Excellent choice for cold sores and herpes simplex. A wonderful bactericide and antimicrobial. Another bacterial infection, meningococcus responds well. A great support to the immune system and a gentle 'pick-me-up' after illness. Has been shown to treat malaria in early stages.

Nervous System: Calming and soothing to the nervous system.

Endocrine System: Applied externally for vaginal itching, discharge or thrush. Thrush of course also being a digestive issue and immune system issue. Helps with gonococcus infection. It is claimed to be regenerative for the hypothalamus.

Respiratory System: All types of mild to moderate respiratory infections can be helped particularly if a bacterial infection, particularly bronchitis. Excellent for a sore throat and tonsilitis. Has been recorded as treating TB. Being a bacterial infection, TB can manifest outside the lungs and on the skin, a condition called scrofula, not often seen these days, but worth a mention I feel. Scrofula presents as inflammation and irritation of the lymph nodes in the neck.

Digestive System: A gentle appetite stimulant which is useful both post infection and for anorexics and those suffering from bulimia. A demulcent (soothing) for intestinal cramps, colic, dyspepsia and flatulence. Helps balance the digestive system in the presence of gingivitis and halitosis. General intestinal infections, bacterial, can be treated successfully. A vermifuge, expels intestinal worms. Has been used to reduce gall stones.

Excretory/Urinary Systems: Bergamot has a very good track record in successfully treating and helping cystitis.

Integumentary/Skin System: It has excellent antiseptic properties. As such it has great success treating eczema and psoriasis. Remembering of course that Bergamot will not suit everyone who has eczema/psoriasis. A 'go-to' oil if there is a shingles (in particular) or chicken pox infection. Great results when treating staphylococcus bacterium, both on the skin and internally. You've probably gathered that Bergamot is an excellent bactericide and as such it makes an effective deodorant.

Used in skin preparations to treat/help oily skin and scalp, boils, rosacea, acne, scalp folliculitis (bacterial) and even abscesses. Often used in preparations to prevent and heal stretch marks and encourages healing of scar tissue. Can also be useful for varicose ulcers.

Dreams and Aspirations: When you want clarity, direction and motivation to 'get the job done'. It helps you to think outside the proverbial box, your imagination. Can be used in meditative and mindfulness practices. Has been said to stimulate our intuition.

Notes:

Mandarin – Summer

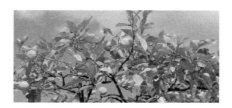

Botanical name: Citrus reticulata
Plant part: Peel
Country of origin: Northern China.
Note: Top
Extraction process: Cold pressed or steam distilled
Known as 'The Child's Oil'

Contraindications: None, other than possible skin irritant to small percentage of people.

Emotional: Very much like Bergamot, Mandarin is uplifting, joyful, encouraging, confidence building, but also brings a sense of peace and 'all is well'. "Don't sweat the small stuff" comes to mind.

Mental: It is sedative to the sympathetic nervous system. Albeit a citrus oil, it can help with sleep issues. It brings mental positivity, a sunny disposition, happy thoughts and is refreshing and revitalising for both the emotions and the mind. A gentle antidepressant, I would suggest not so much strictly an antidepressant but where you are in a 'funk'.

Relationships: Laughter and sandcastles, giggles and ice cream, flitting and fluttering excitement of the social butterfly. Think Wimbledon! The tennis match is on hold due to rain, yet you still smile and laugh at the irony. Excited anticipation knowing that the rain cloud holds a silver lining for the eventual victors. You don't take the interruption to play seriously, as you know it will pass. Mandarin allows the playfulness of the child we all hold within us to radiate and come out to play and splash around in the rain puddles. Has life got a little too heavy or serious? Get the Mandarin out and reconnect with the child within you.

As playful as it is, it is loving, gentle, kind and diplomatic. It will bring integrity and harmony to relationships.

Physical:

Muscular/Skeletal System: Antispasmodic and analgesic to muscular twitches.

Circulatory System: It can improve circulation.

Lymphatic/Immune System:

Nervous System: It can regulate the sympathetic nervous system.

Endocrine System:

Respiratory System: It is antibacterial and antifungal and can help with mild or early onset of upper respiratory infections.

Digestive System: One of the best and effective yet gentle remedies for all types of tummy upsets. It helps promote a sluggish digestion and promotes bile production (cholagogue) where required from the gall bladder to the duodenum, first part of the small intestine. It can help stimulate the appetite during illness or post illness where the appetite is slow to recover. It will also help loss of appetite due to low mood. It is antispasmodic and mildly analgesic so useful where there are stomach cramps due to wind, colic or dyspepsia. It helps aerophagia which is involuntarily swallowing wind. It certainly gets wind moving! It helps stop hiccups if gently inhaled.

Excretory/Urinary Systems:

Integumentary/Skin System: Often used in combination with Neroli Essential Oil in the prevention of stretch marks during pregnancy. Has also been used successfully to treat mycosis which is a fungal infection, such as ringworm or thrush.

Dreams and Aspirations: A lovely oil to help you focus and get back on track with renewed sense of optimism and purpose.

Notes:

Sweet Orange — Autumn

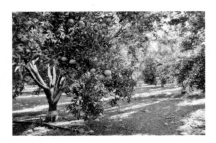

Botanical name: Citrus x sinensis
Plant part: Peel
Country of origin: Southern China, Northeast India, and Myanmar
Note: Top
Extraction process: Cold pressed distillation

Contraindications: Possible skin irritant. Will improve the absorption of Vitamin C supplements. Be aware as it could trigger a bout of diarrhoea.

Emotional: Another citrus oil which brings a lightness of emotions, laughter and happiness. It delivers strength, courage, support and confidence when faced with emotional decisions.

Mental: Sweet Orange marries our mental and emotional decisions when we feel we are at a cross roads. It is refreshing, brings positivity, motivation, creativity and energises your decisions, at the same time calming and relaxing. It makes you take a deep breath, pause and then see things clearly. Often used to treat insomnia. Again, you need to consider what is the trigger for individual insomnia.

Relationships: As the yellow colour of summer fades to the orange hues of autumn, there remain miles of smiles from fond memories past, and the sweet taste of things to come. Autumn is the season of transition, a time of letting go of things past, and preparing for things to come. A season of opposites, of warm days and cooler nights, it is a bridge between our wavering emotions and jumbled up mind. It is the signpost at the numerous crossroads we encounter in our lives and a bridge into our future. Sweet Orange's personality is faithful, honest, stoic, loyal, positive, steadfast, reliable and dependable. It can be dedicated and empathetic and will 'listen to your needs'.

Physical:

Muscular/Skeletal Systems: It is often used for its sedating and anti-inflammatory qualities on tight and sore muscles. It has also been used in the treatment of rickets, but I suspect that has more to do with it helping the absorption of Vitamin C.

Circulatory System: A gentle carminative to the heart (tachycardia) it also helps stimulate a sluggish circulation. It is said to be purifying to the blood (depurative) and claims have been made that it can also reduce cholesterol levels. It can help lower temperature when fever presents.

Lymphatic/Immune System: It helps to absorb Vitamin C from your diet. Please note, it does NOT contain Vitamin C. It is not an antiviral, but its action on Vitamin C levels make it a useful oil to fight off viral infections such as colds, bronchitis in particular and general congestion including the sinuses. A very useful support to our Lymphatic System and Spleen and is a diuretic. It can help reduce fever (febrifuge), shivers and high temperatures.

Nervous System: I would suggest it is soothing to our nervous system, but only because of its effect on our emotions.

Endocrine System:

Respiratory System: Certainly, helps colds and bronchitis.

Digestive System: As with most citruses Sweet Orange works well on all sorts of digestive issues and disturbances including wind, dyspepsia, colic, diarrhoea and constipation, particularly if they are brought on by emotional nervousness like butterflies in the tummy. It stimulates the production of bile where necessary and reputedly helps to break down stored fats in the body. By the same token it is a tonic for the Gall Bladder. It can encourage the appetite, so good for anorexics and those recovering from an illness where the appetite is slow to return.

Excretory/Urinary Systems:

Integumentary/Skin System: In combination with other specific Essential Oils, it can help break down cellulite. Used in facial products for acne, dry skin, mature skin, wrinkles and a good general tonic for the skin. It has also been used alongside Myrrh in the treatment of gingivitis.

Dreams and Aspirations: Has your creativity disappeared? Has your 'get up and go, got up and gone'? Starting to make excuses just to put things off? You need some Sweet Orange!

Notes:

Tangerine – Winter

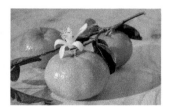

Botanical name: Citrus reticulata
Plant part: Peel
Country of origin: China
Note: Top
Extraction process: Cold pressed extraction

Contraindications: Can cause slight skin irritation in some individuals.

Emotional: Compared to other citrus oils which have a bit of a 'whizz-bang' to them (particularly the range of oranges), Tangerine exudes an air of warmth like a 'hug in a mug' and a warm blanket over your shoulders. It makes you smile. It is emotionally reassuring and calming that all will be well with the world, your world.

Mental: From instilling emotional calm and relaxing, it allows the mind to be refreshed, creative and even inspirational.

Relationships: Imagine the warmth and glow of a winter fire burning in the hearth. The beam of winters sunshine through the window, and the cosiness of being indoors on a cold, dark winters day. Tangerine brings a contented smile of wonderful things to come during those dank and damp months ahead.

It is like an old friend sat beside you on the sofa, which makes you smile and chuckle at silly, childlike moments. But as you turn to look at your friend, you find it is but a child. A child, that holds the wisdom of the ages. Tangerine brings out the wise child within you, "out of the mouths of babes". It makes you want to protect and preserve the child's innocence, to cosset and cherish its personality. Like a child's wisdom, that hits the bull's eye at the first attempt, so too lie the answers in the child within you. Relax in front of that fire, quiet your adult, chattering mind, and let that child whisper you the answer. Learn to trust yourself again.

Physical:

Muscular/Skeletal Systems: Excellent analgesic and antispasmodic to tired and aching limbs. It is also good for tired and aching limbs.

Circulatory System: Because of its warmth, it is useful for cold extremities. An all-round tonic to our circulatory system in particular with our peripheral circulation which means it can be useful in cases such as Raynaud's disease.

Lymphatic/Immune System: A good all-round general tonic.

Nervous System: Soothes the nervous system.

Endocrine System:

Respiratory System: Mildly antiviral it could help at the first signs of an infection e.g., tonsilitis, scratchy throat. It can help fight general respiratory infections.

Digestive System: Digestive disturbances, deals with all manner of gastric complaints and like Mandarin, it is gentle enough to use on children. It is useful during pregnancy because of it helps with the absorption of vitamin C. But please be aware that if you are taking vitamin C supplements alongside the use of this oil, you can reduce your vitamin C intake.

As with other citrus oils Tangerine is no exception when it comes to treating digestive disturbances. Its antispasmodic properties help with stomach ache, wind, flatulence and dyspepsia. It balances either constipation or diarrhoea. It helps stimulate the flow of bile if the liver and/or gall bladder are sluggish. It's a good overall tonic to the digestive system.

Excretory/Urinary Systems:

Integumentary/Skin System: Tangerine can bring a dull complexion back to life due to its action on the vascular system. Stretch marks can be smoothed in conjunction with other oils. Generally, a good skin tonic. A good oil to help clarify and balance the skin. Brings colour and a glow back to dull and 'lifeless' skin. Added to other Essential Oils such as Mandarin and Neroli it helps reduce stretch marks. It has good antiseptic properties and treats mycosis, a bacterial infection such as ringworm or thrush on the skin.

Dreams and Aspirations: While you're sitting there quietly with your mug of tea, enjoying the peace and calm, smelling the Tangerine wafting past you as the rain patters on the window and the wind is blowing, you feel a sense of determination, creativity and focus begin to take hold.

Notes:

The Elements
Lemon – Air

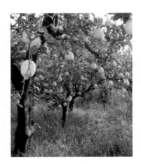

Botanical name: Citrus limon
Part of plant: Peel
Country of origin: Thought to originate in NW India, but in truth, nobody knows for sure.
Note: Top
Distillation process: Steam distilled

Contraindications: Not to be used if undergoing treatment for cancer. Phototoxic as such should not be applied to the skin for 24-48 hours before or after being exposed to sunlight or sunbed, unless you are certain the essential oil has been steam-distilled. Possible skin irritant.

Emotional: There is no doubt about it, Lemon is stimulating, refreshing, uplifting and energising. It certainly puts a zing into you emotionally, mentally and into your step. It is fun and joyful. It brings with it an 'air' of clearing and cleansing.

Mental: It has the same effect on your mind as it does on your emotions. However, you can also add that it is good for memory retention and aids concentration.

Relationships: Look out here comes lemon! Like a blast of fresh air lemon clears and cleanses everything in its path. Like the invisible air, it leaves everything sparkling and glittering in the wake of its torpedo like precision. As it has swept by, it leaves that distinctive fresh smell in its wake. Anything that is ugly or a nuisance dare not raise its head unless it wants to be blasted to kingdom come by this warrior missile! With its sharp, shinny, glinting stainless steel knife-edge, it will cut through the hardest butter. Enough is enough, it is time for a thorough clear out and cleanse!

Physical Just like the element of Air, Lemon quite literally blasts through the systems of the body that need a jolly good 'clear out'.
Muscular/Skeletal System: Lemon is one of the first oils you should consider in a blend for treating rheumatism, arthritis and gout.
Circulatory System: It will lower blood pressure, so useful for hypertension. Very useful in the treatment of varicose veins when combined with other appropriate EO's. Arteriosclerosis, hardening of the arteries responds well. It has also been used in the treatment on anaemia, but I wonder how much of that comes from eating the fruit. It has been used in the treatment of phlebitis. A useful remedy for headaches and migraines if diet induced. It can strengthen the heart and good general tonic to the circulatory system.
Lymphatic/Immune System: Meningococcus, typhus, pneumonia, staphylococcus viruses have all been treated as have general colds and flu and their accompanying symptoms. It helps reduce fever and throat infections. It is also a useful bacteriacide. It has a long reputation as a support to our immune system. It has also been used in the treatment of measles quite effectively.
Nervous System: Excellent on neuralgic pain, yet, it's not an oil many would think of for this. It can stimulate the sympathetic nervous system.

Endocrine System: Male sterility and inflammation of the testicles. Diabetes and headaches and migraines, see above under digestive issues.

Respiratory System: Asthma.

Digestive System: Strengthening and calming for all kinds of digestive disturbances. It helps promote liver activity if digestion is sluggish and helps get the bowels moving in the presence of constipation. It most certainly helps with hyperacidity in the gut if applied to the stomach region. It has helped with diabetes, hypoglycemiant. Will ease headaches and migraines which are diet induced. Can be very useful against heartburn, although peppermint is usually the 'go-to' EO. It is also a vermifuge, expels intestinal worms.

Excretory/Urinary Systems: Useful for urethra infections and helps promote urination. An effective diuretic. Reduces inflammation in the kidneys.

Integumentary/Skin System: Lemon is an excellent antiseptic, styptic and astringent for the skin. Let's just list the kinds of things it is successful in treating: cold sores, herpes, corns, warts and verruca's, cellulite, insect bites, a deodorant, eczema, prevents sclerosis, the stiffening of a tissue, can also therefore help in softening hardened scar tissue or keloid scars, brittle nails and skin parasites.

Dreams and Aspirations In meditative practices it brings focus, direction and clarity.

Notes:

Lime – Earth

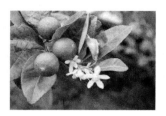

Botanical name: Citrus aurantifolia
Part of plant: Peel
Country of origin: SE Asia
Note: Top
Extraction process: Steam distilled

Contraindications: Not to be used if undergoing treatment for cancer. Phototoxic as such should not be applied to the skin for 24-48 hours before or after being exposed to sunlight or sunbed, unless you are certain the essential oil has been steam-distilled. Possible skin irritant.

Emotional: If cheerful is the middle word to describe Lime, then refreshing, invigorating and strengthening would sit on one side whilst calming, soothing and confidence would sit on the other.

Mental: The emotionally refreshing, invigorating and strengthening aspects of Lime result in determination, focus and creativity. This gives the effect that the oil is considered stimulating, I prefer to think of it as uplifting.

Relationships: If you keep avoiding 'doing' something, to the point of detaching, ignoring and quickly changing the subject, Lime will bring you down to earth and will show you where life has meaning, direction and purpose. Everything has value and a reason for being. The box of jumble has been cleared and sorted, things are a lot clearer now, and you are on a mission!

Physical:

Muscular/Skeletal System: It has been used successfully in the treatment of rheumatism and arthritis and even gout. IT is a first-rate remedy in the presence of asthenia, abnormal physical weakness or lack of energy.

Circulatory System:

Lymphatic/Immune System: A valuable support for the immune system. Helps prevent scurvy (antiscorbutic), allegedly. We know eating the fruit does, but I have yet to see and evidence that the EO does. Unlike a lot of the other citrus oils, Lime is in fact an antiviral. It is also a bacteriacide and makes an excellent disinfectant.

Nervous System:

Endocrine System:

Respiratory System: Can ease coughs, congestion due to mucous, catarrh and sinusitis.

Digestive System: It encourages appetite (aperitif) and is a good all-rounder for general tummy and digestive disorders and upsets. It is a vermifuge, it expels intestinal worms.

Excretory/Urinary Systems: It has good diuretic properties.

Integumentary/Skin System: Lime has excellent antiseptic and astringent properties. Because of its antibacterial qualities it is a useful deodorant. It also helps to stem bleeding. Besides being a vermifuge, it also gets rid of skin parasites.

Dreams and Aspirations: Lime has a long reputation of being able to help our intuition and meditative practices. It will also motivate, strengthen, and encourage you to manifest and bring your plans to fruition. IT will help you through any changes and adjustments you might have to make. It will quieten your mental chatter so you are quiet to listen to your inner voice.

Notes:

Black Pepper – Fire

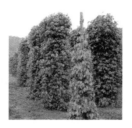

Botanical name: Piper nigrum
Plant part: Peppercorns
Country of origin: India
Note: Middle
Extraction process: Steam distilled

Author's Note: Just a little 'oddity', it has a reputation for quelling cravings associated with quitting smoking and nicotine withdrawal.

Contraindications: Not to be used if pregnant, breast feeding or on babies and children. Not to be used if undergoing treatment for cancer.
Possible skin irritant.

Emotional: Black Pepper will fire you up emotionally when you are feeling like a wet dishcloth. By the same token it will calm down too much heated emotions. It really is a fabulous oil when either of these two extremes present themselves emotionally. Sometimes just a single drop of Black Pepper in a blend is all that is needed to bring back to homeostasis either of these two emotional extremes.

Mental: Black Pepper is a very useful aid when studying as it helps with memory retention. Ideally suited when mental stimulation, stamina and alertness is required. Contrarily, just like its effect on the emotions it is calming and cooling to a 'hot head' that is all over the place.

Relationships: Come out of your angry and frustrated 'fire' by allowing Black Pepper to wash over and thru you. These powerful little peppercorns 'pop' and diffuse the heat in your kitchen. Has your relationship lost its spark? Stoke the fire a bit! Don't all good parties end up in the kitchen as the old saying goes? Black Pepper will fire up or diffuse the excessive fire in your belly and brings back your passion for life.

Physical

Muscular/Skeletal Systems: Black Pepper is probably most well-known, particularly in Sports Massage, for being an excellent remedy for muscular aches, pains and stiffness, tired and aching limbs and particularly where there is muscular stiffness and cold. Very often included in blends for arthritis, rheumatism and gout.

Circulatory System: Excellent for any circulation problems including anaemia and angina.

Lymphatic/Immune System: For the Lymphatic system it is a gentle diuretic. It helps to expel toxins generally through the lymph and immune system and gently supports the spleen. It lowers fever.

Nervous System: It is a wonderful analgesic, (pain killer) in the presence of any kinds of nerve pain and even damage such as in post operation where the skin is itching or tingling due to nerve damage.

Endocrine System: Has a long-standing reputation as an aphrodisiac.

Respiratory System: Supports other oils in the presence of respiratory infections of all sorts. It is an expectorant for coughs, it soothes sore throats, laryngitis and bronchitis.

Digestive System: Black Pepper will stimulate appetite and get a sluggish digestive system going. It can help breaks down fat and is a tonic to the liver, gall bladder and pancreas. It will certainly get constipation moving.

Excretory/Urinary Systems: Antiseptic for urinary tract and bladder infections.

Integumentary/Skin System: Not often considered but Black Pepper is particularly useful for treating chilblains

Dreams and Aspirations: Used in meditative practices, Black Pepper can help our visualisation, intuition, guidance, trust, faith and gives us the strength to see our dreams come to fruition.

Notes:

Grapefruit – Water

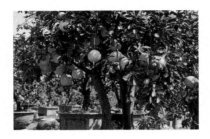

Botanical name: Citrus paradisi
Plant part: Peel
Country of origin: Asia
Note: Top
Extraction process: Steam distilled

Contraindications: Not to be used if on statins, on medication for malaria, lupus or Sjogren's syndrome. The 'jury is still out' in the case of the medication as the essential oil comes from the skin, not the fruit we eat. I would suggest it depends on the individual and proceed with caution if you must use the essential oil.
Possible skin irritant.

Emotional: There is a duality to Grapefruit which is similar to Black Pepper. When we are feeling emotionally exhausted with life and everything is an up-hill struggle, or when we are emotionally being swept along, white water rafting, and all we want to do is scream "Stop! I want to get off!", Grapefruit will bring you back to the 'still water's' and a safe haven.

Mental: Running alongside and parallel to how we might be feeling emotionally as outlined above, is how our mind will be responding as well. Grapefruit returns both the emotional and mental to an even keel. It can help with jet lag and where circadian rhythms have been knocked off kilter suddenly or unexpectedly.

HOWEVER, I would just like to point out that you should be aware of the possibility of an anger release. When either of the two extreme conditions highlighted above present themselves and have been going on for some time, underneath it all, both emotionally and mentally there will be anger, and boy, oh boy, will Grapefruit release that anger.

Refreshing, clarifying, reviving, uplifting, memory retention, positivity, contentment.

Relationships: Everything in life is fine, but suddenly up comes a wonderful little surprise that adds a little zip and zing to your daily routine. You can hear the birds sing and chatter above the daily noises, colours become more vibrant, you can smell the roses and fresh mown grass, your taste buds have become more alive as though you have just had a glass of old-fashioned lemonade, or a sherbet sweet, everything you touch has an ethereal quality.

Whether you are that exhausted salmon trying to leap up river or feel you are white water rafting, Grapefruit will bring you back to calm still waters and enable you to 'go with the flow'.

Life has just become dandy!

Physical:

Muscular/Skeletal Systems: I would suggest with its effect on the nervous system it might help soothe spasms and twitches in the muscles.

Circulatory System: Purifies the blood of toxins.

Haemostatic/styptic: shortens the clotting time of blood/ arrests external bleeding. Can help to reduce high blood pressure, but has no record of lowering low blood pressure any further.

Lymphatic/Immune System: It is antibacterial, antiseptic, antiviral. Should always be considered in a blend when treating cellulite. It is a great Lymphatic system support. A gentle but effective diuretic. Migraine and headaches respond well, as does ear infections.

Nervous System: Migraines headaches jet lag, disruption to sleep patterns due to shift work all respond well to Grapefruit. Damaged or injured nerves e.g., Motor Neurone Disease, can sometimes be repaired. Kurt Schnaubelt claims it repairs the damage to the myelin sheath around our nerves by encouraging new myelin to grow and repair. I can only cite one case where I saw this happen with a client who had been diagnosed with ME. I suggested regular baths in Grapefruit oil. Not only did it repair but completely eradicated any traces of the ME.

Endocrine System: A boon for the adrenals.

Respiratory System: I put ear infections here as it comes under ENT. Helps fight all kinds of respiratory infections and well worth considering in any blend for such conditions.

Digestive System: Grapefruit is a first-rate aid to all types of eating disorders such as anorexia. It has an absolute affinity with the gall bladder and liver. Aids digestion of fats by stimulating bile secretions in the liver and reduces inflammation of and gall stones in the gall bladder. My first 'go-to' oil for gall bladder issues, particularly if there is underlying emotional/mental anger.

Excretory/Urinary Systems: Has been successfully used in some cases of drug withdrawal, particularly when combined with Black Pepper. An excellent diuretic.

Integumentary/Skin System: Almost always used in a blend to treat cellulite. It has excellent antibacterial and antimicrobial properties so useful in the treatment of acne, oily skin, cellulitis, dull skin and generally congested and where toxins have built-up.

Dreams and Aspirations: Once Grapefruit has removed your emotional and mental 'extreme', it becomes far easier to get clarity, focus and inspiration behind your project.

> Grapefruit can release suppressed anger and in quite an explosive way depending on the depth of the anger.

Notes:

May Chang – a little bit of everything!

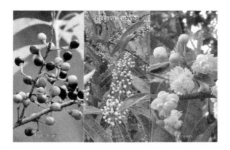

Botanical name: Litsea cubeba (also known by this name)
Part of plant: Fruit
Country of origin: Southern China and SE Asia.
Note: Middle
Extraction process: Steam distilled

Authors Note: I use May Chang especially in the winter months around the home, in burners, to kill off viruses and bacteria before they "get a hold" on members of the family. I also use it down plug holes, wiping down units, cleaning up vomit and even down the loo!

Contraindications: Patients on bupropion antidepressants should avoid it. Possible skin irritant. I would be extremely careful when applying to the skin.

Emotional: May Chang is a happy wee soul, kindly and effectively lifting your spirits when you are in a bit of a flunk. It has a contented air albeit has a sharp perfume.

Mental: Just like its effect on your emotions, May Chang is uplifting to your thought processes and makes you look for the sunshine and not the make-believe cloud that you 'think', just might, appear on the horizon. It is a mentally optimistic oil. It helps with creativity, focus and concentration

Relationships: A little bit of this, a touch of that, a dollop of something else. Sometimes, life is like a cake, we can have the ingredients, they are all blended into a delicious mixture, but the oven won't work! Does your oven need fixing? Are you ready to turn up the heat and cook your cake? May Chang is patiently waiting for you. Take that leap of faith with a smile on your face!

Physical: May Chang is well known to be effective in killing off airborne viruses, bacteria and other pathogens. Pop it in a diffuser at the very first signs of infection.

Muscular/Skeletal Systems:

Circulatory System: It is a tonic for the heart and helps any coronary heart disease, some clinical tests have shown positive responses by coronary heart patients.

Lymphatic/Immune System: Key words associated with May Chang are epidemics and sanitation especially and obviously where viral and bacterial infections abound. Besides killing off these viruses and bacteria May Chang will stimulate, energize and recuperate us when we have low energy during and after times of illness.

Nervous System: Calming and soothing to the nervous system.

Endocrine System: Reputedly helps where there are lactation problems. I can think of other oils for this, but would prefer to use May Chang in a diffuser for obvious reasons.

Respiratory System: Clears stuffed up feeling in the head due to colds and blocked sinuses. Its particular affinity is with respiratory illness e.g., bronchitis, asthma, tonsillitis and chest colds. Perfectly safe oil to diffuse to clear airborne viruses, bacteria and other microbes around children. A first-rate remedy at the earliest signs of respiratory infections.

Digestive System: May Chang stimulates our appetites which is excellent when we are off our food due to illness. Very often a general cold/flu puts us off our food, May Chang is an excellent digestive stimulant in the presence of an infection. It is also said to help with oral thrush, although I have never had the opportunity to verify this.

Excretory/Urinary Systems:

Integumentary/Skin System: For the skin, May Chang will balance oily skin, but only to be used in ***extremely*** small quantities. Personally, I would not use it on the skin for this purpose as there are other gentler oils more suitable, especially for facial skin.

Dreams and Aspirations: Quite simply manifest your dreams into reality!!!!

Notes:

6.

THE FLOWER GARDEN

As I have already mentioned in the previous chapter, our emotions are a sub-conscious 'gut reaction' to a situation, whereas our mental process in evaluating a situation comes from our consciousness. The minute our mental process goes off center or out of balance and our head goes round and round a problem is because our mental body is in conflict with our emotional body. Why does this conflict arise? Two reasons, firstly, we forget to quiet ourselves and reconnect with what our emotions are telling us; and secondly, because of this we have started theorising the situation and allowed fear to colour our thought processes.

Within each aspect of your garden, we have a paradox, or diametrically opposing positive and negative forces at work.

In the emotional garden it is love v. hate.

In the mental garden it is wisdom v. fear.

In the relationships garden it is good company v. loneliness.

In the physical garden it is good health v. ill health.

In the dreams and aspirations garden it is manifestation v. repression, or for those of you spiritually minded light v. dark.

In this chapter I am going to use key words and phrases to help you associate with the oils. Being the Mental aspect of your garden, it will help you decide how and which state of mind you need to be in to be able to resolve your mental conflicts or imbalance to restore clarity and balance to your state of being.

Chamomile – 'The Now'

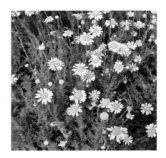

Botanical name: Chamaemelum nobile although it was once scientifically known as Anthemis nobilis.
Plant part: Flowers and buds
Country of origin: 19th century botanist who found some growing by the Roman Coliseum.
Note: Middle
Extraction method: Steam distilled

Author's Note: Please note, this is English Chamomile or Chamomile Roman as it is most commonly known.
I would like to point out that I use Chamomile Roman mostly, it's safer to use on children and I find it's aroma closer to the actual plant than Chamomile German which has a much higher azulene content which makes for the distinctive blue colour of that oil. German Chamomile has more contraindications.

Contraindications: Not at any stage of pregnancy if there has been a history of miscarriage or breakthrough bleeding, otherwise not during first trimester of pregnancy. It can trigger underlying allergies in some.

Emotional: With its calming and relaxing properties it helps focus people's attention on the issue in hand when they keep evading an emotional issue. It encourages stability and gives the feeling of 'centeredness'.

Mental: Hot, disorganized and impatient mental gymnastics are cooled, become organized and patient when challenged.

Relationships: Is your mind refusing to get a grip on your present mental conundrum? Does the answer seem to be 'out there' somewhere, and you just can't reel in the piece of string that is attached to it? Chamomile stops you day dreaming, going off on a tangent, putting things off until tomorrow. It focuses your mind on what needs to be done right now. It brings you into the present in an emotionally calm and rational way. It makes you take a deep breath and settle down to what needs addressing.

Physical:

Muscular/Skeletal System: Analgesic for muscular aches, pains and strains. Chamomile has an affinity with lower back ache like Marjoram.

Circulatory System: Because of its azulene content it helps stimulate the body produce white corpuscles that help fight bacterial infections and possibly help anemia, jaundice and angina.

Lymphatic/Immune System: Anti-inflammatory for Arthritis and rheumatism, fever and influenza. Helps seasonal and non-seasonal allergies.

Nervous System: Facial neuralgia e.g., Bell's Palsy. Neuralgic pain generally. Headaches, teething, toothache, earache and insomnia.

Endocrine System: PMT and PMS, menopause, testicular inflammation, dysmenorrhea, eases period pains and helps regulate the cycle.

Respiratory System:

Digestive System: Peptic ulcers, IBS, intestinal parasites, constipation, diarrhea, nausea, vomiting, gastritis, colitis, flatulence and wind in general.

Excretory/Urinary Systems: Kidney inflammation, cystitis,

Integumentary/Skin System: Acne, abscesses, boils, chicken pox, insect bites, rashes, eczema, psoriasis, dermatitis, burns, cuts, sores, blisters and herpes. Good for the hair. Antiseptic properties and a strong disinfectant.

Dreams And Aspirations: Spiritual awareness, inner peace and security.

Notes:

Geranium – 'Balance'

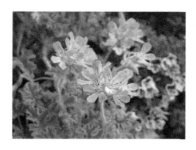

Botanical name: Pelargonium graveolens
Plant part: Leaves
Country of origin: South Africa
Note: Middle
Extraction method: Steam distilled

Author's note: "The first Pelargonium recorded in history was in 1672 when the German botanist, Paul Hermann, collected a sample of *P. cucullatum* he discovered growing on the Table Mountain of South Africa. Various plant collectors, ships surgeons and naturalists who sailed the trade routes around the Cape of Good Hope brought Pelargoniums back from their voyages in the early 17th century. In fact, about 200 of the 250 known species of Pelargonium are native to South Africa, but due to massive hybridization after their introduction to Europe at this time many species today bear little resemblance to their original parentage....... China is now the largest producer of geranium oil, with perhaps Egypt the second most important producer, followed by Morocco, Africa and Reunion. Egyptian geranium oil is considered by experts to be of a better quality than the Chinese oil, whilst Geranium Bourbon (Reunion) is considered superior to all others." Copyright © Quinessence Aromatherapy Ltd 2018. Written by Geoff Lyth.

Contraindications: Not to be used if pregnant, breast feeding or on babies and children. Not to be used by people on blood thinning medication such as warfarin, Not to be used if undergoing treatment for cancer. Possible skin irritant.

Emotional: It is healing, comforting and harmonizing to the emotions.

Mental: Encourages mental flexibility, easing stubborn viewpoints. Promotes a sense of humor and can give feelings of elation before calming back down to a more 'centered' place. Helps to combat depression.

Relationship: Is your mind going in two directions, but both directions seem to give you a solution but with an 'if' attached to them? Well, maybe you need a meeting point between both solutions thus creating a balance. Sometimes one solution wins for you, but the other person becomes the loser. The other solution makes you the loser and the other person the winner – obviously not a choice any of our 'ego' selves would take! Geranium brings a balance to a situation that allows both parties to win, benefit and more importantly move on without any ill feeling or unresolved acrimonious emotions still attached to it.

Physical:

Muscular/Skeletal System: Can help with swelling and joint pain often associated with rheumatism.

Circulatory System: Raynaud's Disease, varicose veins, haemorrhoids, jaundice, a good overall tonic to the circulation, making things more 'fluid', hence the reason why it should not be used if client is taking blood-thinners as Geranium will thin the blood. But it is excellent for hemorrhoids.

Lymphatic/Immune System: fluid retention, swollen ankles, congested lymphatic system, general fatigue and malaise, helps keep infections at bay. Throat and mouth infections respond well.

Nervous System: neuralgia, particularly indicated for facial neuralgia, including Bell's Palsy.

Endocrine System: PMT, PMS and associated cramps, infertility, endometriosis, menopausal symptoms, lack of vaginal secretions particularly during menopause. It can help with congestion in the breasts during monthly cycle and menopause. You could consider combining it with Ylang-Ylang for this as it too has an affinity with breast tissue.

Respiratory System: mouth and throat infections,

Digestive System: gall bladder stones, diabetes, can help to detoxify the liver. Helps clear gastric mucous and eases gastritis and colitis.

Excretory/Urinary Systems: kidney stones, very useful diuretic and a good general tonic for the kidneys. It has been claimed to help with addictions, I would suggest this is both emotional (balance) and to help detoxification. Helps urinary tract infections.

Integumentary/Skin System: nervous and stress related skin disorders, eczema, dermatitis, ulcers, shingles, herpes, ringworm, head lice, chilblains. Good for wounds and helps form scar tissue generally. Acne, bruises, minor burns, balances sebum and getting sluggish, congested and dull skin moving and a good insect repellent. Apparently helps with gum infections, alveolar pyorrhea particularly.

Dreams And Aspirations: Strength, perseverance, determination and accomplishment.

Notes:

Hyacinth - 'Journey away'

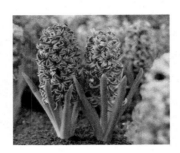

Botanical name: Hyacinthus orientalis
Plant part: Flowers
Country of origin: Eastern Mediterranean and said to be Syrian in origin.
Note: Middle
Extraction process: Solvent extraction making it an Absolute

Author's Note: Sadly, not used much in Aromatherapy, which is a shame, as I have always found just a drop of this oil in a blend, particularly where the client is over-fraught and focused on negativity works wonders.

Contraindications: Not to be used if pregnant, breast feeding or on babies and children. Classified as a narcotic and hypnotic, use in tiniest amounts and with care. Not to be used if undergoing treatment for oestrogen-related cancers.

Emotions: It improves self-esteem, feelings of self-worth and is calming. Very useful at times of grief or loss of any sort.

Mental: Although regarded as bringing mental persistence, positivity, relieving stress and anxiety I feel this comes about by 'journeying away' so you can get a bird's eye view as it were, of the situation in hand. It allows you to 'step away' and see the 'bigger picture' of what is going on. A very useful antidepressant.

Relationships: Have you allowed yourself to become so embroiled in a situation that you just can't see the wood for the trees? Is there just 'too much information' involved and you have become bogged down? It's time for a new perspective and angle on the situation, along with some clarification as to what is really important. The only way to do this is to 'Journey Away' and see the situation from a higher perspective, an eagle's eye view, so you can see the whole picture.

Hyacinth allows you to be forgiving and trusting, but will also make you very aware when something is not right, not serving your highest purpose, and if you are being deceived. Hyacinth will enable you to be a good listener to other people's problems and situations. It will allow you to exude an air of gentle independence, and keep you detached so that you do not become emotionally involved and can therefore help from a place of wise pragmatism. It will also, through your independent and detached air, mean that others will recognize your need to be alone at times, so that you can have the space to breathe.

I also call it the 'therapist's oil'. It allows us to step back from our clients to asses them professionally and objectively when we find ourselves getting emotionally embroiled with and too empathetic with our client's needs.

Physical: Now, what can we say about the physical properties of Hyacinth? Well, it's effects on the emotional and mental bodies and their 'knock-on' effect to our relationships moving us into a more positive place will immediately alleviate physical discomfort. If there was ever an oil which clearly shows that by releasing underlying emotional and mental negativities has this wonderful effect on alleviating physical symptoms, this is the oil. In combination with Neroli, you have a very heady but effective release mechanism.

Muscular/Skeletal Systems:

Circulatory System: It is said to have styptic properties.

Lymphatic/Immune System: Mildly antiseptic.

Nervous System: I would suggest its effect on the mental and emotional will have an indirect action on calming the overall nervous system. Helps with addictions, but again I think this goes back to its effect on the mind and emotions.

Endocrine System: It is said to be an aphrodisiac and I can see why when it releases underlying worries and anxieties.

Respiratory System: I would again suggest that its effect on the mental and emotional will have an indirect action by calming the breathing when there is a shortness of breath.

Digestive System: I would also suggest because of its effect on the mental and emotional calming the nervous system, it will then have a indirect effect on the Vagus Nerve and thus calming a nervous tummy and accompanying symptoms.

Excretory/Urinary Systems:

Integumentary/Skin System: Mainly used in perfumery. It does have some antiseptic properties so could be a useful adjunct to skin conditions which are exacerbated by anxiety and stress such as rosacea.

Dreams and Aspirations: As already mentioned, Hyacinth is a hypnotic oil and can be very sedating and can take your abilities as far as vision and prophecy in your meditation and self-hypnosis practices, if you wish to explore that aspect. The oil will connect you with your divine self, and bring the realization that there is 'much twix heaven and earth'. That you need not question what or why, but to accept there are greater forces at work than we can explain. In other words, it can help open you up to be a pure channel from the highest source, and communicate the message through words or healing to its destination.

Notes:

Immortelle – 'Journey Within'

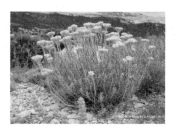

Botanical name: Helichrysum Italicum/Helichrysum officianalis, some suppliers call it Helichrysum
Plant part: Flowers
Country of origin: Mediterranean countries
Note: Middle
Extraction process: Steam distilled

Author's Note: It has a nickname of 'the wounded healer' or 'for wounds that will not heal' and is also known as Everlasting. The price of this oil has gone up about threefold in the past 10 years. One reason for this is that a well-known skincare brand became aware of the massive benefits that this oil gives. The best oil comes from Corsica where it is now cost-effective for distillers to collect wild-growing flowers from the high mountains using helicopters apparently! I have to say Corsican Immortelle is something very special. It keeps for a very long time and I am graced to have been gifted a bottle of organic, wild harvested and distilled by an artisan distiller from Corsica several years ago and it is just as beautiful as the day my student gifted it to me.

Contraindications: Not to be used if on blood thinning medication such as warfarin.

Emotions: It is warming, calming and comforting to our emotions. It holds us gently in its essence as it digs deep into your soul. It will leave no stone un-turned as it restores your inner strength. Do not be surprised if you have a sudden bout of inexplicable crying or a fit of giggles as it releases negativities without bringing the issues to the surface. Whether it is tears or giggles, it leaves you feeling refreshed and cleansed. I have seen this happen to several clients over the years and I always warn clients that they might experience one of these emotional out-pouring. But I have to say, it is very few and far between. It lifts depression, lethargy, and soothes nervous exhaustion.

Mental: Helps with memory recall and comprehension. It is clarifying, and brings patience with self and others. Particularly helpful with stress-related disorders such as insomnia.

Relationships: It will bring about a calm acceptance of life and thus patience and understanding. It releases the positive inner child. It will help you leave the problems of the past and help you face a 'new tomorrow'. It will help you learn the lessons in everything that occurs in your life both your successes and your mistakes. It will help you contact and acknowledge your inner child/guide/guardian/angel/soul self. It will give you the strength and perseverance at times of difficulty. It will open your heart to be receptive to all the joys of life and make the opening of your heart safe to do so.

Being a powerful transformational oil, it will bring out your ultimate capacity and capabilities. Immortelle is an indispensable companion when personal problems need to be addressed and worked out. Its buffering action helps you at this time as facing your problems and situations inevitably brings about changes, and it is not the situation, but the fear of the change which stands in your way of moving forward in your life. It will aid you to look inside yourself for your truth, for you already hold the answers within.

Physical:

Muscular/Skeletal Systems: Its anti-inflammatory properties help rheumatism, general aches and pains, arthritis, polyarthritis and pelvic pains.

Circulatory System: It can help to regulate blood pressure. It is a blood purifier, a blood decongestant and as such haematomas or thrombosis, for which it is widely used in modern Clinical Aromatherapy. Please do not try to use it for this purpose on yourself or if you are not a Clinical Aromatherapist. It enhances arterial circulation and can help prevent coronary problems. I think this aspect is due to its deep effect on our emotions (see above). It also enhances arterial circulation.

Lymphatic/Immune System: It is one of the most important oils we can use today to strengthen our immune system as our primary defense system to wellbeing. A great Lymphatic cleanser and a great detoxifier of all our various systems. It is also a great support to our spleen which is the 'cross-over' point between the Lymphatic and Circulatory Systems.

Its chemistry shows it is THE strongest anticongestive known in nature.

It is very effective against viral and bacterial infections.

Nervous System: Soothes and calms the nervous system.

Endocrine System: Regulates irregular periods, eases menstrual cramps. Helps treat goiter (usually overactive thyroid). Helps alleviate headaches and migraines.

Respiratory System: All sorts of respiratory problems can be helped: asthma, bronchitis, coughs, flu, helps remove mucous from the lungs and the sinuses.

Digestive System: Cleanser and decongestive for the liver, gall bladder and pancreas. Helps treat candida. Migraines/headaches particularly if food related.

Excretory/Urinary Systems: Cleansing and tonifying to the kidneys. Very effective in treating cystitis.

Integumentary/Skin System: Wonderful skin purifier and regenerative. Eczema, psoriasis, acne, abscesses, sun burn, bruises, inflammation of gums, herpes, all respond well to Immortelle. As Lavender is to burns, Immortelle is to wounds, cuts and grazes.

Dreams and Aspirations: Frustrating, isn't it? The answer is there on the tip of your tongue. You know it's starring you right in the face! Darn it's annoying! You just need to calm yourself, quiet down your enthusiasm, and 'Journey Within'.
Quiet now...hush...EUREKA"!
Immortelle opens the feminine, intuitive, right-hand side of the brain. It will release deeply rooted emotions, thus clearing the way to more intuitive insights into life. So be prepared for a fit of unexplainable giggles, or a good cry that feels oh, so good!

Notes:

Jasmine – 'Acceptance'

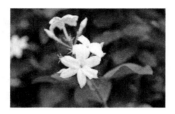

Botanical name: Jasminum sambac
Plant part: Flowers
Country of origin: Jasmine originates from the Himalayas.
Note: Middle to base
Extraction process: Solvent extracted making it an Absolute.
Extraction method: Steam distilled

Contraindications: Not to be used if pregnant, breast feeding or on babies and children.

Emotional: Jasmine can have a euphoric effect on the emotions. It helps promote self-confidence, self-esteem, optimism, bringing feelings of happiness and joy. It has relaxing properties which encourage a sense of peace. Along with Hyacinth an excellent remedy for therapists who get too embroiled emotionally with their clients, thus keeping them objective and detached.

Mental: Mentally Jasmine is inspirational. It has a quiet wisdom. It is fearless, brings mental positivity, assertiveness, creativity and harmony. Next to Neroli, Jasmine is an excellent remedy for depression.

Relationships: Jasmine brings out the beauty from within. Its archetypal female being Mother Earth, giver of life. It will enable you to become comfortable and confident with who you really are. Jasmine has a sense of humour and fun. It will bring together your heart and soul, so that you can be in acceptance of all things, so that you can also, through gentleness, allow that which does not help or serve you to be released from your life without causing you pain or anguish - a respect that all things have the simple right to just be.

Jasmine brings back and restores balance and grace when life just seems to be that little bit too difficult, and gives you confidence through new possibilities, by a single change in viewpoint, to see you through these times. It will open you up to your very soul and will diminish the fear you might have in facing who you really are. Because you must never forget, that in essence, we are all wonderful people within, and Jasmine helps you see this, and accept yourself and others as perfect being.

Physical:

Muscular/Skeletal Systems: General back pain, joint and muscle pain.

Circulatory System:

Lymphatic/Immune System:

Nervous System:

Endocrine System: Uterine tonic, menstrual problems, hormonal balancer, frigidity, impotence and premature ejaculation, and allegedly increases the number of sperm, could be considered a good adjunct to Sandalwood in this case. Excellent to help during delivery of a baby and post-partum to help against baby blues. Like Dill it does help with the production and flow of breast milk, but should be used very sparingly so as not to taint the milk. Also helps vaginal infections.

Respiratory System: Good for bronchitis, coughs and some allergies. At first sign of flu like symptoms combine with Ginger in a bath.

Digestive System:

Excretory/Urinary Systems:

Integumentary/Skin System: Can help dermatitis, eczema, dry and/or irritable skin. Particularly good for mature skin and can soften hard scars, keloids.

Dreams and Aspirations: This oil will also bring the angelic realms closer to you, and through this, your unconditional love of all things will resonate back through the universe. But your intent must be pure of heart. It will bring greater harmony into your life. It will enhance your intuition. Jasmine, throughout history has long been associated with the Goddess of the Moon, and in many traditions especially those with shamanistic roots the moon is regarded as female. Isis, the Egyptian Mother Goddess has strong links with Jasmine, and was regarded as the keeper of secrets of fertility, magic and healing.

Notes:

Lavender – 'Calm'

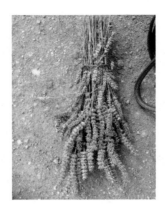

Botanical Name: Lavendula angustifolia (English Lavender)
Plant part: Flowers and stems
Countries of origin: Mediterranean, Middle East and India
Note: Middle
Extraction method: Steam distilled

Author's note: I would suggest that Lavender is particularly effective when there are underlying emotional root causes.

Contraindications: Not at any stage of pregnancy if there has been a history of miscarriage or breakthrough bleeding, otherwise not during first trimester of pregnancy. It can lower blood pressure, take care if you have low blood pressure. Not to be used if undergoing treatment for cancer. Do not use if taking preparations containing Iodine or Iron is being taken. **English Lavender** has higher Linalool content. It can trigger underlying allergies in some.

Emotional: Lavender is kind and gentle on the emotions, instilling feelings of peace, acceptance and comfort. Calms feelings of anger and frustration.

Mental: Mentally it brings vitality, clarity and balance. Another good oil for depression, suggested for manic depression. Used often to treat insomnia, but remember it is an adaptogen oil so time of day and dosage must be taken into consideration.

Relationships: When you seem to be on a boat adrift in a ragging sea, Lavender brings calm security and tranquility. The storm abates and you find yourself in a safe haven of comfort. You are no longer heading for 'burn-out', your panic even hysteria, shock, fears and nightmares are finally over as a gentle state of acceptance blankets you.

Physical:

Muscular/Skeletal Systems: Lavender has pain and anti-inflammatory properties and is therefore good for muscular sprains, strains and sharp or stabbing rheumatic pain), lumbago, rheumatism, particularly when combined with Marjoram, all respond exceptionally well. Together they have a beautiful symbiotic relationship.

Circulatory System: It lowers high blood pressure very effectively and calms palpitations. Regulates, sedates and helps strengthen the heart. Caution if using for a period of time with low blood pressure as it can lower it even further.

Lymphatic/Immune System: It is a powerful antiseptic. It also contains natural antihistamine.

Nervous System: Headaches and migraines are greatly helped, particularly if they are stress induced. It has also been known to cure tinnitus. If you suffer from tinnitus, try putting just one drop of oil behind your ear stroking it in, in a downward motion towards your jaw daily. It relieves tooth ache and neuralgia, although not to be applied directly to the tooth ache! Stimulates and strengthens the nervous system, but also subdues what is known as the cerebro-spinal pathway of the nervous system. Indicated for sciatica, nervous tension, shock and vertigo.

Endocrine System: It can be used for scanty periods. Massaged into the lower back during childbirth will reduce pain and speed up delivery. PMT/PMS have long been known to respond well to Lavender. Helps with labour pains, speeds up delivery and helps expel placenta/afterbirth.

Respiratory System: Asthma, bronchitis, catarrh, halitosis, laryngitis, tuberculosis, throat infections, whooping cough and possibly asthma, if it is **not** allergy induced, are just some conditions of the respiratory system that are helped by this oil. It can also help keep a viral infection down due to its antiviral properties.

Digestive System: Nausea due to imbalance or infection in the ear or sea sickness are relieved. Digestive cramps, colic, dyspepsia, nausea and flatulence. Has an affinity with the spleen, think more on the underlying emotional root cause being anger here. Also helps in the production of bile thus aiding in the digestion of fats. It helps to stimulate the appetite, so good for anorexia and people who are slow to regain their appetite after an illness.

Excretory/Urinary Systems: Mild diuretic and good for kidney inflammation. One to consider for the treatment of cystitis. I would align this more with its effect if the client is 'pissed off' emotionally. A gentle diuretic. Is gentle on kidney inflammation.

Integumentary/Skin System: All-round good skin tonic for all sorts of skin conditions: wound healing and in particular burns. Also, because of antihistamine properties helps with pruritis (itchy skin) and reactions to insect bites for example. Athlete's foot, abscesses, acne, allergies (Lavender contains natural antihistamine), boils, carbuncles, bruises, insect bites, inflammation, wounds stings, psoriasis, ringworm, scabies, sores, acne, sunburn, and most famously of all, burns. It has been used in the treatment of alopecia. Athlete's foot, abscesses, acne, allergies (Lavender contains natural antihistamine), boils, carbuncles, bruises, insect bites, inflammation, wounds stings, psoriasis, ringworm, scabies, sores, acne, sunburn, and most famously of all, burns. It has been used in the treatment of alopecia.

Dreams And Aspirations: Awareness, growth, meditation and visualization.

Notes:

Melissa – 'Setting Boundaries'

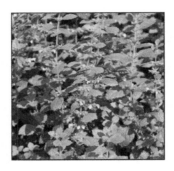

Botanical name: Melissa officinalis
Plant parts: Leaves/flowers/buds
Country of origin: Greece
Note: Top to middle
Extraction method: Steam distilled

Author's Note: I have used Melissa ever since I first qualified over 30 years ago. I have always been surprised that it is not used more by Aromatherapists, but this seems to be changing, thankfully. Also known as Lemon Balm or Bee Balm

Contraindications: Not to be used if pregnant, breast feeding or on babies and children. Not to be used if you have glaucoma, or diagnosed with prostatic hyperplasia. Patients on bupropion antidepressants should avoid it. People who are diabetic must be extremely careful when using this oil. Possible skin irritant.

Emotional: Calming, uplifting, peace, self-worth, relaxing, revitalizing.
"Like a beam of light on a dark winter's day, melissa softens extreme emotions, eases resentment, gladdens the heart and engages the soul in its own graceful rhythm," Robbi Zeck.

Gabriel Mojay recommends Melissa "for people who are easily traumatised by confrontation. They often manifest their strength by attempting to contain, rather than respond to and express their feelings of hurt and anger." I totally agree with Mojay's description here. People who are affected and respond this way draw in their boundaries closer and become what could be perceived as stubborn almost to the point of intransigence.

Keim Loughran & Bull explain that Melissa oil helps us release emotional blocks and heal the wounds caused by the death of a loved one. It teaches us that death is a part of life, without interfering in the natural grief process.

Mental: Generally, and overall, it restores positivity, mental strength and courage. It is revitalizing to the mind, memory, wisdom and restores enthusiasm. Helps insomnia, sleep disorders, general nervousness, stress, and anxiety-related symptoms.

Herbalist John Evelyn (1620 -1706) described Melissa as the ruler of the brain, strengthening the memory, removing melancholy and depression.

A double-blind, placebo-controlled trial confirmed that topical application of Melissa oil significantly reduced agitation in severe dementia patients.

Lavender is often used to calm Alzheimer's patients. Trials have shown Melissa has a more profound effect than Lavender and clearly helps with 'sun-downer' anger and extreme anxiety that accompanies it.

Recent research indicates that cholinesterase is a main contributor to dementia. Melissa oil demonstrated high acetylcholinesterase inhibitory activity, meaning it may be effective for treating Alzheimer's disease. Let's hope they do more research!

Besides Alzheimer's there have been positive results using Melissa for ADD/ADHD.

Relationships: Ever feel that sometimes everybody wants, wants, wants, and you've been saying "yes, yes, yes", just to be the good guy? Then lo and behold some of your "yes's" have rebounded and you have had egg on your face? Time to put on the Mr. Nice Guy brakes, slow down your runaway train and consider everything individually. Melissa won't turn you into a negative, miserable sour puss, quite the contrary. It will allow you to set boundaries which will mean that when you say "yes" an even better result ensues for all concerned.

Television, computers, noise pollution, advertising, even other people, all these things attack our personal boundaries, if you let them. This is known as social conditioning to which most of us have fallen into. This constant daily bombardment makes your efforts to keep your boundaries more and more exhausting. In other words, this oil will afford you the protection from outside stimuli. All this bombardment weakens your nervous system resulting in stress, insomnia, anxiety and also a loss of personal direction and control of your own life. It is a wonderful defense shield in that it keeps out these 'negativities', yet allows in the positives.

Physical:

Muscular/Skeletal Systems:

Circulatory System: Lowers high blood pressure, slows rapid heartbeat, nervous palpitations and attacks of lightheadedness and dizziness. Avicenna recommended Melissa for strengthening the heart.

Lymphatic/Immune System: An in vitro study confirmed that Melissa oil had excellent antibacterial activity when used on its own and when used with standard antibiotics. Melissa oil displayed very high antibacterial activity against four bacterial strains responsible for nosocomial infections. A nosocomial infection is an infection you get while you're in the hospital for another reason.

Nervous System: Avicenna also recommended Melissa for "neuralgic affectations and nervous headaches." Said to help tinnitus.

Endocrine System: It regulates periods, aids menstrual pain, is a uterine tonic and helps with all sorts of menopausal symptoms. Also said to help epilepsy.

Respiratory System: A massively anti-viral and anti-bacterial essential oil which is often overlooked. It has proven results with asthma and allergies.

Digestive System: Melissa oil regulates the digestive system, relieving cramps, reduces flatulence and stimulates the gall bladder and liver. It settles nausea, vomiting, dyspepsia, indigestion, food induced headaches and migraines, dysentery and candida. It can also help to stimulate appetite. An in vitro study found that Melissa oil may play an important role on diabetes.

Excretory/Urinary Systems:

Integumentary/Skin System: It calms insect bites. Treats fungal infections, viral skin infections, particularly Herpes and Candida, see above. Greek physicians used Melissa to treat wounds. Studies in Germany have found Melissa oil to possess antiviral properties against *Herpes simplex* and *Herpes zoster*. Dr Wabner suggests using an undiluted blend of rose and melissa oil directly onto the herpes lesions. He states that the herpes lesions often disappear within one or two days.

Dreams and Aspirations: This is another oil that has an affinity with your heart, and through its protective mechanism keeps your heart space sacred and pure, yet it allows you to be safely sensitive to messages, or inner guidance, that you receive. It acts as a filtration system and will allow in only that will serve your highest purpose and good. This is again an oil which not only restores balanced aspects in your physical, mental, emotional and spiritual being, but it will help you to keep the balance through its intrinsic 'protective' nature. Melissa has the ability to reach the very roots of your psyche, the inner child. Worwood explains that Melissa oil is a spiritual conduit. She describes the oil as encouraging strength and having a revitalising effect that is especially appreciated before meditation or prayer.

Melissa represents femininity and maternity, and through this restores tranquility, simplicity of heart and provides you with spiritual strength. It has a very high vibratory light frequency and because of this its energy travels far. The energies it can bring you come from a distance one cannot begin to imagine. It is a spiritual channel in itself, it is therefore a wonderful oil to help you prepare for meditation and prayer.

Notes:

Neroli – 'Bringer of Light'

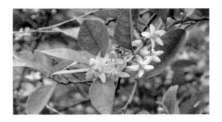

Botanical name: Citrus aurantium/Citrus aurantium var. amara (commonly known as sweet and not to be confused with Citrus v. bigaradia which is bitter)
Plant part: Blossoms
Country of origin: Tunisia
Note: Middle
Extraction method: Steam distilled

Contraindications: Not to be used if undergoing treatment for cancer.

Emotional: Neroli is known as the King of anti-depressant oils. It brings optimism. It can be very tranquillising, relaxing, stabilising, regenerating, protective, calming, joyful and euphoric to the emotions. It brings contentment, a sense of self-assurance and peace.

Mental: Neroli brings mental strength, fortitude, courage, creativity, balance, assertiveness, stability and wisdom. It is well known for treating insomnia and shock, but I suspect this has more to do with the underlying emotions it helps with. Will help insomnia where the root cause is depression. Massive antidepressant, best there is.

Relationships: The light is on but nobody is home? No, this is worse, the light is off and the occupant has up and left! You had enough, went into overload, blew a fuse and went into complete meltdown. Result? Total shut down and you couldn't care less about anything. It's taking all your energy just to operate on autopilot. Even if you've not quite reached this point, but can feel yourself nose diving in this direction, it's time stop, ask for help, and get the light within you switched back on.

Neroli enables you to see the light within any dark. It will open you to see some goodness in even the worst person, even yourself, and you will draw this light out of any person or situation. Neroli gives you the freedom of spirit, allowing your own light to glow and make you non-judgmental of others lifestyles.

Physical:

Muscular/Skeletal Systems: It has analgesic and antispasmodic properties. It can ease muscular cramps, but I suspect this is more due to its effect on our emotions and mind.

Circulatory System: Regulates heartbeat, tachycardia, and purifier. Can lower blood pressure in some when high blood pressure is presenting. Helps haemorrhoids, varicose veins and phlebitis. It is an excellent overall circulatory tonic. Helps purify the blood.

Lymphatic/Immune System: Antibacterial, antiparasitic, antifungal properties.

Nervous System: Helps stop headaches, yawning, insomnia due to its soporific (induces tiredness or sleep) properties. It has a direct calming action on the Sympathetic and Central Nervous Systems. Vertigo and general neuralgia respond well due to its calming effect on the CNS.

Endocrine System: Helps PMS/PMT and menopausal symptoms. It is a gentle aphrodisiac, by easing underlying frigidity.

Respiratory System: Helps stop bouts of yawning! Can be a good antiviral for early stages of all types of lung infections.

Digestive System: Great for flatulence, colitis, liver-pancreas deficiency and stomach cramps An all-round digestive stimulant. Treats diarrhoea and digestive headaches. Will treat bacterial and parasitic infections of the digestive system particularly hook worm and lamblia.

Excretory/Urinary Systems:

Integumentary/Skin System: A first-rate oil for inflamed skin, thread veins, stretch marks, regenerates skin cells so good for dry, sensitive and mature skins, and softening scar tissue due to its cell regenerative properties. A natural deodorant.

Dreams and Aspirations: Like Melissa, Neroli has a very high vibratory rate and as such can take you to the angelic realms if you so wish, and will bring you back in a state of purity, peace and love. Neroli will reveal the truth in and behind any situation or person. Neroli will connect you with your divine self.

It has an affinity with female energy (Yin), even though Neroli's energy is more Yang, and will help with any stages of transition and changes you go through. As such, it is invaluable as you discover your inner truth and the changes this will inevitably bring about as you proceed on your spiritual self-discovery and recovery of your soul purpose.

Notes:

Rose – 'Serene Centeredness'

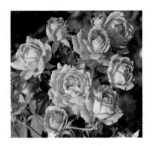

Botanical name: Rose damascena
Plant parts: Flowers
Country of origin: Central Asia
Note: Middle
Extraction method: Solvent extraction making it an Absolute

Contraindications: Not to be used if pregnant, breast feeding or on babies and children. Not to be used if undergoing treatment for cancer.

Emotional: Promotes feelings of confidence, joy, happiness and contentment.

Mental: Motivational oil, promoting co-operation, completeness and patience, Depression, jealousy, resentment and grief in particular respond well.

Relationships: Rose has an affinity with our heart, it gladdens our heart, it makes our heart sing, it returns us to 'centeredness'. So, it is no surprise that it's feelings of serenity encapsulate our hearts.

When everything around us is in a state of hubbub, when there seems to be no joy and compassion, when all around us is taking us from a state of grace to a state of flux and turmoil, rose will quiet us down, and allows us to see that there is goodness and love and a silver lining in all things.

Physical:

Muscular/Skeletal Systems:

Circulatory System: Helps to stimulates blood circulation, toning to the heart and capillaries. Helps treat angina and jaundice.

Lymphatic/Immune System: Rose has antiviral and antibacterial as well as anti-inflammatory properties.

Nervous System: Very calming to the nervous system, bringing that complete sense of serenity to your being.

Endocrine System: For the ladies: PMT, increases vaginal secretions particularly useful during menopause. Regulates menstrual cycle. Toning for the uterus. For the gentlemen: increases semen, frigidity and impotence. For both: an aphrodisiac. Stimulates the brain to produce dopamine, so could be indicated not just for depression but also Parkinson's disease.

Respiratory System: Soothes sore throats and coughs. A gentle expectorant. Excellent for chronic bronchitis. Tuberculosis and asthma have both been successfully treated with Rose.

Digestive System: Helps to clear the alimentary canal. It is a gentle remedy for nausea, vomiting and mild/gentle laxative for constipation. Supports a nervous tummy during emotional upsets. Allegedly helps hangovers!

Excretory/Urinary Systems:

Integumentary/Skin System: Nourishing and moisturizing for all skin types. Promotes wound healing and scar formation. Antiseptic for skin problems. Reduces broken capillaries.

Dreams And Aspirations: Awakening, inner vision, euphoria.

By reconnecting to our 'serene centeredness', our hearts, our mind stills and we see past all the turmoil and have the ability to love almost any situation better.

Notes:

The following two oils work in a sort of tandem. What this means is that although both oils have their distinct personalities of course, I would strongly recommend that you smell both oils whilst mentally focusing on the games your mind is playing on you. Then go with the oil that smells the best! Both oils can have male and female qualities, but this does not mean that if you are thinking in a masculine way and feel that you need more of a female perspective that using Ylang-Ylang will temper your 'masculinity'. The opposite could happen and it could fire up your masculinity even more. Smell is best in both these oils cases!

Tagetes – 'Divine Masculine'

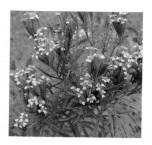

Botanical name: Tagetes minuta
Plant parts: Flowers and leaves
Country of origin: Southern South America
Note: Middle
Extraction method: Steam distilled

Contraindications: Some say it is phototoxic, but I believe this is for its cousin, Marigold. Possible skin irritant.

Emotional: Calming and relieving to erratic emotions promoting steadfastness and a better grip on them.

Mental: Brings clarity, perseverance and focus to our thoughts.

Relationships: Tagetes is connected to the left, analytical side of our brain. Often thought of as our masculine brain. Sometimes we need our thinking brain ramped up a bit to make sense of all the information input. This is not the same as memory recall and helping our brains to study like Rosemary or Basil will do. This is deeper, this is getting into and dissecting the nitty gritty of the information we have at hand.

It literally gets to the root of the problem we are trying to fathom, and keeps you grounded during the process. Yet, it will still connect us to the etheric information data bank. Einstein once said all the answers are out there in the universe, we just need to reach out and connect to it.

It brings empathy, and can help us to recognize narcissists.

Physical: A very powerful oil and should be used sparingly in a blend.

Muscular/Skeletal Systems: Anti-inflammatory and analgesic properties help muscular aches and pains.

Circulatory System: Can help to lower high blood pressure.

Lymphatic/Immune System: Parasitic infestation and resistant fungal infections.

Nervous System:

Endocrine System:

Respiratory System: Ear, sinus, throat and chest infections. Helps to remove mucous congestion of the chest, sinuses and the digestive tract. I've used it to treat croup very quickly for my son.

Digestive System: Will help treat Candida mycosis of the gut.

Excretory/Urinary Systems:

Integumentary/Skin System: Well-known for reducing inflammation and pain of bunions, gout and carbuncles. Also used in the treatment of chilblains, calluses, corns, warts, athletes' foot, and fungal infections of our feet.

Dreams And Aspirations: Helps us achieve our dreams and aspirations by keeping a clear and focused mind, our feet on the ground without getting carried away, and join the dots and facts to make us achieve our dreams and aspirations in a pragmatic and organized way. Tagetes has an affinity with our throat, in spiritual terms this is our throat chakra. This is where we take information in and where we regurgitate information from. This is why so many students often get sore throats and tonsillitis during exam time. They take the information in and then have to regurgitate it, so putting their throats under a lot of stress. Now that I have explained what Tagetes does, and as you will see from its attributes to the physical body, it makes it an invaluable tool for those studying to keep the mind clear and therefore not compromise or put our immune system under stress.

Notes:

Ylang-Ylang – 'Divine Feminine'

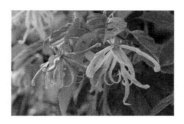

Botanical name: Cananga odorata var genuina
Plant parts: Flowers
Country of origin: countries surrounding the Indian Ocean
Note: Middle to base
Extraction method: Steam distilled

Author's Note: All Essential Oils are what is known as 'complete' oils, meaning the plant material goes through a single extraction process. Ylang-Ylang is not what is known as a 'complete' essential oil. It can go through several extraction processes giving us different qualities or 'levels' of Ylang-Ylang, so be very careful when you purchase. Some disreputable suppliers will sell the lower levels of Ylang-Ylang at the same price as the more expensive 'complete' Ylang-Ylang.

Contraindications: Lowers blood pressure, care should be taken if you have low blood pressure. It reduces tachycardia and can stabilize arrythmia, so would be advisable not to use if you are on heart regulating medications. Possible skin irritant. May cause nausea or headaches in high concentrations or prolonged use.

Emotional: Raises low self-confidence and low self-esteem, promoting an air of assured calm.

Mental: Mentally it is uplifting, promotes enthusiasm. Helps with insomnia due to its sedative properties. A valuable antidepressant, although the very heady aroma will not be appealing to some.

Relationships: Ylang-Ylang connects us to the right, intuitive, feminine side of our brain. When we can't quite grasp the answer, we need being hidden in the depths of our mind we become anxious, angry and frustrated. This is not like our emotional body experiencing these feelings, this is clearly in your head where you feel like you are 'banging your head against a brick wall'. Ylang-Ylang calms this mental anxiety and frustration, relaxes our breathing, reduces our blood pressure and thus allows the free flow of mental clarity.

Once the negative mind set is released, joy, calm and enthusiasm follow resulting in a free-flowing mind that is happy and contented.

Physical:

Muscular/Skeletal Systems:

Circulatory System: Lowers blood pressure, tachycardia (rapid heart-beat), palpitations,

Lymphatic/Immune System:

Nervous System: Relaxing and sedative properties to our nervous system, particularly through the vagus nerve. But this should be short term use. Prolonged use of Ylang-Ylang could have the opposite effect, which indeed it does, to a very few people, who have an adverse reaction to Ylang-Ylang. I have seen it affect a fellow Aromatherapist where his breathing became shallow, pulse rate elevated and became very light headed. In severe reactions he had been known to completely pass out. The only essential oil he had a reaction to even in a blend. He would smell and react to Ylang-Ylang a mile off!

Endocrine System: balances hormones, aphrodisiac, impotence and frigidity. Regulates adrenalin flow. A tonic for the womb. Reputedly helps to keep the breasts firm, but also clears recurrent cysts in the breast. I can vouch for this through clinic experience with a client.

Respiratory System: Calms hyperpnoea (rapid breathing). It helps fight general infections of the respiratory tract.

Digestive System: Infections of the gut respond well. It is antispasmodic helping to smooth out cramping and returning normal peristalsis to the digestive system. I feel this is more due to its sedating effect on our Vagus Nerve.

Excretory/Urinary Systems:

Integumentary/Skin System: Balancing to both oily and dry skin. Has been used in hair products to stimulate hair growth.

Dreams And Aspirations: Let's go of self-judgment which self-sabotages us achieving our goals.

Notes:

7.

THE ARBOUR – RELATIONSHIPS

In Native American tradition, trees represent our relationships, not just with Mother Nature, but with ourselves, our family, specific people, our job, our environment, and with life generally. I have assigned the 'personalities' of different famous people to represent each individual tree. So, if a situation or person makes you feel that you wish you could be more like the Dalai Lama: calm, logical and eloquent, or maybe you need more of Eleanor Roosevelt's attitude and temperament: roll up your sleeves and just get on with it, to improve or enhance a relationship or situation, then all you will have to do is find the corresponding tree!

If any of the famous people I have chosen are unfamiliar to you, please don't worry. The ensuing descriptions alone should be enough to make you think of somebody that is familiar to you and fits the bill. So please go ahead, and add your own choice of person/personality if it sits more comfortably within the description I have written.

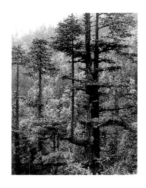

Botanical name: Cedrus deodara
Plant part: Wood
Country of origin: Himalaya
Note: Base
Extraction method: Steam distilled

Contraindications: Currently it is best to follow the same contraindications of the more popular Cedarwood Atlas, until we know more if it is a safer alternative. Not to be used if pregnant, breast feeding or on babies and children. Not to be used if undergoing treatment for cancer. Can cause severe thirst therefore not suitable for those with kidney disorders. Possible skin irritant.

Emotional: Think of the Dalai Lama. He exudes emotional strength, stability, confidence. integrity, and courage. His personality is one of warmth, calmness, dignity, self-knowing and harmonious. Oh, to have this emotional balance of the Dalai Lama!

Mental: This Cedarwood will strengthen your mental resilience and fortitude. It helps with memory recall. Encourages concentration and focus which can be to the point of being steadfast and persevering, until the job in hand is done. An organised mind shows a wise mind.

Relationships: Calm wisdom of the ages in serene centeredness and grace, that's the Dalai Lama is it not? If you feel a quiet, still, integrity is required in dealing with a relationship, then visualise yourself as the Dalai Lama.

Unlike the other Cedarwood oils, the Himalayan variety not only has a distinctly different aroma, it also has a much more profound effect on your psyche and spirituality. It brings clarity and a sense of connectedness with everyone and everything that is in this physical world and 'other worlds'. This particular Cedarwood strengthens the transforming power of your will, as opposed to your ego, and restores spiritual certainty in your relationships. It will manifest your thoughts into reality, so be careful of what and how you think and wish for, both in your relationships and otherwise! It will bring strength of spirit to any difficult situation and help you resonate and be in harmony with the forces and cycles of nature, which affect all your relationships. Being an ancient oil, it has a long memory and will help you with past life recall if you call on its energies to help you with this. With being of a dignified nature it will bring grace into all your varied relationships.

Physical: Cedarwood has a reputation for moving chronic and hard to shift ailments.

Muscular/Skeletal System: Rheumatism and arthritis respond well.

Circulatory System:

Lymphatic/Immune System: Any glandular problems, it kicks starts the Lymphatic System to remove toxins and waste.

Nervous System: It has a calming the nervous system, but I feel this is because of its effect on our emotions and mind.

Endocrine System: An aphrodisiac. Allegedly helps sexual asthenia also known as erectile dysfunction.

Respiratory System: Bronchitis, catarrh and coughs respond well. However, be very careful if you are going to use it to dry up mucous, it could leave you with a very dry cough, and that hurts more than a wet cough. I speak from personal experience.

Digestive System:

Excretory/Urinary Systems: Has a toning effect on kidney disorders, bladder problems and urinary tract infections such as cystitis. A useful diuretic, particularly when combined with Cypress.

Integumentary/Skin System: Good for hair loss, dandruff and a greasy scalp. Has been used successfully to treat acne, oily skin, psoriasis and dermatitis. It is well known for wound healing on skin abscess.

Dreams and Aspirations: A great and well-respected oil for meditative manifestation practices. Even without meditative practice it keeps your mind focused with quiet and resolute determination.

Notes:

Cypress – Peter Ustinov (Stephen Fry)

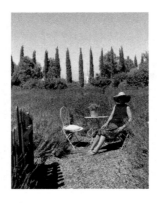

Me, in Cyprus, taken by my son.

Botanical name: Cupressus Sempervirens
Plant part: Needles and twigs
Country of Origin: Pangea!
Note: Middle
Extraction method: Steam distillation

Author's Note: Country of origin: Pangea! 280-230 million years ago, the continent we now know as North America was continuous with Africa, South America, and Europe. They all existed as a single continent called Pangea. The tree can be traced back 12 million years in the UK. The Cypress as we know it, was probably first utilized in Persia (Iran), Syria or Cyprus. Its name may derive from Cyprus, although this is not a certainty, nor is there any specific historical reference to this affect. There are many different types of Cypress trees, many due to cross-breeding. One Bald Cypress tree (Taxodium distichum) growing along the Black River in the state of North Carolina in the USA is at least 2,624 years old as of 2018, a new study has found. The oldest living cypress is the Sarv-e-Abarkooh in Iran's Yazd Province. Its age is estimated to be approximately 4,000 years old. Fascinating history to these majestic trees which grow to a height 115ft tall or more.

Contraindications: Not to be used if pregnant, breast feeding in the presence of mastitis or on babies and children. Not to be used if undergoing treatment for oestrogen-related cancers.

Emotional and Mental: Very difficult to separate the emotional from the mental with Cypress. Imagine if you will, a great Uncle type of personality, somebody who has a comforting air, a quiet confidence and has found inner peace. "Been there, done that, worn the T-shirt, wrote the book" type of person. They are 'worldly wise', well read, intelligent but also witty because they see the lightness in life and don't see mountains. They understand you. They make you feel calm, re-assured. This is what Cypress will bring to you.

We know there are two key words with Cypress, bridge and excess. Where there is an excess of emotions and mental activity, Cypress brings stillness, stability, calm, clear thinking and even inspiration and understanding. The inspiration and understanding are your bridge from where you are emotionally or mentally out of the cycle and to where you need to be.

We also know Cypress is the master when it comes to grief. It allows us to remember happier times and see the perceived loss as a bridge to your loved ones continued journey. It also helps those who know they are passing but are filled with fear and trepidation and naturally do their best to cling to life. No wonder we see them so often in British cemeteries.

Very talkative people, who keep changing subjects, we've all met one, is showing signs of mental and emotional stress. Cypress has been successfully used to release both and calm the person down and bring them more into focus.

Relationships: Cypress has a sense of humour, it chuckles at the irony, paradox and incongruity of life. "Oh well, here we go! What do you expect? Life is full of little surprises and inconsistencies!"

If a relationship, for example your work, seems to be going through a state of continuously changing tack and this is becoming infuriating as you can't seem to see what is coming next, then chuckle out loud and say "well, there you go!" Cypress is a life raft when all around you is flotsam and unknown, unchartered territory; it carries you through and over the bobbing and jostling sea of humanity to a calm port. It acts like a bridge from the past or present into your future.

Physical: Key word with Cypress is 'excess', of any kind.

Muscular/Skeletal Systems: Some rheumatism sufferers find relief from the use of Cypress. It is a sudorific and a febrifuge thus helping with cramping of the muscles too. Helps with asthenia, abnormal physical weakness or lack of energy.

Circulatory System: It is a haemostatic: stops nose bleeds and haemorrhages. Being a vasoconstrictor, it reduces varicose veins and piles/haemorrhoids. It reputedly strengthens veins and arteries and has been used in the treatment of thread veins quite successfully. Sudorific: promotes sweating. Febrifuge: reduces fever.

Lymphatic/Immune System: A well-known remedy for cellulitis and oedema. It comes into its own where there is excess of any kind. In fact, 'excess' could be Cypress' key word. Allegedly helps in the treatment of malaria.

Nervous System: Because of its 'personality' it is balancing and a demulcent to the nervous system.

Endocrine System: Being a hormonal balancer, it is useful for all aspects of PMT, PMS and the menopause, particularly when there are hot flushes. Particularly good for ovarian dysfunction, and reduces pain and heavy periods. Allegedly helps treat prostatic tumours.

Respiratory System: Very good for coughs, whooping cough, asthma, bronchitis, pleurisy tuberculosis, malaria, which are all respiratory problems that respond well to Cypress.

Digestive System: A great tonic to the liver. Can help dissolve gall stones.

Excretory/Urinary Systems: Well-known for its diuretic properties and the treatment of oedema. Can help break down kidney stones. It has proven results with incontinence and bed wetting too, young or old.

Integumentary/Skin System: For the skin, it is useful for mature skin where loss of moisture increases wrinkles. Sweaty (particularly feet, but check thyroid function) and oily skin are also helped. Also helps scar formation and breaks down cellulite and treat cellulitis.

Dreams And Aspirations: Using Cypress in your meditative practices to manifest your dreams and aspirations will bring you inner wisdom, patience and trust in the process. It will bring you inspiration to think outside the box and prevent you from self-sabotaging. It also has an air of incorruptibility, thus preventing others putting you off your intentions.

Notes:

Eucalyptus – Bruce Lee/Steven Segal

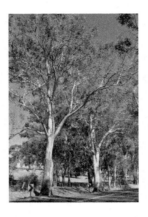

Botanical name: Eucalyptus globulus
Also known as Eucalyptus Blue Gum
Plant part: Leaves
Country of origin: Australia
Note: Middle
Extraction process: Steam distilled

Contraindications: Not to be used during the first trimester of pregnancy. Personally, I would use other safer alternatives such as Niaouli. Not to be used if undergoing treatment for cancer. Not to be used if you have high blood pressure, or have epilepsy. Avoid using if you are also taking homeopathic remedies. Not to be used on children under the age of 8 years. Personally, I prefer not to use it on pre-pubescent children. Possible skin irritant.

Emotional: Just like anyone who practices the Martial Arts, Eucalyptus brings an emotional balance and calm. There is an inner stillness to the emotions allowing for the mental attributes to come through.

Mental: Leading on from the emotional balance and calm, Eucalyptus brings concentration, focus and determination.

Relationships: Cool, calm and collected with an air of self-assuredness that if somebody crosses your line, you can strike back twice as fast and twice as hard, think of a scorpion, you have a sting in your tail.

If you take the lid off a bottle of Eucalyptus and let it's smell waft about, it will take the heat out of the situation, thus calming it down. But if you get a little to close and sniff the bottle again, it will bite your head off. So, you need to take the heat out of the situation, and then assume the pose, legs slightly apart and firmly anchored, hands loosely clasped together and make eye contact. Oh, the ponytail is optional!

Eucalyptus brings self-assuredness and confidence.

Physical:

Muscular/Skeletal System: Often used in blends to help muscular aches and pains and rheumatism.

Circulatory System: It is a hemostatic: stops bleeding and hemorrhage. Long used to treat migraines. Lowers fever and temperature very quickly. Has also been known to treat angina and malaria.

Lymphatic/Immune System:

Nervous System: Helps stop neuralgic pain.

Endocrine System: Has been used in the treatment of gonorrhea.

Respiratory System: Throat and ear infections including Scarlet Fever, otitis, rhinopharyngitis, sinusitis, all respond well. It helps stuffy colds, coughs, eases and loosens off congestion. Helps flu and asthma symptoms, although I'd go carefully in the presence of asthma. Diseases such as tuberculosis, typhoid, diphtheria have all been successfully treated. Apparently can be effective against hay-fever symptoms.

Digestive System: Can help: dysentery and diabetes. It is anti-parasitic. Stems diarrhea. Can help dissolve gall stones. Pyorrhea: inflammation of the gums.

Excretory/Urinary Systems: Can help cystitis, nephritis and general bladder inflammation.

Integumentary/Skin System: Helps scar formation and helps heal wounds including ulcers. Anti-fungal, anti-bacterial and anti-parasitic. Deodorising action because it can kill off those pesky smelling bacteria. Can help soothe the itch of Chicken Pox although I would prefer it in hydrosol form for children. Herpes responds well. It has also been used on minor burns, but it will never better Lavender for burns in my view.

Dreams And Aspirations: Looping back to what Eucalyptus does for us emotionally and mentally, it keeps us balanced, centered, focused and brings rational and logical thinking to manifest our dreams and aspirations.

Notes:

Juniper – Eleanor Roosevelt

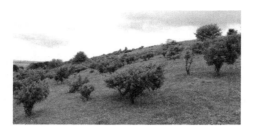

Botanical name: Juniperus communis
Plant part: Berries or leaf, should be clearly indicated.
Country of origin: Europe and NE Asia.
Note: Middle
Extraction method: Steam distilled

Contraindications: Not to be used if pregnant, breast feeding or on babies and children. Not to be used if there are kidney problems, or have been on long-term steroids in past seven years. Not to be used if undergoing treatment for cancer.

Emotional: The key word here is "blockages". This means that whether it is mental, emotional or a physical blockage, Juniper will clear it almost immediately. For example, we have all walked into a room and felt "you could cut the atmosphere with a knife" – a quick waft of Juniper very quickly clears it. It is of great support in challenging or difficult situations.

Mental: Mentally Juniper brings strength to our mental processes. By clearing mental 'blockages' it brings sincerity to your words and deeds, but still keeping your verbal filter in place! In other words, it is very diplomatic but will 'hit the nail on the head' as they say. So yes, in some cases people can't 'handle the truth'. It can be mildly sleep inducing, but this I believe to be when mental stress is cleared and the physical body needs to rest and recuperate, probably because of its direct effect on our nervous system too.

Relationships: I apologise for my rudeness, "but cut the crap, cut to the quick, children's eyes don't see all that shit." Perhaps, maybe, and I mean no disrespect, but today dear Eleanor would use such frank words with you to stop pussy-footing around, stop making mountains out of molehills and make you roll up your sleeves and get on with it. And the children? Well, don't they just have a natural and uninhibited ability to see everything in its simplest form? They have not been conditioned by society, they are still innocent and see things for what they really are. "Out of the mouths of babes".

Juniper clears the blockages, obstacles and confusion, emotional, mental, physical and even spiritual levels. "You can cut the atmosphere with a knife," well, next time it happens, just take the lid off your Juniper oil and………. BAM, it's gone. So, if it is mental clarity you need to get to the core of the situation, then call on Eleanor.

Physical:

Muscular/Skeletal System: Juniper has a long-standing reputation for helping arthritis, rheumatism and gout. Asthenia: general weakness, lack of strength and energy in the limbs.

Circulatory System: An excellent remedy for piles when combined with Cypress and Frankincense. Reputedly a blood purifier. A sudorific, it encourages sweating when required. It is helpful for pericarditis, but I can't find anything about myocarditis.

Lymphatic/Immune System: It is excellent for throwing off poisons – especially where disease carrying insects are prolific. Breaks down cellulitis, particularly when combined with Cypress. It is a major detoxifier to the whole body.

Nervous System: Calming and relieving to the whole nervous system and in particular it seems to have an affinity with sciatica. Strengthens the nerves generally. Good for dental neuralgia and facial paralysis such as Bell's Palsy in particular.

Endocrine System: It regulates periods and eases period pains. It can help reduce an enlarged prostate, thus making urination easier. But please remember it is contraindicated in the presence of cancer.

Respiratory System: Expectorant for congestion and excess mucous. Treats rhinitis and sinusitis.

Digestive System: A brilliant regulator for the appetite, especially where obesity is a problem. A tonic for the liver and especially in the treatment of cirrhosis. If you are feeling drowsy and sleepy, Juniper can relieve this if the condition has been brought on by waste overload in the small intestine, also check the Ileocecal Valve – a simple foot bath should suffice in this case. It helps regulate the appetite and stimulates metabolism. Said to help cirrhosis of the liver. Used to help break down and eliminate gall stones. Can help with diabetes. Clears mucous from the intestines.

Excretory/Urinary Systems: A very effective diuretic (blockage) and lack of urination. Invaluable for cystitis, especially when combines with Bergamot. Fluid retention (strangury) in particular can benefit from the use of Juniper. A first rate "detoxifier" of the body, enhanced when combined with Geranium. cystitis, strangury, kidney stones, fluid retention. Helps eliminate uric and oxalic acids.

Integumentary/Skin System: For the skin, oily and congested skins benefit, as does seborrhoea of the scalp. Acne, blocked pores, dermatitis, weeping eczema, psoriasis, cellulite, ulcers and swellings all respond well. It is wound healing and helps scar formation.

Dreams And Aspirations: Juniper is often associated with our 3rd eye, or our intuition for those not familiar with the chakra's. As such it brings 'inner vision', enlightenment and inspiration. By removing blockages, whether they be emotional, mental or physical, Juniper will clear the way to new ideas and approaches to your dreams and aspirations.

Notes:

Myrtle — Jesus/Christ energy

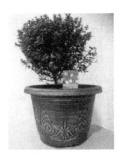

My small Myrtle tree, taken by me.

Botanical name: Myrtus communis
Plant parts: Leaves
Country of origin: probably Persia or Afghanistan.
Note: Middle
Extraction method: Steam distilled

Author's Note: In a study, scientists inoculated fresh tomatoes and iceberg lettuce with a nalidixic acid resistant strain of Salmonella. Then they used a cleaning solution containing essential oil of myrtle to test if it would kill the bacteria. They found that washing with myrtle leaf oil caused a significant reduction in bacteria. The results suggest that the use of myrtle oil can be an alternative to the use of chlorine or synthetic disinfectants on fruits and vegetables. (Appendix 1.)

Contraindications: Avoid during pregnancy although looking at the chemistry I believe this to be more applicable to Lemon Myrtle or Green Myrtle. Over-use may cause damage to mucus membrane/tissues.

Emotional: The key phrase to remember about Myrtle is "Love it better".

Emotionally it can soothe and dissipate feelings of anger. It is for those people who are not happy with themselves or have self-destructive, self-sabotaging behaviour. It is sedative, uplifting, comforting effect on the emotions and mind, and brings acceptance and harmony. When going through difficult times, Myrtle helps with looking at brighter times ahead it becomes your 'friend in need'. Not just a 'companion oil for the dying', it also helps the living to let go not just the loss of a family member or friend, but also let go of 'that which no longer serves us'.

It will also help people with addictions, not just chemical addictions, but unhealthy emotional, mental and relationship 'addictions'.

Mental: Myrtle brings mental strength and empowerment. It creates mental and emotional space for forgiveness. It brings mental acuity and drive. Helpful to those who are not happy with themselves or have self-destructive, self-sabotaging behaviour.

Relationships: Agape, philein and eros? It's all Greek to me, we have one word for all these and it is love. Love has many, many forms, hence the Greek love of self, love of others, sexual love, love of Mother Nature, even love of God. Love is the key word to all of Jesus' teachings. Now don't worry, I am not about to get all religious on you. But I do want to point out one aspect of this 'love principal' that we often forget. Allowing others to love you, everyone should have someone who loves them; it is something we all, each and every one of us need as much as the air we breathe to get through life. It is a very rare gift we are given when someone is in love with us. It is even more special when we allow ourselves to <u>be</u> loved. Whether the giver or receiver, love is something which surpasses all other emotions, it supports us and motivates us. It negates any negativity that life throws at us. It turns problems and demands made of us into situations and opportunities.

To love and more importantly allow ourselves to be loved gives us the freedom to be all we can be, soar ever upwards, on and through life; until the day comes when we can look back and say "I loved life." Very few of us reach the end of our time and can say this because we allowed our life to be dictated by fear, worry, and basically self-doubt. We build false walls and defenses in the hope of stopping any pain or grief hurting us. If we allow this and don't give ourselves permission to love and be loved, then our lives will only have been an illusion of reality.

Remember this, you are beautiful just as you are. When somebody loves you, they have seen the beauty within you and the love follows. Beauty first, love follows.

Physical:

Muscular/Skeletal Systems: For the muscular/skeletal systems, chemistry wise being an anti-inflammatory, it is particularly effective for aches and pains in the knees and shoulders. This is particularly interesting when we are talking about 'love it better' and moving forwards. Our knees represent our ego, either too much ego that needs constant feeding or because you have the type of ego that finds it difficult to accept compliments, both can create problems in the knees. As to shoulders, we carry the weight of everybody else's problems and forget to address our own first. See how 'love it better' fits in here?

Circulatory System: Reduces blood congestion and indicated for haemorrhoids and varicose veins. Treats hemorrhoids and general pelvic congestion due to blood 'pooling'. Works especially well on bruises, particularly if combined with Marjoram and/or Immortelle.

Anti-parasitic: Myrtle oil has been traditionally used in Iran for the treatment of Malaria. Malaria is a parasitic disease of the blood which is passed to human beings by mosquitoes. Scientists administered Myrtle oil to mice that had been infected with Malaria and found that the treatment resulted in an 84% suppression of parasitic activity after four days of treatment. The treatment was not toxic to the mice, and researchers believed that this treatment offered promise for human cases of Malaria.

Lymphatic/Immune System: Reduces lymphatic congestion and enlarged lymph nodes. Although not much is written about Myrtle and our lymphatic system, in fact, you will be hard pushed to find anything, I am of the strong belief it gets the lymphatics moving again because of its effect on our emotions and mind.

Nervous System: It is very neuroprotective.

Endocrine System:

Respiratory System: Clears congestion in the sinuses. For the body, one of the most important uses is for clearing chest disorders, catarrh, similar to the effects of Eucalyptus, and keeps infection down generally. A relatively mild oil, therefore a preferable choice for children's chest complaints. It was only in the last century that the therapeutic properties of Myrtle were properly investigated. A gentleman by the name of M. Linarix judged Myrtle the best tolerated of all the balsamic plants. He judged Myrtle's most important uses is for clearing chest disorders, catarrh and the sinuses, similar to the effects of Eucalyptus. According to Wanda Sellar, Myrtle is effective against pulmonary diseases particularly when night sweats are also presenting.

A relatively mild oil, therefore a preferable choice for children's chest complaints, particularly before bedtime because of its gently sedating qualities.

Digestive System: The drying and binding properties of Myrtle make it useful for treating diarrhoea and dysentery. Dioscorides would prescribe a wine in which the Myrtle leaves had been macerated. According to his writings, this concoction fortified the stomach and was effective for pulmonary and bladder infections, and for those who were spitting blood. The drying and binding properties of Myrtle make it useful for treating diarrhoea and dysentery. It has been used to treat peptic ulcer. It also protects the liver (hepatoprotective).

It is claimed to be anti-diabetic. Myrtle leaves as well as the essential oil obtained from the leaves are used to lower the blood glucose level in type-2 diabetic patients in Turkish folk medicine. A study worked with groups of diabetic and non-diabetic rabbits. They measured the effects of single and multiple doses of myrtle oil on blood sugar levels for both groups. The non-diabetic rabbits did not experience a change in blood sugar levels after being given oral doses of the essential oil. However, the diabetic rabbits had a 51% reduction in blood sugar levels which appeared after 4 hours. The repeated administration of myrtle oil once per day to the diabetic rabbits maintained the lower blood sugar levels during the week-long study.

Excretory/Urinary Systems: It is indicated for pelvic congestion. I suspect this has more to do with our Sacral Chakra, represented by 'I am'. If we can't love ourselves (love it better), then congestion of all kinds will occur in the pelvis. Myrtle is also noted for its regulation of the genito-urethra system e.g., haemorrhoids and acts as an antiseptic for cystitis, bladder inflammation and urethritis.

Integumentary/Skin System: For the skin, Myrtle will strengthen and cleanse congested skin, it can alleviate acne and blemishes and works especially well on bruises, particularly if combined with Marjoram and/or Immortelle.

Can also relieve psoriasis. I have seen Myrtle work well with psoriasis sufferers when Myrtle is used with the intent of investigating why it is they 'can't live in their own skin'...they do not love themselves or have something they really don't like about themselves or a situation, which often as not stems back to childhood, the healing and 'loving themselves' starts to happen quickly. I can't say it cleared any case completely, but it certainly helped the symptoms.

Mouth and other ulcers. Warts are a contagious skin disease, but Myrtle seems to eradicate them.

Myrtle is also a natural deodorant. Sometime during the 16th century, what we would consider a floral water or hydrosol today, Myrtle was known as 'eau d'angles' or, Angel Water.

(Appendix: 2. 3. 4. 5. 6. 7.)

Dreams And Aspirations: Myrtle has the ability to bring enlightenment, inspiration and vision to your dreams and aspirations. Myrtle can cleanse your 'inner being' bringing peace and stillness to the job in hand.

Notes:

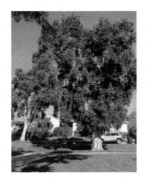

Botanical name: Melaleuca quinquenervia
Plant part: Leaves
Country of origin: Australia and Malaya
Note: Middle
Extraction process: Steam distilled

Author's Note: Everyone who uses Essential Oils should have Niaouli in their family medicine cabinet! Niaouli is also sometimes known as the Broad-Leaved Paperbark Tree or the Paper Bark Tea Tree

Contraindications: None known.

Emotional: Emotionally, Niaouli helps to 'cut the ties that bind' and 'can't please all the folk all of the time'. More about this in the relationships section.

Mental: Niaouli is stimulating, clarifying, invigorating, reviving and focuses our mind.

Relationships: Mother Theresa was in effect attacked on two fronts. Firstly, in her home country of India she became vilified for drawing international attention to their orphans. Eventually as her fame grew, this little lady from India was scorned by the west for flying all over the world at the behest of governments and the rich and famous when people thought she should have stayed at home and not joined the 'jet set' to garner more donations for her charity. She couldn't win whichever way she turned.

But, just like Niaouli, she found the will and the way to heal, to fix and improve the children's lives. But not just the children directly, she also found a way to heal adults too by opening their hearts to compassion and understanding. She went back to what was important to her, the children.

When a relationship isn't working because it is imploding and destroying itself, when it's clear it has come to an end, somebody has to find the will and the way to heal the situation, but to also move on. When it's clear both parties are just flogging a dead horse as they say. Maybe it's a narcissistic relationship? Then it's time to heal yourself and just walk away. This is an oil for empaths.

Physical: Same botanical family as Tea-Tree but with more of the effects of Eucalyptus, but is more sedative than stimulating and is safe to use on children.

Muscular/Skeletal System: I have firsthand experience of treating my mother's osteomyelitis with Niaouli. Again, Balz says Niaouli will treat arthrosis, often referred to as osteoarthritis as well as rheumatic polyarthritis.

Circulatory System: Rodolphe Balz cites Niaouli will treat diseases such as Viral hepatitis and malaria. It is a hypotensive oil, i.e., it will lower high blood pressure but has no effect on low blood pressure. It increases localized circulation when needed. It will help stimulate our white blood cells and antibodies in our Lymphatic System when fighting an infection.

Lymphatic/Immune System: It will help stimulate our antibodies when fighting an infection.

Nervous System: Neuralgia.

Endocrine System:

Respiratory System: Its main effect is on the respiratory system, laryngitis, catarrh, sinusitis, whooping cough, asthma, pneumonia, influenza, tuberculosis and bronchitis.

Digestive System: Flatulence, indigestion and nausea. Parasitic enterocolitis.

Excretory/Urinary Systems: Bladder and Urethra inflammation and infection.

Integumentary/Skin System: Fights infections of all kinds, including those on the skin.

Dreams And Aspirations: Niaouli will most certainly bring a sense of accomplishment to your dreams and aspirations through focus, determination and prevention of being 'side-tracked' and trying to please everyone else except yourself. Niaouli, like Cardamom has the ability to connect us with our guides, whether they be ancestral, personal guides and even angelic realm.

Every time I smell Niaouli my attention is always taken to my Crown Chakra. It's like a 'light bulb' that seems to just 'switch on' when my focus is on its vibration and energetics.

Notes:

Petitgrain – John Lennon

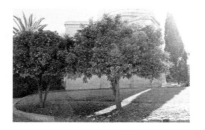

Botanical name: Citrus aurantium
Plant part: Leaves and sometimes twigs are included
Country of origin: The Moors of North Africa first introduced it to Spain, but orange trees originated in China
Note: Middle
Extraction method: Steam distilled

Contraindications: No known contra-indications.

Emotional: John Lennon was ever the optimistic, a glass half full type of person. It has relaxing and stabilizing effects on our emotions.

Mental: It is uplifting, joyful, playful and brings mental strength.

Relationships: If John Lennon were alive today this would be his oil. Yes, John was sad and disappointed in humanity, but Petitgrain would have lifted that as did John. He became a humanitarian, a peace maker. He had no ego in the traditional sense of the word. Yes, he had addictions, I'm not talking of his substance abuse, I am talking about his addiction to world peace and Yoko.
You see, Petitgrain removes any ego, it gives us healthy, happy and positive addictions. By the same token it will help us let go of bad or negative addictions. Addictions to people that don't actually bring out the best in us.

Petitgrain uplifts our relationships, it lifts them out of a stale quagmire and challenges us to investigate our inner vision, to look beyond the current situation and see something better. It helps us find our inner confidence and a way to express ourselves clearly and eloquently. It brings peace and harmony to a relationship.

Physical:

Muscular/Skeletal System: Eases muscle spasms, but I suspect this is because of its effect on the nervous system.

Circulatory System: Tachycardia and arrythmia can be helped.

Lymphatic/Immune System: An excellent immune-stimulant and support.

Nervous System: Sedates an overactive nervous system. Helps vegetative dystonia.

Endocrine System:

Respiratory System: Can be very useful in fighting off infections of the respiratory tract.

Digestive System: It has antispasmodic properties which calm a nervous stomach, dyspepsia and flatulence.

Excretory/Urinary Systems:

Integumentary/Skin System: Can be beneficial against boils, acne and general pimples.

Dreams And Aspirations: Once you focus on your dream or

aspiration it will bring determination, confidence and inspiration for ideas you might not thought about, some 'outside the box' ideas.

Notes:

Rosewood – Princess Diana

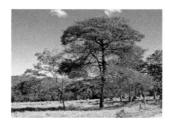

Botanical name: Aniba rosaeaodora
Sometimes referred to as Bois de Rose
Plant part: Wood
Country of origin: South America
Note: Middle
Extraction method: Steam distilled

Contraindications: No known contra-indications.

Emotional: Rosewood is a very comforting oil. It makes you feel safe, whole and complete emotionally. It is non-judgmental and thus allows you to feel secure in who you are regardless of internal or external influences. It is emotionally compassionate and graceful.

Mental: It balances a mind which keeps flitting from one scenario or situation to another. It helps you find the words to express yourself both emotionally and intellectually whether you are speaking to one person or a group of people. It stops the self-blame cycle and restores belief in yourself.

Relationships: Rosewood is your 'go-to' oil if you have been the victim of a narcissistic relationship, abusive relationship, domineering relationship, any kind of relationship where you have been the victim of predatorial abuse and bullying. Princess Diana's life was plagued from an early age with abuse. She was a 'victim' in her parent's divorce which saw the beginnings of her self-abuse with bulimia and anorexia. This led on to her marriage, where again she was stifled and controlled. Somewhere "enough is enough" hit home, and we saw this beautiful woman blossom into the Princess of hearts, who most of us loved and admired.

What is abuse? Abuse is the invasion of your space whether that be emotional, mental or physical. Rosewood gives you the strength and courage to speak from the heart. To recognize that abuse and reclaim yourself and be able to walk tall and proud and become a stronger, courageous and most importantly loving person, not just to others, including your antagonist, but more importantly to love yourself.

Self-loathing is abuse of self, where we have lost love of self. So, when your relationship issue is with yourself reach for Rosewood. When dealing with clients where there has been self or external relationship abuse, Rosewood is my 'go to' oil. It usually gets combined with Frankincense to allow the client to release the past. It then sometimes moves on to be combined with Sandalwood and Linaloe when they are ready to move on into the future. One of the citrus/fruit oils is usually combined to support where the client **wants** to feel emotionally, and again this citrus/emotional oil will also change as progress is made.

Physical: Any chronic (long term) complaints.

Muscular/Skeletal Systems: Analgesic for muscular aches and pains, arthritis, rheumatism and very possibly fibromyalgia. Treats asthenia which is a weakness and lethargy in the limbs.

Circulatory System: Can encourage sweating when fighting off an infection.

Lymphatic/Immune System: Long standing complaints with the immune system respond well. Antiviral, antimicrobe properties. One of its best effects is on our immune and lymphatic system, keeping it healthy and moving and helps the cleaning out process after infection.

Nervous System: Good for jet lag. Calms the nervous system.

Endocrine System: A well-known aphrodisiac, restoring libido and helps impotence and frigidity. Invaluable for those who have suffered sexual and other abuse. Treats vaginitis due to candida.

Respiratory System: Calms ticklish coughs. Particularly good on viruses and antiseptic for the throat. Infections in the ear/nose/throat and bronchial lung areas. Effective against flu and coronaviruses.

Digestive System: Helps nauseous headaches. I would suggest because of Rosewood's calming effect on the nervous system, I'm thinking in particular of the Vagus Nerve here, that Rosewood could help with a nervous tummy at the very least.

Excretory/Urinary Systems:

Integumentary/Skin System: Useful healer for cuts and wounds, dry skin, sensitive and inflamed skin. Beneficial to all skin types including the young, pimples and acne, and the old, combats ageing and wrinkles and dehydrated skin. Treats mycosis which is an infection caused by any fungus that invades the tissues, causing superficial, subcutaneous, or systemic disease and can be life-threatening. I can attest to it being an excellent natural deodorant and insect repellent.

Dreams And Aspirations: Rosewood will give you determination, fortitude and perseverance to get your dreams and aspirations done.

Notes:

Sandalwood – Ghandi

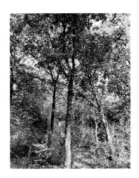

Botanical name: Santalum album
Plant part: Wood
Country of origin: Mysore region of India where the best
Sandalwood still comes from
Note: Base
Extraction method: Steam distilled

Contraindications: Avoid in cases of diagnosed clinical depression, as it may lower your mood further particularly if you are on antidepressant medication.

Emotional: Sandalwood is calming, it slows down erratic and racing emotions. It has a sensitive air; it listens to you and provides the emotional stability you need.

Mental: It is a wise old owl, that sits in its tree serenely, peacefully and quietly observing all around him. He has insight into the problem and when he sees the 'target' he swoops down and removes it.

Relationships: Sandalwood allows us to move on into the future with clarity, strength and fortitude. It allows us to let go of feelings of isolation, loneliness, stubbornness and obsession, thus bringing harmony into our relationships. It enables us to bring words of co-operation into a relationship and let's go of conflict. It will help you bring inspiration, insights and new ideas to the table and thus a win win situation for everyone. Sandalwood is an expert chess player, and plays the long game. It's in no rush to achieve its goal and will guide the relationship quietly and gently to a harmonious place of benefit to all involved. It will teach you to be gentle on yourself, to take baby steps, if necessary, but each step will be confident, assured and in the right direction. Its goal is unity.

Physical:

Muscular/Skeletal System:
Circulatory System: Reduces blood congestion in cases of venous stasis. Venous stasis is a problem with the veins, usually in the lower legs, that keeps blood from moving through very well. As more fluid and pressure builds up, some of the blood leaks out of the veins and into the skin.
Lymphatic/Immune System:
Nervous System:
Endocrine System: Helps frigidity, impotence, re-educates sperm, prostatitis, gonorrhea and is a well-known aphrodisiac.
Respiratory System: Sinusitis, laryngitis, sore throat, bronchitis, dry cough, pneumonia and catarrh, all respond well.
Digestive System: For the digestive system it helps heartburn, diarrhea and gastritis.
Excretory/Urinary Systems: An antiseptic for cystitis. A good diuretic.
Integumentary/Skin System: Excellent for more mature skin, but also beneficial to dry, irritable, sensitive and inflamed skin. Can remove skin tags when used daily. As a cell regenerator it is useful in healing wounds and cuts. A natural deodorant.

Dreams And Aspirations: Sandalwood encourages you to be trusting of your thoughts and ideas. It raises your self-esteem; it is also insightful for new ideas and plans to bring your dreams and aspirations to fruition.

Notes:

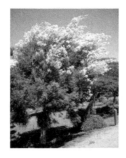

(Think of single-handed yachtsmen)

Botanical name: Melaleuca alternifolia
Plant part: Leaves
Country of origin: Australia
Note: Middle
Extraction method: Steam distilled

Contraindications: Possible skin irritant to small percentage of people.

Emotional: One of Tea-Tree's well-known emotional attributes is in the treatment of trauma, grief and shock. In extreme cases it can act like the old-fashioned smelling salts, for those of you old enough to remember them! For this, it has to be used as soon as possible to be dramatically effective.

Mental: Following on from its emotional attributes, as our brain will immediately flip into 'survival mode' when confronted with trauma, grief and shock, it will allay the mental panic, fear and worry and snap you back into rational, logical and calm thinking. Emotionally and mentally combined, when you feel you are at the bottom of your barrel with no more emotional or mental energy to give, when all you want to do is cry and give up in despair, Tea-Tree comes to the rescue.

I am happy to share my own personal experience here with you to give you a better picture and understanding. When I was driving for a crucial meeting with my solicitor, I had to pull my car into a layby as I suddenly felt totally overwhelmed, I had absolutely no fight left in me. My now ex was a solicitor and chronic alcoholic, he right royally put me through the wringer. I sat in the car literally bawling my eyes out, totally emotionally and mentally done in. Suddenly I could smell Tea-Tree fill the car. I had no Tea-Tree on me. Oh, my goodness, the more I inhaled the 'energy' of Tea-Tree my tears stopped, my resolve strengthened, my determination became immense. I suddenly found the 'warrior' inside of myself. I was not under any circumstance going to let him continue to beat me into an emotional and mental pulp. Boy oh boy! Did my meeting with my solicitor go amazingly well. That day in the car with dear Tea-Tree not only gave me the strength and resolve at that particular moment, but it also shone the light on truths.

Relationships: These men and women know themselves to the depths of their souls. They are constantly challenged and find that extra strength, determination, fortitude and resilience when most of us would have reached the bottom of our own barrel and given up.

Tea-Tree will keep you protected, your mind clear and objective in a confusing and seemingly hopeless relationship. When all seems lost, Tea-Tree will give you the insight, strength of mind, body and soul to see it through, whether that be to resolve the situation or to walk away with yourself intact.

Physical:

Muscular/Skeletal System:

Circulatory System: Will help re-address candida imbalance and associated symptoms in the gut and vaginal. Viral and parasitic infections of the gut.

Lymphatic/Immune System: Flu, colds, glandular fever all respond well. It is a well-known immune supporter. Stimulates white blood cell production to fight off infections. A highly antiseptic, antiviral, antibacterial oil. It also contains some pro-biotic properties. A series of Lymphatic massages with Tea-Tree before major surgery will support all the systems of the body, and because of its reviving properties it will help overcome the shock/trauma of the operation.

Nervous System:

Endocrine System:

Respiratory System: A long list of infections: catarrh, tonsillitis, bronchitis, gum infections, tooth abscess, pyorrhea, gingivitis. Otitis media is inflammation or infection located in the middle ear. Otitis media can occur as a result of a cold, sore throat, or respiratory infection.

Digestive System: Will help re-address candida imbalance and associated symptoms in the gut and vaginal. Viral and parasitic infections of the gut.

Excretory/Urinary Systems: Treats cystitis.

Integumentary/Skin System: It is good for cold sores, chicken pox, insect bites, boils and carbuncles, shingles, warts, and athlete's foot. Can protect against radiation burns when undergoing cancer treatment, as a preventative. HOWEVER, this MUST be discussed with the oncologist. Can help pruritis and vaginal itching. Helps a dry and dandruff prone scalp.

Dreams And Aspirations: What can I say any differently to what I have already said about Tea-Tree in the emotional, mental and relationships sections other than to reiterate it brings hope, fortitude, protection, clarity and determination.

Notes:

8.

THE HERB GARDEN - PHYSICAL

These gifts of Mother Nature were at one time in gardening history regarded somewhat as weeds by some!! Yes, indeed they were, and were plucked out as quickly as weeds are today. You see herbs would grow as freely as weeds do today. They were everywhere, accessible at all times. But they had lost their value, as modern allopathic medicine became the norm; we had other 'medicines'. Neither were they aesthetically as pleasing as other plants. "Aha, but what about good old Lavender?" I hear some of you ask. Lavender, although thought of as a herb; it looks very similar to Rosemary, until Rosemary grows to its full height of five to six feet; is in fact a flower!

The herb garden represents our physical well-being. By physical I mean tangible, reactive and quantifiable symptoms. From aches and pains to digestive disturbances to sleepless nights. These are all measurable occurrences, which take us away from our normal state of being. Behind most of these physical ailments are emotional issues. Whatever the underlying emotional issues are, we can call them a stress. Stress puts pressure or blockage on the physical body, causing it to malfunction. When that malfunction is allowed to continue it manifests as a pain or discomfort, which in turn causes more distress in itself. So begins the downward spiral of physical ill health. This in turn has an outward projection to other aspect of your life such as your family or your job. This is why, when you have a physical situation going on, you will also need to look at other parts of your garden for the healing root cause of your physical discomfiture. In the meantime, if you can ease the physical, it will allow you the space to look at its root cause.

Starting at your head and working down to your toes, let's see what each of these herb oils are good for.

Angelica – 'Courage of your convictions'

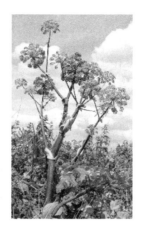

Botanical name: Angelica sinensis/officianalis (root), Angelica archangelica (seed)
(Also known as Wild Celery)
Plant part: Root & Seed
Country of origin: Africa. Most comes from France.
Note: Middle
Extraction method: Steam distilled

Authors note: Please note it is the essential oil *generally* I am describing below. Angelica can grow to over 6 feet in height and the main stem can be as thick as an arm! Probably not what you imagined! The root oil is very grounding, whereas the archangelica, as the name implies, allegedly has more spiritual connotations. There are records to show that Angelica was used in the Middle Ages to fight the Bubonic Plague! There are also some conflicting reports that it was the Vikings around 900AD who were the first to utilize Angelica as an herb, introducing it to the rest of Europe.

Contraindications: **Angelica Root (Angelica sinensis):** Not to be used in pregnancy or whilst breast feeding. This also implies that the root should not be used on children or babies. People with diabetes, high blood pressure, cysts, tumours, undergoing treatment for or still in remission from cancer should not use it. Avoid if on blood thinning medication. There is scientific research showing Angelica Root being an anti-coagulant. It may cause insomnia in some people. The root is highly phototoxic, as such should not be applied to the skin for 24-48 hours before or after being exposed to sunlight or sunbed.

Angelica Seed (Angelica archangelica): No known contraindications, some say same contraindications as the root. HOWEVER, I would err on the side of caution and avoid in pregnancy, breast feeding, using on babies and children and undergoing treatment for cancer. It is however far less phototoxic than the root.

Emotional: Angelica brings comfort, stamina and strength where there is emotional nervousness, anxiety, instability, exhaustion where they are related to a traumatic event. This also suggests it may have therapeutic benefits for those with post-traumatic stress disorder (PTSD) or those dealing with feelings of hopelessness, and to alleviate patterns of negative behavior. Susanne Fischer-Rizzi writes that Angelica is for those who are afraid, timid, weak or who lack perseverance and have a tough time making decisions.

Mental: Angelica is indicated for a tired mind, to relieve stress, tension and fatigue and can help you to keep going when feeling 'faint-hearted'. It brings concentration, incentive, focus and is grounding. It is good for insomnia where the root cause is mental stress. It lessens memories of traumatic memories and events, (see above for PTSD).

Relationships: For this part I used Angelica Seed (Angelica archangelica).

First, I saw a pair of men's legs bound in skins and leather straps. For some reason these legs made me think of Vikings. I looked it up and indeed there are reports of Vikings using Angelica back in 900AD. I looked up Anglo-Saxon footwear, because of the dates 450-1066AD. Nothing that resembled this footwear, they actually had shoes! OK, maybe I was over-thinking and trying to validate what I saw. So, I left it alone for a while. One thing that proved was, it certainly brings focus and concentration to get to the 'root cause' as it were.

Right, back in I went. I saw more of this gentleman now. He was huge! His arms were across his barrel chest, he was dark haired with a beard, grinning with the most immaculate set of white teeth! There was a fearlessness and fearsomeness to the oil. Angelica encourages you to stand your ground, to assert and to express your truth and confidence, and can assist in strengthening your resolve and to follow through with your convictions.

Then it dawned on me! Not only does Angelica do what I have said above, but this beaming, huge 'manifestation' was of Archangel Metatron. So, perhaps Angelica does connect you to the 'spirit realms' after all!

Physical:

Muscular/Skeletal Systems: Well-known for treating rheumatism, arthritis, gout, joint and muscular aches and pains.

Circulatory System: Helps red blood cell production when a person is anaemic. Helps to boost the circulation to warm up cold extremities. But by the same token it has febrifugal properties which means it can also reduce temperature. It will induce sweating when toxins are present and need eliminating. Has been used to calm palpitations and tachycardia. It strengthens the heart and stimulates the circulation generally. Has been claimed to be an anticoagulant which is very possible as it helps to disperse bruises.

Lymphatic/Immune System: Helps to restore and strengthen the immune and lymphatic systems bandwidth after illness. Patricia Davis, in her Aromatherapy A-Z book, also states that it may be beneficial for people suffering with M.E. (Chronic Fatigue). Said to be a tonic for the spleen.

Nervous System: A nervine oil which helps sciatica, headaches, migraines and tooth ache.

Endocrine System: Helps both male and female infertility issues. For men it can increase the production of sperm. Stimulates production of oestrogen thus easing irregular periods, heavy mensuration and period pains. It will also help expel the placenta.

Respiratory System: In its herbal form, it has been used for centuries in Europe for the common cold, feverish colds, bronchitis and chronic coughs - particularly dry, irritating coughs and pleurisy. It is also indicated for asthma. The same holds true for the essential oil. It is also said to relieve anosmia, restoring the loss of smell.

Digestive System: Angelica can help combat all types of stomach issues including: indigestion, flatulence, dyspepsia, stomach ulcers, nausea, constipation, general digestive pain and colic. It can be especially useful where digestive problems are stress-related resulting in headaches or migraines. May help with anorexia nervosa and general loss of appetite. Said to be a tonic for the liver.

Excretory/Urinary Systems: As a urinary antiseptic, Angelica is helpful on cystitis, fluid retention and kidney inflammation.

Integumentary/Skin System: Fungal growths eczema and psoriasis can respond well. It can also help to tone, rejuvenate and revitalise a dull, dry, lacklustre complexion and restore the skin's microbial balance.

Dreams And Aspirations: It is suggested that it connects us with our Guardian Angel and other spiritual guides, by creating a 'communication bridge' between ourselves and them, hence the reason it is often called 'holy spirit oil' or 'oil of angels'. Angelica, it is said, helps us hone the spiritual gift of keeping our perspective clear—seeing ourselves and the world around us "as it really is."

Although I have never tried using it for this specific spiritual or meditative practices on its own before now, I have always been skeptical of its ability to do this because of its smell. I find it very clarifying and clearing and not in the least a 'spiritual' smell, if there is such a thing. Well, as you have just read above, Angelica proved me wrong!

Notes:

Basil – 'Words have power'/Integrity

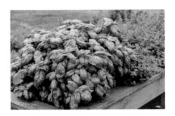

Botanical name: Ocimum basilicum
Plant part: Leaves, flowers/buds
Country of origin: India
Note: Top
Extraction method: Steam distilled

Contraindications: Not to be used if pregnant, breast feeding or on babies and children. Not to be used if undergoing treatment for a hormonal/oestrogen cancer. Possible skin irritant to a few.

Emotional: Emotionally, Basil is both stimulating and soothing. It will treat the extreme negative emotions from hysteria, fainting and depression, to encouraging calm, positivity and assertiveness.

Mental: It energizes the mind encouraging concentration and memory recall while, at the same time, relieves mental anxiety, fears, depression, doubts, mental fatigue and brain fog and insomnia and lightens our mental burdens.

Relationships: I first saw an elder statesman making a speech from a podium. The 'visual' was in black and white and made me think of rousing speeches made by the likes of Churchill during the war, or maybe JFK. Basil is an orator, a great communicator with integrity and carefully considered words.
I could immediately hear Basil say "trust me". My head/brain felt it had been cleared and defragged of any useless clutter, I felt focused. Then my shoulders relaxed as did my breathing, real 'chill' but completely 'in the present' feeling. What next?

Well, Basil appears to enjoy a good friendly chat with you. It draws your attention away from whatever/whoever is causing you angst and distress and reminds you that you have personal integrity, self-esteem and power and you don't have to accept or acknowledge the behavior of others towards you. Like Melissa, it can set boundaries if required, but Basil is a teacher and it would rather you learn for yourself how to put your own boundaries in place.

It does not tolerate fools i.e., the aggressor, instead focusing your attention on yourself, your strengths and the positivity's you have in your life. However, if you have been putting yourself down, it will give you a stern speech without the wagging finger. Carefully chosen words which will reconnect you to your own integrity and truth. It won't allow you to say what you *think* the other party wants to hear; he will teach you diplomacy, truth and integrity, not just towards others but to yourself too. "To thine own self be true". Basil will teach you to take note of the way you speak to and about yourself and will kick your butt to notice when you are down-talking yourself. Remember your words have power, use them wisely.

Physical:

Muscular/Skeletal System: Muscular aches and pains, gout and cramps. Can restore strength in the presence of asthenia. Helps rheumatism, arthritis and polyarthritis.

Circulatory System: Can reduce blood congestion in the veins and therefore increase blood flow. In a bath, even a drop or two produces an interesting sensation of tiny pin pricks as it increases circulation to the capillaries just under the skin.

Lymphatic/Immune System: Protects against infection from bacterial and viral pathogens. Can help prevent allergic reactions when they are stress induced.

Nervous System: Sedating to the nervous system generally. Headaches, migraines, earache, and neurological pain generally respond well to Basil.

Endocrine System: Imitates oestrogen hormone, as such, may help with conception difficulties, menstrual problems, engorgement of breasts and helps expel placenta. Indicated for sluggish and depleted adrenals. Said to help with prostate problems, but this should always be medically investigated and determined first.

Respiratory System: Bronchitis, coughs, flu, asthma, emphysema, whooping cough. nasal polyps, allergies, sinus congestion and rhinitis all respond well to Basil. It restores lost sense of smell due to viral infection or mucous build up.

Digestive System: Helps dyspepsia, flatulence, nausea, vomiting, hiccups, gastric cramps. Fights viral hepatitis and food poisoning.

Excretory/Urinary Systems: Has an antiseptic action on kidney infections.

Integumentary/Skin System: Acne, insect bites, dull congested skin, cellulite, alopecia, herpes virus and shingles can all be helped with Basil.

Dreams And Aspirations: Basil restores strength, belief, purpose, decisiveness and enthusiasm to your dreams and aspirations. Scott Cunningham (Magical Aromatherapy) suggests it is good for bringing in abundance, and not just the monetary kind. Avarice will back fire! Basil can be very helpful when you are at a crossroads in life or going through changes, including physical ones such as the menopause. He supports you in overcoming any doubt, worry or anxiety allowing you to trust in yourself and will renew your zest and enthusiasm for life.

Notes:

Cardamom/Cardamon – 'Appetite for life'

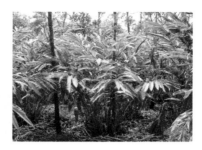

Botanical name: Elettaria cardamomum
Plant part: Seed
Country of origin: India
Note: Middle
Extraction method: Steam distilled

Author's Note: Cardamom is in the ginger family. It has many of the same properties, but is less of an irritant. As you will see, I have bolded 'strap lines' to each of the systems of the body Cardamom helps with. Not had this with any other EO. This is a very clear and direct oil, but gentle with it. You could say 'in your face', but with a gentle smile, like your granny telling you what is and what isn't. I personally love Cardamom and wish more therapists would get to know her better.

Contraindications: Do not use if you have stomach ulcers. Possible skin irritant.

Emotional: Cardamom encourages enthusiasm, confidence and, here comes that word again, courage. It lifts emotional fatigue and stress and restores an appetite for life where apathy has taken hold. She (I feel female energies) expels feelings of fear, of being stuck, of freezing because of others' opinions, and gives us feelings of courage, stamina, patience and strength.

Mental: When there's mental fatigue, it brings concentration. Where there's confusion it is invigorating, and where there is stress Cardamom is uplifting.

Relationships: The first impression I had with Cardamom is that it is as straight as a die, no messing about, a 'let's get on with it then' attitude. It does this with a feeling of encouragement and support. It will also pick you up when you stumble or fall.

I felt it connect my 'I will' (solar plexus) to my 'I am' (sacral). I could feel my solar plexus almost sigh with relief, that I was not going to be influenced by external sources. I could feel myself being just me. If you feel like saying "stuff it, they can like it or lump it" then reach for Cardamom for support and balance that you won't over shoot the mark and not let ego creep in.

Physical:

Muscular/Skeletal System:

Circulatory System: Warms the body where there is cold. *'Cold hands, warm heart'.*

Lymphatic/Immune System: Supports the immune system. *'Go with the flow'.*

Nervous System: Headaches and possibly migraines, particularly if brought on by diet. *'Stop banging your head against a brick wall!'*

Endocrine System: A well-known aphrodisiac, which also helps impotence and sexual dysfunction. For the ladies it helps PMT. *'No comment'.*

Respiratory System: Helps make coughs more productive on mucous. *'Get it off your chest'.*

Digestive System: It treats colic, dyspepsia, indigestion, heartburn, a laxative, helps anorexia and stimulates the appetite after an illness. It treats halitosis (bad breath) which is due to digestive imbalance. It increases the production of bile to break down fats in the gut and liver. Cardamom is useful for nausea, even in pregnancy. Finally, it encourages the flow of saliva. *'Appetite for life'.*

Excretory/Urinary Systems: A useful diuretic where the problem is passing urine. *'Let it go'.*

Integumentary/Skin System:

Dreams And Aspirations: Cardamom is strongly associated with the Earth element and Mother Earth energies. It strengthens our ability to see the opportunities before us and gives us the motivation and direction to pursue them. It allows us to give generously and live openly and happily with our 'appetite for life'.

Notes:

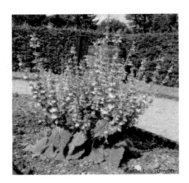

Botanical name: Salvia sclarea
Plant part: Leaves, flowers, buds
Country of origin: Southern Europe
Note: Middle
Extraction method: Middle

Author's note: Linalyl acetate is present, albeit at lower levels, in other essential oils e.g., Lavender, Petitgrain, Bergamot. Linalyl acetate is an ester known for its calming properties, Clary-Sage has between 60-70% probably making it the EO that contains the highest amount of this lovely calming ester.

It was referred to as "clear-eye" by the famous herbalist Nicholas Culpeper in his "Complete Herbal" (1653).

Note the flowerheads of the French Clary-Sage shown below. Do they not invoke feelings of the divine intuitive woman?

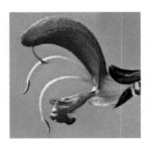

Many of the aromatic plants that can be found in your herb garden, including Clary, belong to the Lamiaceae family. Labiatae, labia in Latin, was the original name of this family and reflected the fact that the flowers typically have petals fused into an upper lip and lower lip.

Contraindications: Not to be used if pregnant, breast feeding or on babies and children. It can lower blood pressure, so take care if you have low blood pressure as it could lower it further. Do not use within 24 hours of consuming alcohol, it can result in night terrors. Do not use if taking iron supplements. Not to be used if undergoing treatment for cancer or oestrogen-related cancers. It can be very intoxicating so great care with using machinery or driving for example after using it on its own.

Emotional: It is an oil of calm, tranquility, restoration and balance and can help treat/alleviate depression and bring joy and happiness in its stead. It can release anger, aggression and inconsistent emotions like spontaneous or outbreaks of hysteria.

Mental: It is grounding and inspires confidence, revitalizes a tired mind. Quietens a chattering mind.

Relationships: I could immediately feel the soothing effects quite literally in my brain. As though it had been defragged and re-booted with more memory space being made available. All the 'rubbish' had gone into the 'recycle bin', gosh it felt good!
I then saw a 'wise old woman', akin to a hedge witch, but she was young, not old. I could see her standing there with a bonnet on her head, a trug over her arm with herbs in it, wearing a long dress and white apron. She beckoned me, "Come over here and learn something new." I could see the flowering fronds of the Clary-Sage in her trug. "There's great power in all these plants. You must use them wisely" she said, as she extended her free arm over all the other plants. "But Clary is the mother to all these other herbs. They are her children. She nurtures them. Teaches them secrets to keep them safe. If you talk with Clary, she will tell you which plant will help with what ails you. She is a friend to you if you honor her. If you too become her student, she will grant you freedom of mind and spirit to learn about the healing arts." Wow! I've always liked Clary, saved me from numerous migraines, but I have a new found respect for her now.

Physical:

Muscular/Skeletal System: Muscular aches and pains and asthenia, muscular fatigue, respond well to its use.

Circulatory System: Lowers High Blood Pressure. Massively effective against migraines, it is the first oil I reach for when I feel one coming on or a migraine has caught me unawares and it has worked each time without fail.

Lymphatic/Immune System:

Nervous System: Relaxes nervous tension and stress and can therefore alleviate headaches and migraines. The migraines I can vouch for. It has a direct effect on the central nervous system and has been used to help in alcohol and drug withdrawal.

Endocrine System: It is a hormonal balancer, therefore eases amenorrhea, dysmenorrhea, hot flashes, night sweats, menstrual pain and regulates menstrual flow, but be aware it can induce heavy bleeding too. Treats PMT and PMS. Helps male and female infertility, impotence and frigidity. Excellent for post-natal depression and labour pains being a uterine tonic. Where there is an excess of estrogen which is linked to several women's cancers, Clary Sage can moderate excessive estrogen production.

Respiratory System: Been known to treat Tuberculosis, asthma and whooping cough with some success. Sore throats and bronchial infections generally will respond to Clary.

Digestive System: It is a kind demulcent on the gut easing gastric spasms, wind and colic.

Excretory/Urinary Systems: Indicated for kidney infections and where there is excessive perspiration.

Integumentary/Skin System: Acne, boils, dandruff, ulcers, skin inflammation, hair loss and dry or mature skin all respond to the use of Clary-Sage. It is also a natural deodorant. It has some cell regenerating properties.

Dreams And Aspirations: An inspirational oil, which can bring feelings of euphoria, through clear perspective that instils confidence and belief in the future. Clary sage feeds the soul and helps us get through rough times. It has also been said to encourage vivid dreams and assist with dream recall. Said to enhance psychic ability. Well, that's good if we need to connect through the hedge witch!

Notes:

Dill – 'Smile'

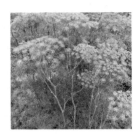

Botanical name: Anethum gravolens
Plant part: Seed
Country of origin: Mediterranean and SE Europe
Note: Middle
Extraction method: Steam distilled

Contraindications: Not to be used if pregnant, breast feeding or on babies and children, but can ease childbirth. Phototoxic as such should not be applied to the skin for 24-48 hours before or after being exposed to sunlight or sunbed. Not to be used if undergoing treatment for oestrogen-related cancers. Possible skin irritant.

Emotional/Mental: The most important aspect of Dill is that just a gentle inhalation of this oil never fails to put a smile on your face. It is the perfect oil to use when you just want 'your own space'. Use it on those occasions where you feel you would just want to disappear into a room, close the door, and when you re-appear all will be well in the world. When everything around you are jangling your nerves and you just want to yell in frustration. When life takes you out of your comfort zone, knocks you off your centred place, reach for Dill! Mentally, it is exactly the same as Dill's effect on our emotions but added that things are illogical and don't make any sense.

Relationships: I've never yet met anyone who, on smelling Dill, doesn't break out in a grin or at the very least a small smile. Dill came over as a happy, playful and a little bit cheeky child that you can't help but smile and laugh at their antics.

Just like a child, Dill is innocent and doesn't understand the 'ways of the world'. When something they don't understand happens and throws them off kilter, they become upset and just want to retreat from the World and close their bedroom door. As adults, sometimes life throws such a wobbler nothing seems to make sense even. Too much happening at once and all your neat boxes have tumbled off the shelf and everything is mixed up and a mess. At that point of frustration, you just want some quiet space to re-group.

Dill affords you this. It's the Greta Garbo "I want to be alone" of the Essential Oils. We can't always, as adults, just retreat to our personal space and shut the door, and when you reappear you will be fine. Just smelling Dill and imagining it getting out into your aura will help to keep others away from you. It gives you an invisible space to be safe while de-frazzling your nerves whilst you get on with your daily tasks. Just smile!

Physical:

Muscular/Skeletal Systems:

Circulatory System: Dill is also a mild way to cleanse the blood as it does with the liver. Helps ease digestive headaches.

Lymphatic/Immune System: Stems excess sweating. GC-MS analysis of the essential oil shows it having highly antimicrobial properties, antimicrobial being a blanket term for fungi, protozoa, viruses and bacteria.

Nervous System: No direct effect on this system has been reported to date, although I would suggest its effect on the mental and emotional will have an indirect action. The autonomic nervous system controls such things as heartbeat, the function of our kidneys, the flow of hormones, and blood pressure, think Vagus Nerve in particular. We have been taught in the past that we have no conscious control of these functions. I would disagree! Studies and common sense both indicate that this is not entirely true. For example, army snipers are taught to emotionally/mentally slow their breathing and thus their heartrate and sharpen the acuity of their vision as they prepare to make their shots. In the nerves and impulses of this area of the nervous system, Dill brings sustenance, strength, and calmness. Other benefits of Dill essential oil include calming headaches whether they be digestive or stress induced.

Endocrine System: Stems excess sweating, so might be useful for the endocrine system for menopausal sweats. Helps childbirth and increases lactation/mother's milk. Also useful in cases of dysmenorrhea, hence the reason it is contraindicated in pregnancy.

Respiratory System: Bronchial ailments and asthmatic symptoms can be alleviated, but I feel this is again due more to its actions on the emotional and mental.

Digestive System: Well-known, both in its herbal and EO format, to treat wind, dyspepsia, flatulence, constipation, hiccups, indigestion and colic. Most of us have heard of Gripe Water used for babies, young children and even adults alike. Pharma couldn't call it Dill Water now could they. A sluggish colon is often the result of emotions such frustration and intermittent depression or repression of emotions. Dill's action on the digestive system can help lift the frustrations and depression and bring buried emotions to the surface where they can be processed. Dill supports pancreatic functions, helping to normalize glucose and insulin levels. Physically, glucose and insulin stabilize energy levels to remain steady. Clinical tests have shown there are no glucose spikes followed by periods of abnormally low glucose levels with the use of Dill. I would also add here that diabetes mind/body connection is "when all sweetness has gone from life". This effect of the aroma of Dill is almost instantaneous and brings that smile to your face replacing emotional and mental frustrations and anger. Dill is also a mild way to cleanse and detox the liver.

Excretory/Urinary Systems: A good diuretic.

Integumentary/Skin System: Helps to heal wounds.

Dreams and Aspirations: As I have already outlined above about the "I want to be alone" aspect of Dill, it makes an excellent meditation tool where you particularly need to just re-organize, re-group and put things back in their boxes. Perfect for that quick 10 minute 'switch off'.

Notes:

Fennel – 'Fortitude'

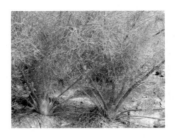

Botanical name: Foeniculum vulgare
Plant part: Seed
Country of origin: Southern Mediterranean
Note: Top/Middle
Extraction method: Steam distilled

Contraindications: Not to be used if pregnant, breast feeding or on babies and children. Not to be used if undergoing treatment for cancer. Not to be used if you have endometriosis, epilepsy or taking warfarin or other blood thinning drugs. Experts disagree about the use of Fennel with kidney problems and kidney stones. Some texts list Fennel as strongly contra-indicated for these conditions, while others say that Fennel is specific for these ailments. I prefer to use something else for these ailments. Over-use, (I know we could say this about any oil, but it is important here in particular), and it can become toxic. Possible skin irritant.

Emotional: It is calming to emotions which are driven by the fear of failure. It brings strength and fortitude to get through what needs to be done with calm emotions.

Mental: Fennel connects your mind to your emotions by unlocking the feelings behind your thoughts. By bringing in this mental clarity you might find yourself being enlightened that your thoughts did not match your emotions. You could say it decongests the mind. By doing this, Fennel gives you motivation and perseverance, together they give you fortitude. As Robbi Zeck, wrote in her book The Blossoming Heart: Aromatherapy for Healing and Transformation "The sweetness of Fennel assists in completing things that are unfinished or requiring further attention in your life... Fennel keeps your mind concentrated on a particular direction and accesses the quiet containment of continuity." In other words, mental and emotional fortitude. Very similar to Ginger in this respect and together they make a good 'pairing'.

Relationships: I've always associated Fennel with Roman Soldiers, their discipline, training, mental analysis, imaginative engineering, ahead of their time, great fortitude, team work and a few other things too. But their negative traits were not so good. Poverty was rife, with multiple families living and sleeping in one room with no jobs most of the time for example.

The first thing I experienced on my journey to get to know Fennel up close and personal was how it immediately calmed my whole body. I sat and enjoyed the relaxing sensations, then suddenly BAM, I was sitting on the ground watching Roman Soldiers marching past me. As I smiled to myself, I thought "give me a break, that's MY association with Fennel, I need and want to get to know YOU!"

I saw the gentle fronds of Fennel wafting quietly in the wind filling the surrounding air with its scent. I felt myself getting lighter and begin to float above the scene I was being shown. A sense of all knowing, seeing the bigger picture, discovering 'outside the box' solutions and serene calmness.

I felt it working through my 3rd eye and lightening up my Crown Chakra. No surprise there as it is associated with spirituality. But I also felt it in my Throat Chakra. In this chakra I felt it helps you discover what you want to say and then accurately express it to others in a positive way. It is also a protective oil and can stop you from being harmed by someone else's negative words as well as thoughts and deeds. Here come those Roman Soldiers! It made me feel that I was 'carrying the truth and the light'.

I was then swept back to Greek or Egyptian times and had the sense that Fennel was used in healing practices then. I felt there was ancient knowledge stored in its energy, something we don't know about yet. I did check and indeed, it was used by both cultures and was regarded as a sacred plant by the Greeks. Their mythology says the Fennel bulb was used to catch the godly fire by Prometheus to bring it here for mortals. Hmmmmm, reflective of our connection with the 'divine'? There is a healing secret to Fennel!

Physical:

Muscular/Skeletal System: It helps rheumatism and can give relief to sore or tight muscles, mainly through its clearing-out of toxins waste and build up, but not so much arthritis. Asthenia, which is a weakness in arms and legs will be fortified and strengthened.

Circulatory System:

Lymphatic/Immune System: It gets the lymph moving where it has stagnated thus useful for fluid retention and lymph issues. It helps fight parasitic infections generally, not just in the gut.

Nervous System: It is calming to all aspects of the nervous system.

Endocrine System: A huge influence on the reproductive hormones because it imitates oestrogen, it treats menstrual problems such as menstrual cramps, PMT/PMS, infertility issues, and menopause generally. It increases milk in nursing mothers. But it should not be used if endometriosis is presenting.

Respiratory System: Indicated and successfully treats bronchitis, whooping cough and asthma.

Digestive System: Typically treats colic, dyspepsia, flatulence, hiccough, constipation, nausea, indigestion, vomiting, IBS, gastrointestinal spasms, parasitic infections, gout and pyorrhea. Hangovers respond well to Fennel. Has been successfully used to help people who are anorexic, and conversely those who are obese. *The seeds were carried by Roman soldiers on long marches to chew when they didn't have time to stop and have a meal.* It is also hepatic, meaning a tonic for the liver.

Excretory/Urinary Systems: As already mentioned that Fennel is good for fluid retention in the cells it is also a diuretic to the Urinary System. It is said to clear kidney stones, but please see the contraindications again for my view.

Integumentary/Skin System: It helps cellulitis, bruises, insect bites, fades bruising, dull, oily, and mature complexions.

Dreams And Aspirations: Fear of failure is often the root cause of procrastination. Fennel, with its impact on creativity and confidence, can help us get started on a project we have been putting off.

Notes:

Ginger – 'Courage'

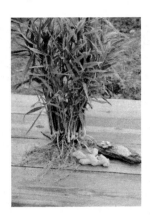

Botanical name: Zingiber officinale
Plant part: Root
Country of origin: South-eastern Asia
Note: Middle/Base
Extraction method: Steam distilled

Author's Note: Major Constituents: camphene, beta-sesquiphellandrene, zingiberene, curcumene, gingerin, gingenol, gingerone. There can be a significant variation in the main constituents depending on where the ginger is grown and distilled. The colour of the rhizome varies from buff to dark brown according to the soil and climatic conditions it's grown under. This may affect the aroma and could possibly influence the therapeutic actions.

Ginger mixed with Lime is a nice combination. I enjoy the combination for the emotional, mental and physical lift it provides. This mixture also disinfects and purifies while leaving a uniquely pleasant aroma behind.

Scott Cunningham in his fabulous book Magical Aromatherapy cite that it influences how we relate to money and how we feel about our material possessions. Also, that Ginger is indicated for the usually dynamic individual who has lost drive and ambition and has become apathetic and confused.

Contraindications: Not to be used if pregnant, breast feeding or on babies and children. Do not use if you have stomach ulcers. Some people are allergic to Ginger, so the essential oil must be avoided as well. Very possible skin irritant. I would suggest localised treatment only, as it will raise temperature.

Emotional: A warming oil which brings emotional optimism and sedates nervous exhaustion. The emotional impact of Ginger is absolutely uncompromising. It insists on burning away illusions and mis-perceptions and replacing them with clarity and vision.

Mental: Has been reported to help with memory issues. It certainly does help with both emotional and mental fatigue. There is a quiet but solid sense of courage with Ginger.

Relationships: Ginger won't let up letting you know that you have great power to change your reality with your mind. It will not tolerate mental or emotional self-sabotage. Although the oil isn't challenging me, the aroma is acceptable, I still can't help but feel the word 'bully' is appropriate here. By this I mean it will tackle you, it's like a dog with a bone and won't let go. By the same token there is an underlying air of empathy with a hint of "it's for your own good". You see, Ginger knows you, your strengths and your weaknesses and only wants to bring out those strengths that you keep prevaricating yourself with.

Work WITH Ginger and it will stand by your side and not just have your back.

Physical:

Muscular/Skeletal Systems: Has a very consistent history in treating arthritis and rheumatism because of its warming properties. But I would suggest ginger tea is better for this as the EO can inflame both conditions where heat aggravates said conditions. Plai would be a better alternative. It certainly helps with cramps both muscular and digestive, sprains, muscle spasm and general aches and pains in the muscles. Can be very effective on lower backache like its counterpart Marjoram which has the same affinity, so would be very effective in combination. Personally, I find Marjoram on its own to be enough.

Circulatory System: It does help with symptoms of angina by relaxing the heart muscles. It is warming to a poor circulation where there is cold. Helps to improve capillary strength.

Lymphatic/Immune System:

Nervous System:

Endocrine System: It has aphrodisiac properties, and can help improve impotence in both males and females.

Respiratory System: We all know how the root/herb of Ginger helps with catarrh, flu symptoms, sore throat, general congestion, stops a runny nose and eases sinusitis, so does the EO.

Digestive System: Improves loss of appetite particularly after illness. Well known remedy for nausea and motion/travel sickness. It will also help with flatulence, diarrhea, indigestion and hangovers. It has a long-standing reputation for treating scurvy. Scurvy is the caused by a vitamin C deficiency, where there has been a deficiency for as little as 3 months. Not usually common these days, but it does still happen. It can lead to anemia, debility, exhaustion, spontaneous bleeding, pain in the limbs, and especially the legs, swelling in some parts of the body, and sometimes ulceration of the gums and loss of teeth. With these symptoms it is well worth checking out your client's diet. Scurvy has been known since ancient Greek and Egyptian times.

Excretory/Urinary Systems:

Integumentary/Skin System: It helps chilblains and sores, but I would caution against direct application and use around the affected area. Excellent for bruises and carbuncles. Brings a glow back to a dull or tired complexions.

Dreams And Aspirations: Ginger will work with you, even with baby steps, if necessary, by reassuring you each step of the way, but it will not let up. See it as your friend, not a hard task master and your dreams and aspirations will soon become a reality.

Notes:

Marjoram – 'Perseverance'/'Badgering'

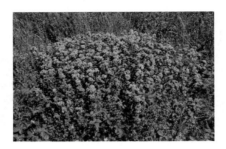

Botanical name: Origanum majorana
Do not confuse with Spanish Marjoram (Thymus mastichina)
Plant part: Leaves, flowers and buds
Country of origin: Mediterranean regions particularly Cyprus
Note: Middle
Extraction method: Steam distilled

Author's note: This oil should be in everyone's first aid kit. In ancient times, Marjoram was said to increase the lifespan. Marjoram was known as the "herb of happiness" to the early Romans and "joy of the mountain" to the Greeks.
Lavender and Marjoram work particularly well together, almost like a symbiotic relationship.

Contraindications: Not to be used if pregnant, breast feeding or on babies and children. Low blood pressure, with care.
*Please note that Marjoram is the only oil that is an anaphrodisiac! Maybe this is why some say Marjoram should not be used on those who are depressed, hmmmmm looking at its personality I would disagree. Prolonged use can dull the senses and cause drowsiness and high doses can be stupefying. Possible skin irritant.

Emotional: She is calming, comforting and warming in the presence of grief, sadness, hysteria and stops any accompanying tears. Not by masking these emotions, but by bringing the acceptance or realization that such feelings are due to a natural process. It moves you forward through this, not around it. Calming, comforting and warming it relieves anxiety, stress-related conditions and perhaps deeper psychological traumas. It can strengthen the mind and helps to confront issues.

Mental: Marjoram is quieting to obsessive worry where negative thoughts circle repetitively in the brain hour after hour, rather like Cape Verbena or White Chestnut from the Bach Flower Remedies. In its wake it brings cheerfulness, balance, self-assurance, focus, direction, encouraging support and strength. A very well-known and effective remedy for insomnia. But I would caution, that depending on the level of either emotional or mental stress that its sedative action could happen almost immediately, even during the day! Comforting during grief and loneliness as it warms the emotions and can help calm hyperactivity.

Relationships: The first thing that I saw was a badger! In Native American traditions and according to Jamie Sams "Badger is willing to persist." That is very much the impression Marjoram gave me. She will never give up and she will keep on going until the issue is resolved.

She feels like a good and wise friend who will stick with you through thick and thin. She is full of integrity and sincerity. She will point out where you are going wrong with kind compassion and is very tolerant.

Marjoram will also help rid you of thoughts/emotions which are negative and detrimental and which just keep going round and round in your head. She will show you what you have been hanging on to for far too long and will help you let go. This maybe a relationship that's not working or some task or goal you set yourself.

There is a sense of clarity and logic to Marjoram and because of these traits, it is very difficult to argue against her!

Physical:

Muscular/Skeletal Systems: A localised application and massage may help with rheumatic aches and pains and swollen joints that feel cold and stiff due to its positive effect on the circulatory system. It is anti-inflammatory, warming, analgesic and sedative. Marjoram has an affinity with lumbago (particularly in the lower back area when connected to digestive problems or digestive disorders), and lower back ache generally and a boon for muscular aches and pains, muscular spasms, rheumatism, arthritis, sprains and strains. It can and does ease headaches that are caused by muscle tension or lack of circulation.

Circulatory System: It dilates the arteries and capillaries allowing easier flow of blood, thus bringing warmth. Effective for after-sports massage. Tonic for the heart as it lowers blood pressure and eases heart palpitations. See, it wants to bring this system back to its natural order.

Lymphatic/Immune System: Antibacterial properties helps the immune system fight infection.

Nervous System: The relaxing properties of Marjoram make it beneficial for treating headaches, migraines and insomnia. All stress related conditions. Marjoram has a calming effect on the sympathetic nervous system but stimulates the parasympathetic nervous system. A vagotonic: overactivity or irritability of the vagus nerve, adversely affecting function of the blood vessels, stomach, and muscles. Allegedly helps with vegetative dystonia.

Endocrine System: Apparently will regulate overactive thyroid. Now to the Endocrine System and it just keeps going. It treats amenorrhea, leucorrhea and dysmenorrhea. Treats every single menstrual and menopausal symptom you could possibly think of. Can regulate the menstrual cycle and relieve painful periods. Depending on your point of view, it is also an anaphrodisiac, meaning it quells sexual desire because it has a lessening action on both emotional response and physical sensation. I can vouch for this having used it on my first husband!

Respiratory System: Sinusitis and a runny nose respond well. Otitis: infection of the inner ear. It has also been noted to relieve chest infections as well as colds and that stuffed-up feeling. Marjoram is one of the best oils for treating chest conditions such as asthma, although some say it shouldn't be used with asthmatics, coughing, whooping cough and bronchitis. It relaxes your breathing.

Digestive System: Its efficacy continues with gastrointestinal disorders such as colic, dyspepsia, constipation, flatulence, indigestion, irritable bowel syndrome, diverticulosis and eradicates intestinal parasites. Soothes the digestive system – relieving stomach cramps and can aid in clearing toxins from the body. Has potential to be effective against sea-sickness. Infections of the digestive tract, nausea and vomiting.

Excretory/Urinary Systems: Helps to clear toxins out of the body. Relieves water retention.

Integumentary/Skin System: First class remedy on bruises, but will also be effective on burns, chilblains, cold sores, ringworm, shingles, sunburn and neutralizing and eradicating tick bites.

Dreams And Aspirations: Do you sometimes give up just before attaining your goal? Ha! Marjoram will keep you going until you've covered the whole 9 yards! She brings perseverance and courage to get the job done.

Notes:

Peppermint – 'Focus'

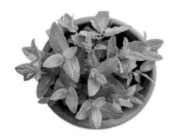

Botanical name: Mentha piperata
Plant part: Leaves
Country of origin: Northern Africa and the Mediterranean
Note: Top
Extraction method: Steam distilled

Author's Note: This oil is also known to effectively repel ants, aphids, beetles, caterpillars, fleas, flies, mosquitoes and lice. I can absolutely vouch for deterring ants! Grows to around 100cm with underground runners. It rarely seeds as it is a hybrid except in Japan where it seeds freely, which is why I wonder why the Hakka (Japanese Peppermint) 'feels' much gentler as it has not been 'restricted'. Peppermint is thought to be a hybrid between spearmint (Mentha spicata) and water mint (Mentha aquatica).

Contraindications: Not to be used if pregnant, breast feeding or on babies and children. Not to be used if you have epilepsy, Petit Mal, heart disease or cardiac fibrillation. Do not use if you have a fever as it will raise temperature even further. It is a neurotoxic if over used. Not to be used if undergoing treatment for oestrogen-related cancers.
Possible skin irritant. Not to be used if you are taking homeopathic remedies.

Emotional: It calms the emotions where they have become overheated, such as anger. A good pick me up where there is emotional exhaustion. I kept hearing the words "It is what it is and I am what I am. I'll just have to get on with it".

Mental: Increases focus, attention, alertness and concentration. It can soothe mental fatigue, depression and hysteria. One Dr. Dembar of the University of Cincinnati discovered in a research study that inhaling Peppermint oil increased the mental accuracy of the students tested by up to 28%. No wonder it enhances our ability to "digest" new ideas and impressions.

Relationships: Maybe it's because I use Peppermint to remove ants, and that's pretty much all I use it for personally, it didn't come as any surprise that I saw the ants marching in a straight line as they do, but they were huge, massive! I felt like I was in the film Antz! I didn't get it at first, then the light bulb moment struck. The Ants in the film woke up to what was really going on around them, rebelled, stuck to their guns and changed the society. Peppermint really connects us to our dreams and aspirations so we can bring it all into the now. Have a look in the Dreams and Aspirations chapter and marry the two descriptions together.

Physical: Peppermint Essential Oil contains menthol. Menthol induces a cooling sensation, and use of Peppermint Oil in a body mist or even in the diffuser can help to cool you down. Peppermint should be avoided before bedtime. Peppermint, like Lavender, is soothing in small amounts and strongly stimulating in larger amounts. Small doses warm and tend to relax while large or frequent doses cool and tend to stimulate.

Muscular/Skeletal System: It is pretty much a given oil in foot preparations for aching feet and sore muscles in general and in many rheumatic pharmaceutical preparations, and for good reason!

Circulatory System: It stimulates and increases circulation. For the heart it reduces palpitations.

Lymphatic/Immune System: It will treat colds and flu as many bacterial, fungal, and viral infections are destroyed by it.

Nervous System: Being an anti-inflammatory to the nerves, it treats neuralgia, headaches, migraines, toothache, vertigo and revives fainting. Said to help nerve regeneration, but I have yet to find a science paper to verify this.

Endocrine System: It has been successful in treating mastitis, but I wouldn't encourage its use if there is ongoing breast feeding as it will taint the milk. Peppermint oil is stimulating to the uterus and helps with painful periods. For men, it is anti-inflammatory to the prostate. For both sexes it can be an aphrodisiac.

Respiratory System: Peppermint has treated tuberculosis, bronchitis, dry coughs, pneumonia, asthma, sinusitis and halitosis.

Digestive System: It has a long list of treating the digestive system: food poisoning, vomiting, constipation, diarrhea, flatulence, colic, gall stones, nausea, mouth or gum infections, halitosis, liver problems, and travel sickness. It restores the sense of taste by stimulating the trigeminal nerve. Oddly, inhaling Peppermint oil can also curb the appetite.

Excretory/Urinary Systems:

Integumentary/Skin System: Listed as effective on pruritis, dermatitis, ringworm, skin inflammation, sunburn, scabies, acne and hives. Although, I have to say, I have never used it for a skin condition. I can see why the cited conditions would benefit from it though.

Dreams And Aspirations: Keim and Bull write that peppermint promotes healthy self-esteem, integrity and ethics and helps us to discover our hidden gifts and strengths. I agree with them. Compare to Archangel Jophiel's oil Elemi: when something is out there but don't know what it is.

Notes:

Rosemary – 'Memory'

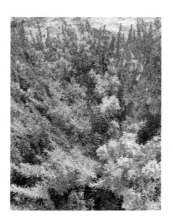

Photo taken by me in Cyprus

Botanical name: Rosmarinus officianalis
The proper botanical name for Rosemary is now *Salvia Rosmarinus*. However, you may still often see *Rosmarinus officinalis* used until more people and companies update their literature, posts and botanical references.
Plant part: Leaves and flowers
Country of origin: Around the Mediterranean
Note: Middle
Extraction method: Steam distilled

Author's Note: Major Constituents: There are 3 chemotypes, 1,8 cineole, camphor and verbenone. The amount of each constituent varies with the chemotype but all include 1.8 cineole, alpha-pinene, camphor, alpha-pinene, borneol, borynl acetate. Rosemary 1,8 cineole chemotype is warming and stimulating The North African climate is responsible for this outstanding Rosemary ct cineole. This is the Rosemary preferred in massage blends to increase circulation, soothe muscular aches, pains and treat headaches.
Rosemary essential oil was first distilled in the 13th century.

Contraindications: Not to be used if pregnant, breast feeding or on babies and children. Not to be used if you have epilepsy, Petit Mal or have high blood pressure. People who are diabetic must be extremely careful when using this oil. Possible skin irritant. Not to be used if you are taking homeopathic remedies.

Emotional/Mental: Let's look at Rosemary's effect on our emotions and mind in tandem as it is very difficult to separate the two as Rosemary is one of those oils that affects both simultaneously.

It is excellent for poor memory, therefore uplifting to frustrated emotions.

It aids concentration thus reviving to the emotions.

It brings mental clarity thus stimulating emotional creativity.

In both cases it treats emotional and mental exhaustion.

Relationships: Oh goodness! Rosemary is most definitely a tall, elegant, elderly lady with a walking stick! In came the Dowager Duchess of Grantham from Downton Abbey TV series! Yes, she was there, both hands resting on her stick (She doesn't really need it, it's a prop. She's more likely to shake it at you than use it to help her walk!), with her head turned slightly over her shoulder, looking me square in the eye as though to say "Now get on with it!".

Duchess Rosemary will not tolerate bad manners, weak-will, ego, laziness, excuses, apathy, forgetfulness, over-zealousness, excitability, idle chatter and dullards. She will however almost demand diplomacy, assuredness, humility, energy, accomplishment, creativity, memory, calm, logic, truth, strength and gentility of character.

Duchess Rosemary has a very long memory, so you had best be honoring all her positive traits, or that stick will be shaken or tapped on the floor to remind you if you have strayed off the path.

Physical:

Muscular/Skeletal System: Rosemary is well known for treating arthritis, rheumatism, gout, strained, cramping and aching muscles and back pain.

Circulatory System: Rosemary assists with a long list of circulatory problems: poor circulation, arteriosclerosis, varicose veins, migraines, headaches, and low blood pressure. Rosemary balances heart function such as palpitations, and energizes the solar plexus. It reputedly helps hypercholesterolemia, removing cholesterol build up in the venous system.

Lymphatic/Immune System: Breaks down cellulite, and stimulates the lymph where there is fluid retention in the cells.

Nervous System: Very effective against any Neuralgic pain including migraines, headaches and vertigo.

Helps to regrow damaged nerves apparently. A compound in Rosemary called carnosic acid (also found in Sage), has been found to stimulate nerve growth, meaning that Rosemary helps build and repair the nervous system, strengthening it to cope better with stresses. This immediately made me think about Grapefruit and how Schnaubelt cites it will repair the melanin sheath around nerves. So, I went digging to see if carnosic acid was present in Grapefruit as well.

I found this research paper titled "Combination of grapefruit and rosemary extracts has skin protective effect through MMPs, MAPKs, and the NF-kB signalling pathway in vitro and in vivo UVB-exposed model" Not exactly what I was looking for, but it does say carnosic acid is in both, still an interesting read. (Appendix 8.)

Endocrine System: Second to none on period pains and menstrual mood swings. Has been used with some success on menopausal sweats.

Respiratory System: A good remedy for colds, asthma, bronchitis, influenza, sinusitis.

Digestive System: Its main actions focus on hepatic disorders: viral hepatitis, cirrhosis, jaundice, overindulgence in food or drink, and hangovers. For the rest of the digestive system, it treats flatulence, colitis, dyspepsia, intestinal infections and breaks down gall stones. Is useful in weight loss and obesity when used alongside a healthy diet.

Excretory/Urinary Systems:

Integumentary/Skin System: The astringent properties of Rosemary make it effective for oily and dull skin, tightening saggy areas of skin, acne, dermatitis, eczema, scabies and lice. Rosemary is used to minimize gray in the hair of brunettes, dandruff and hair loss.

Dreams And Aspirations: As mentioned in the Relationships section, Rosemary reminds you of who you are, what your dreams are and she supports you with a sense of conviction, pride and determination.

Notes:

Sage – 'Wise-One'/Wisdom

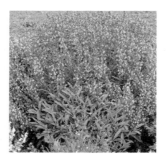

Botanical name: Salvia lavendulaefolia/Salvia officianalis
Essential oil that is steam distilled specifically from the
plant *Salvia officinalis* is referred to by several common names
including *Common Sage,* and *Dalmatian Sage.*
Plant part: Leaves and sometimes also flowers
Country of origin: Mediterranean regions
Note: Middle
Extraction method: Steam distilled

Author's Note: **Dalmatian Sage** (Salvia officianalis) Essential Oil
contains approximately 25-50% thujone, a ketone that requires
greater care and has more limited use.
Spanish Sage (Salvia lavendulaefolia) Essential Oil contains
primarily Oxides (particularly 1,8 Cineole), Ketones (particularly
Camphor) and Monoterpenes. Spanish Sage has some beautiful
Lavender undertones. These notes are every bit as evident as the
properties that are reminiscent of Sage, giving this oil a unique
character and aroma. This is the Sage I am writing about.

White Sage Essential Oil is steam distilled from Salvia apiana, an aromatic shrub that is native to the Southwestern United States. White sage is revered by Native Americans for its wellness, spiritual and energetic applications. It is considered by Native Americans to be a powerful plant that helps to cleanse a space of negativity. It is commonly used in smudge sticks. Use White Sage Essential Oil very mindfully as the supply of oil from ethical sources is quite limited. This is a precious essential oil, refrain from using it for other applications in order to conserve the oil for emotional and particularly spiritual work.

Sage has long been considered the "master healer". I've always seen sage as the epitome of a Native American Medicine Man.

Contraindications: Not to be used if pregnant, breast feeding or on babies and children. Not to be used if you have epilepsy, Petit Mal or high blood pressure. Not to be used if undergoing treatment for oestrogen-related cancers. Possible skin irritant. Excessive inhalation can cause vertigo.

Emotional: It helps to ground nervous emotions yet is uplifting where there is emotional exhaustion.

Mental: It alleviates depression and grief. Improves memory and has been reported as improving memory loss too. It brings mental perseverance. Calming and eases mental fatigue and tiredness without being too stimulating when we need a 'pick-me-up' during the day.

Relationships: I've already alluded to Sage being the epitome of a Native American Medicine Man/Woman, I was not disappointed. There he was, legs apart, firmly planted, arms crossed across his chest wearing a war bonnet looking me firmly in the eye totally indefatigable. Please note a Medicine Man/Woman is NOT the same as a shaman, but nor are they mutually exclusive of each other. Medicine Men (for brevity) would utilize healing herbs, and ceremony which included sweat lodges, chanting, prayers, drums and rattles in their healing practices.

A healing ceremony would usually begin with the Medicine Man preparing himself with cleansing of the physical body, attention to diet (some would eat no meat for 3 days before) and connecting to the sun spirit and star people. Then he would begin the ceremony proper by burning Sage to clear the atmosphere around the recipient from any negative influences that might surround them, which would block any healing intentions. Sage would also offer protection from any external influences. But it would also enable the Medicine Man to maintain his connection to spirit. Smudging with white sage in particular, is a practice westerner's have adopted.

Back to the oil. Once I moved past the 'symbolism' I was shown it became very clear that Sage is the Yang to Clary-Sage's Yin. This is what I have written about Clary, "But Clary is the mother to all these other herbs. They are her children. She nurtures them. Teaches them secrets to keep them safe. If you talk with Clary, she will tell you which plant will help with what ails you. She is a friend to you if you honor her. If you too become her student, she will grant you freedom of mind and spirit to learn about the healing arts.". Just change the mother and she to father and he. Along with the male wisdom of Sage, comes a very powerful, indefatigable, protective energy as opposed to Clary's gentle, mutable, shielding energy.

Physical:

Muscular/Skeletal System: Besides being very effective on general muscular and joint aches and pains, it is also very effective on fibrositis, fibromyalgia, stiff neck (torticollis) and palsy.

Circulatory System:

Lymphatic/Immune System: Sage is useful for most glandular disorders, any complaint related to lymph congestion. Sage also clears away cellular debris and strengthens cell wall integrity. Fights viral infections, bacterial infections, especially staph, strep, and pseudomonas and a powerful antifungal.

Nervous System: Helps headaches and disorders related to nerve deterioration or prolonged nervous stress.

Endocrine System: This Essential Oil imitates oestrogen. As such it aids conception, helps menopausal symptoms, particularly hot flashes and night sweats. For menopausal symptoms I always suggest sage herbal capsules as a much safer alternative if the EO is contraindicated. A hydrosol of Sage sprayed on the body has also proven to be effective for some. Very effective on period pains. Sage is believed to contain constituents that stimulate the secretion of progesterone-testosterone and keep their activities balanced. It helps to stop the flow of milk in nursing mothers. It can be an adrenal stimulant where there is adrenal fatigue due to stress.

Respiratory System: It treats colds, catarrh, bronchitis, sore throat, coughs, and other respiratory infections.

Digestive System: It helps with the loss of appetite, constipation, gingivitis, general digestive upsets, reduces candida and helpful for inflammations of the mouth, tongue, and throat.

Excretory/Urinary Systems: A very useful diuretic.

Integumentary/Skin System: Stems bleeding from cuts. Helps dermatitis and psoriasis. Sage is used to minimize gray in the hair of brunettes, I can vouch for this. It also helps dandruff, hair loss, skin conditions such as acne, it firms tissues and treats herpes.

Dreams And Aspirations: Sage cleanses the energy grid and strengthens its ability to protect us from negative influences. Sage has a positive influence on intuition, bringing clarity and vision to our souls if we will take the time to ponder and listen.

Notes:

Spearmint – 'Lighten-Up'

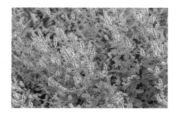

Botanical name: Mentha spicata
Plant part: Leaves and sometimes flowers too
Country of origin: Europe
Note: Top/Middle
Extraction method: Steam distilled

Author's Note: The Romans introduced spearmint into Britain where it was used it to stop milk from curdling.
In medieval times it was used to heal sore gums and whiten teeth.
Mentha comes from the Greek meaning mint or the Latin mente meaning thought.
Spearmint is thought to be the oldest of the mints and named Spere Mynte in the 16th century.

Contraindications: Might neutralise homeopathic remedies if used within 20 minutes of taking a homeopathic remedy. Other than this caution, Spearmint is pretty much a safe oil.

Emotional/Mental: Here's another oil that deals with both emotional and mental exhaustion in a gentle, kind, almost childlike way, allowing your heart to smile and mind to feel content.

Relationships: There is an innocent playfulness to Spearmint. A childlike quality of being immersed in the moment and just dancing, laughing and celebrating life. It asks you to be innocent, vulnerable, feel the emotions of the child within you and 'lighten-up', stop looking at the world with cynical eyes. Focus on the goodness around you. It will help you walk away, nay, even reject anything and anyone who is negative to your happy spirit with a simple flip of your hand. You won't have time for any negativity, depressing thoughts, you will be too busy embracing life, then feel your energy levels soar!

Physical: Many a time, Spearmint is treated as nothing more than a milder form of Peppermint, but these two essential oils have very different chemical components and very different therapeutic actions. Spearmint oil is a pleasant alternative to citrus oils for treating mental fatigue, depression, and eating disorders. Spearmint helps to restore normal function to the organs and systems of the body by repairing damage that has been done to cells, tissues, and nerves.

Muscular/Skeletal System: Gently eases muscle cramps, can be used for growing pains in children.

Circulatory System: Improves blood circulation not just for warming, but also cooling where necessary. I much prefer Spearmint in foot preparations than Peppermint in the heat of summer.

Lymphatic/Immune System: Helps fight fever and infections. Its mildly stimulating properties make it a great tonic oil following an illness.

Nervous System: Works on vertigo, nervous convulsions. headache, migraine and brain neurasthenia which is a condition that is characterized especially by physical and mental exhaustion usually with accompanying symptoms (such as headache and irritability), is of unknown cause but is often associated with depression or emotional stress, and is sometimes considered similar to or identical with chronic fatigue syndrome.

Endocrine System: Controls over abundance of breast milk, but use with caution and extremely diluted as it could taint the milk.

Respiratory System: Helps bronchitis, catarrh, asthma spasmodic cough and sinusitis and gentle enough to help children.

Digestive System: Treats colic, nausea, vomiting, dyspepsia, flatulence, hiccups, abdominal cramps and spasms, bad breath travel sickness. It can stimulate the appetite, whereas Peppermint can stymie it. Ideal for children's emotionally upset tummy, a safer and gentler alternative to Peppermint. Spearmint can be diluted in water and used as a mouth wash. Spearmint, swished regularly in the mouth, allegedly helps repair the enamel on the teeth. Spearmint is said to help the body burn fat. Good for hepatobiliary (liver) disorders.

Excretory/Urinary Systems:

Integumentary/Skin System: Acne, dermatitis, scabies wounds, injuries, relieves itching, dermatitis and congested or greasy skin all respond well. Research has shown spearmint to be effective against bacteria and fungi and so could be considered in a blend for infected skin.

Dreams and Aspirations: Going beyond what I have said about the childlike quality of Spearmint, when it comes to your dreams and aspirations, it will connect you to the energies of the fairy and elemental realms to help you manifest. Sometimes we need to just stop 'adulting' and let the creative and inspirational 'child' run lose, you'd be surprised at the simplistic yet so pertinent ideas that will get your imaginative juices flowing.

"Smell of rain, smell of spearmint, smell of soil.

And smell of boughs that are wet of gentle spring rain and shining clean"

Ali Shariati

Notes:

Thyme — 'Decisiveness'

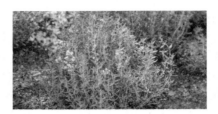

Botanical name: Thymus vulgaris, also known as White Thyme
Thyme Linalol higher in linalol than White Thyme
Plant part: Leaves and sometimes flowers are included
Country of origin: Southern Mediterranean and North Africa
Note: Middle
Extraction method: Steam distilled

Author's Note: Historically, fresh and dried Thyme as well as the essential oil have been used to help ward off bacteria and viruses. Of the most commonly available Thyme Essential Oils, Thyme ct linalol tends to be amongst the most gentle and safe while Thyme ct thymol contains more thymol and can be a more potent antibacterial/antiviral oil.

Thyme was a strewing herb in ancient Britain and was included in the posies carried by judges and kings to protect them from disease in public.

Thyme was used with clove, lemon and chamomile essential oils as a disinfectant and antiseptic in hospitals until World War I.

Philippe Mailhebiau writes that Sweet Thyme is very helpful for children suffering psychic problems due to parental lack of understanding and conflicts and who are unbalanced by family disharmony, due to its strong anti-depressive and stimulating effect on the psyche.

Constituent and safety information varies depending on the specific chemotype of Thyme Oil used.

Contraindications:

Thyme (Thymus vulgaris, also known as White Thyme): Not to be used if pregnant, breast feeding or on babies and children. Nor is it to be used if you have high blood pressure, epilepsy or hypothyroidism. Possible skin irritant.

Thyme Linalool (higher in linalool than White Thyme): Same as above until more research is done, although it is regarded as a safer alternative and doesn't seem to have the same effect on high blood pressure. This is the Thyme I am writing about here.

Emotional: Thyme is such an energising, joyful, courageous and warming oil to our emotions.

Mental: Much like Sage, Thyme aids memory and concentration, removes mental blockages. It is mentally invigorating resulting in decisiveness. It is specific for physical exhaustion, especially when there seems to be a lack of mental direction and motivation more than physical overwork.

Relationships: The first impression was of one of those southern black 'mamas' from old Hollywood films, with a headscarf tied on her head, one hand on hip and animatedly wagging her finger at me saying, "I'm not taking any of your nonsense ya hear? Oh no, no siree! I'm not messin' here!" Absolute frankness, unequivocally laying down the T&C's! But Thyme is doing this for your own good. She comes from a place of tolerance, support and sensitivity. She's analytical and can work out the logistics of what needs to be done even if that means finding a fresh perspective or a new way of doing something. Thyme can give us strength, self-confidence, and will power.

Physical:

Muscular/Skeletal Systems: Gout, rheumatism, arthritis, muscle aches, arthritis, rheumatic pain all respond to its anti-inflammatory properties.

Circulatory System: Warming and stimulates white blood cell production to fight off infections. It improves poor circulation, warms cold hands and feet, reduces bruises and stems nosebleeds.

Lymphatic/Immune System: There is nothing like Thyme to kill the strep or Staphylococcus virus. An absolute boon for killing off virus and bacterial infections.

Maggie Tisserand in her book "Aromatherapy v MRSA", identifies Thyme as one of the three key essential oils that have the potential to combat MRSA, the other 2 being Tea-Tree and Manuka. Thyme came out on top and why am I not surprised? The antiseptic and antiviral properties of Thyme are strong enough to handle most situations. Thyme is even recommended, applied diluted along the spine, for such ailments as spinal meningitis. Thyme, along with killing the invading microbes, aids lymphatic drainage and urine output, and strengthens the immune system generally. It will also help cellulite and oedema. I still can't think of a better anti-viral/bacterial EO.

Nervous System: Stimulates the CNS, alleviates sciatica, nerve pain generally and chronic fatigue.

Endocrine System: Inflammation of the vagina, uterus, cervix and fallopian caused by candida and/or staphylococci and eases birthing. Viral prostate inflammation. Allegedly an aphrodisiac!

Respiratory System: Inflammation of the mucous membranes of the mouth and nose, sinusitis, otitis, sore throats, tonsillitis, laryngitis, pharyngitis, flu, colds, coughs, bronchitis, asthma, whooping cough, pneumonia and pleurisy (I can vouch for both of those!), tuberculosis, upper respiratory tract infections, and eliminates phlegm. It is THE go-to oil to kill viruses and bacteria, particularly strep and staphylococcus, dead in 20 minutes!

Digestive System: Will treat dyspepsia, wind and diarrhea, bacterial enterocolitis caused by E. coli bacteria. Stomachic for gastritis, bacterial, viral and candida caused enterocolitis, parasitic caused colitis.

Wind is an indication of poorly digested food. Poorly digested food can interfere with the ICV (Ileocecal Valve) amongst other things and can affect your sleep, raise your blood pressure, become a threat to your cardiovascular system, cause severe stomach aches, cramps, diarrhoea and vomiting, as well as headaches and nausea.

Excretory/Urinary Systems: Thyme treats candida causing cystitis and bladder inflammation and Kidney tuberculosis.

Integumentary/Skin System: Helps dandruff, dermatitis, eczema, psoriasis, shingles, abscess, acne, cuts, bruises, cellulite, carbuncles, boils, insect bites, head lice, oily skin scabies warts, mycosis and infected pimples.

Dreams And Aspirations: I can do no better para-phrase Robbi Zeck who writes that Thyme activates a vital force for the positive use of willpower. It strengthens your resolve and assists in breaking negative patterns or habits. Thyme brings in a dynamic quality of energy that is needed by the physical body to maintain willpower, (refer back to my last sentence in the mental section) and instills a greater sense of empowerment and strong belief in oneself.

We all need more "Thyme" (pun not intended) not because of its powerful cleansing properties which also clear the person from blocked or stuck emotions but mainly because it is the oil of releasing and forgiveness which we all need more of in our lives. Thyme digs deep within our soul for unresolved negativity and old, stagnant feelings. It brings to the surface toxic emotions of hate, rage, anger and resentment, which cause the heart to close. Thyme empties our soul of all negativity and leaves the heart wide open.

Thyme teaches us that "it's time to move forward and let go". As we forgive, we release ourselves from emotional bondage. Thyme transforms hate and anger into love and forgiveness.

Notes:

Yarrow – 'Harmony'

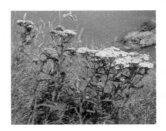

Botanical name: Achillea millefolium
Also known as Devil's Nettle
Plant part: Leaves and sometimes flowers are included
Country of origin: Native to Northern hemisphere
Note: Middle
Extraction method: Steam distilled

Author's Note: We all know the story of Achilles being dipped into a tea of Yarrow to protect him, but it was his ankle that led to his death when an arrow pierced his Achille's Tendon. Throughout the remainder of the Trojan war, and wars to follow, Yarrow was used to stop bleeding from the wounds of soldiers. Yarrow leaves have been used in many battlefields to treat injured soldiers, which led to the commonly used nicknames, "soldier's woundwort" or "warrior plant". Fossilized Yarrow pollen has been discovered in Iraq at Neanderthal burial caves dating from 60,000 years ago. Yarrow has been around for some considerable time by the looks of it.

Contraindications: Not to be used if pregnant, breast feeding or on babies and children. Not to be used if you have epilepsy, Petit Mal or running a fever. Not to be used if undergoing treatment for cancer. Patients on bupropion antidepressants should proceed with caution.
Possible skin irritant. Prolonged use may cause headaches.

Emotional: Robbi Zeck tells us that Yarrow Essential Oil helps to bring about balance and stability. "Yarrow stabilizes polar opposites within the body and is useful during times of major life changes, when emotional equilibrium needs greater support.", (The Blossoming Heart: Aromatherapy for Healing and Transformation). What we sometimes refer to as 'centering'.

Mental: A beneficial remedy for insomnia where the mind before bed, won't sit still, so restoring calm and balance to an overactive mind. During the day, it gently clears the clutter and restores focus and attention.

Relationships: I rather like the smell of Yarrow these days, I wasn't keen in the past. There's an older lady feel to Yarrow when I inhale it. An older lady who is wise because of her years. She's seen it all and reflects on how foolish she was, many a time in her younger days, for allowing situations and events making her blood boil. As it transpired, they weren't worth the agitation they caused.

I feel her gently showing me how to step back and look at the bigger picture then ask me "Is it really worth getting all het up about it?" She'll also ask you to look inwardly at yourself and re-asses those times which have left you still feeling anger, pain and bitterness when you reflect back on your past.

I felt harmony, a balance. I found myself looking at anything myself or others around me which had or still does cause me malcontent, with new eyes.

Physical: Yarrow will be a deep blue colour because of its azezulene content. It is this chemical component that works directly on the blood and circulation.

Muscular/Skeletal System: Alleviates back ache, rheumatic pain, arthritis, inflamed/injured muscles and muscular cramps.

Circulatory System: Hemorrhoids and varicose veins can be reduced. It is a well-known styptic, stops bleeding. Yarrow has a direct effect on the bone marrow and stimulates blood renewal, particularly red blood cells and can enhance the coagulation of the blood. Known to reduce hypertension, high blood pressure, but can stabilize low blood pressure too.

Lymphatic/Immune System: Yarrow is gently diaphoretic and a febrifuge. When you are ill, the use of Yarrow holds the fever from getting dangerously high and stimulates perspiration. Fever and perspiration are the body's way of killing the microbes and then carrying them out of the system.

Nervous System: Can ease and resolve headaches.

Endocrine System: Yarrow is an excellent oil for the female reproductive system. It has a mild hormonal action making this oil important in the treatment of menstrual cramps, ovarian cysts, menopausal problems including sweats, prolapse and uterine fibroid tumors. Susanne Fischer-Rizzi considers Yarrow the perfect oil for times of major life changes such as mid-life crisis and menopause because it helps reconcile opposing forces when we are feeling torn.

Respiratory System: Used in the early stages of colds, respiratory infections generally and congestion.

Digestive System: Yarrow improves the digestion by stimulating the secretion of bile and restoring the liver. It helps to restore other organs of the digestive system thus easing bouts of colic, flatulence, sluggish digestion, diarrhea, constipation and indigestion. It encourages appetite. It successfully treats hemorrhoids.

Excretory/Urinary Systems:

Integumentary/Skin System: Yarrow can be applied neat to close a wound, for this reason it is also known as Soldier's Woundwort in some texts. Interestingly, and in light of it being known as Soldier's Woundwort, it is recorded that Achilles tended his soldier's wounds with yarrow during the war with Troy. Yarrow's antiseptic properties are strong enough to prevent infection too. Yarrow also contains astringent properties which causes the tightening of tissues as afore mentioned for wound healing. But this also makes Yarrow very helpful for such things as: hair loss, dandruff, chapped hands, cuts, acne, burns, eczema, rashes, inflammations, improves scars, helps set the teeth firmly into the gums and firm up areas of sagging skin. Oily skin and acne are also successfully treated.

Dreams And Aspirations: In Chinese folklore, the aroma of Yarrow is said to bring about the meeting of Heaven and Earth in our lives. It can increase your intuition, and improves your ability to dream and apparently have visions. However, whilst you might have your 'heads in the clouds', it is also a very grounding oil, helping to keep both feet firmly on the ground so you aren't totally 'away with the fairies'.

Notes:

9.

THE EXOTICS AND GRASSES – OUR DREAMS AND ASPIRATIONS

"If man could pass through Paradise in a dream, and have a flower presented to him as a pledge that his soul had really been there, and if he found that flower in his hand when he awake. Aye, and what then?"

R.S. Coleridge

We all have private conversations with ourselves where we discuss the merits of a new idea, a change of career, even what we would do if we won the lottery. Sometimes though, we have situations where we find ourselves praying for a positive outcome to a situation with the help of unseen helpers, guides and even God. Whatever these internal communications are, they have one thing in common, they have not yet manifested in your physical reality. It does not matter whether the internal babbling is with yourself or somebody out with yourself, your dreams, aspirations and hopes, will remain in that 'other world' until you get the right 'energy' behind what your dream is before it will manifest. Whether you want to believe that you are trying to talk and communicate with your inner self, a guardian angel, spirit guide or God himself for help and assistance in manifesting your dream, or reaching a decision, is personal to yourself. But what you do need is the right energy behind what you want to bring into reality. For this purpose, I have allocated the 'energy' of the Archangels to each of the essential oils.

As this part of your garden is more spiritual as it deals with your soul purpose, the true you, it follows that this is also a prayer and meditation part of your garden. You must remember that prayer is to ask, and meditation is to listen for the answer.

Nurture your garden, manifest your dreams and aspirations......

Myrrh – Archangel Melkizadek

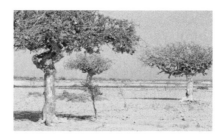

Botanical name: Commiphora myrrha
Plant part: Resin
Country of origin: North East Africa, Arabian Peninsula and India
Note: Base
Extraction method: Steam distillation

Contraindications: Not to be used if pregnant, breast feeding or on babies and children. Not to be used if undergoing treatment for oestrogen-related cancers.

Emotions: Myrrh has a cooling, calming effect on the emotions and brings a sense of peace. It is very similar to Spikenard (Metatron) here, in by it helps you be resilient, courageous and strong. These two oils would combine well together for emotional and mental support.

Mental: Where Spikenard brings mental courage, strength, determination and fortitude, Myrrh brings positivity, acceptance, is uplifting and energising. Again, a perfect marriage between both oils.

Relationships: **Melkizadek is the mental General in Chief.** She is the all-knowing Archangel; she knows everything about everything, a venerable encyclopedia. She even knows everything about you! So, if you are stuck, or not sure about where your life should be going, ask for Melkizadek's energies to help you. Everything she knows is balanced with wisdom and this is where Myrrh comes into its own.

Myrrh is all about supporting you to have the confidence to move forwards and communicate your intention and direction clearly and succinctly to others.

Together they will bring you that "Aha!" moment, when that missing piece of the jigsaw falls into place where previously you felt deflated, ambivalent, disheartened. When that "Aha!" moment hits there will be no stopping you!

*You might have noticed that I have referred to Melkizadek as a she and Metatron as a he. I did say Metatron is the connection to Divine Masculine, well, Melkizadek is the connection to the Divine Feminine, as I said, a perfect marriage.

Physical:

Muscular/Skeletal Systems: Myrrh has anti-inflammatory and analgesic properties therefore helps relax sore, painful and tight muscles.

Circulatory System: A well-known remedy to help reduce hemorrhoids. There is evidence to show it can help lower cholesterol. It stimulates the production of white blood cells in the bone marrow to fight infection.

Lymphatic/ Immune System: Myrrh supports the immune system, by helping to treat oral and vaginal thrush, glandular fever, viral/parasitic infections generally.

Nervous System:

Endocrine System: Myrrh help regulate scanty periods and leucorrhea. As already mentioned, it helps with vaginal thrush. Rodolphe Balz says Myrrh can regulate a hyper thyroid gland. I have no in clinic evidence to support this.

Respiratory System: As with all resin oils, Myrrh is no exception when it comes to respiratory ailments which include: bronchitis, sore throats, colds, catarrh, pharyngitis, coughs, glandular fever and asthma. Be careful with trying to dry out a cough, it could leave you with a dry cough. All mouth and gum disorders including pyorrhea and gingivitis.

Digestive System: Some research suggests it lowers blood sugar levels therefore could be useful for diabetics. It helps stem diarrhea and flatulence. Halitosis, hepatitis (liver is part of digestive system) and thrush start in the gut and Myrrh has a long history of helping all of them. It can stimulate the appetite, particularly after an intestinal parasitic infection.

Excretory/Urinary System: Inflammation of the urinary tract including the bladder.

Integumentary/Skin System: Excellent results can be achieved when used on boils, weeping eczema, athlete's foot, skin ulcers and bed sores. Has a drying action on any weeping or wet skin sores. A natural deodorizer.

Dreams and Aspirations:

Question: **Do other people's opinions end up confusing and deflating you?**

Answer: **The only opinion that matters is your own when your emotions and mind are in harmony.**

Myrrh and Melkizadek will help manifest your dreams, if they are meant for you. If your dream is not meant for you, together they will point you in the right direction. They will open you up to receive their guidance and restore your belief in yourself. They will support the manifestation of your dreams into reality. Myrrh keeps you grounded so you don't get carried away, and supports you when you are ready to verbalise and communicate your dreams to others.

Notes:

Spikenard – Archangel Metatron

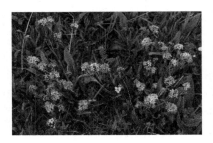

Botanical name: Nardostachys jatamansi
Plant part: Roots
Country of origin: Northern India and Nepal
Note: Base
Extraction method: Steam distilled

Author's Note: Also known as Nard oil or Muskroot.

Contraindications: Not to be used if pregnant or on babies and children or by nursing mothers. Not to be used if undergoing treatment for oestrogen-related cancers.

Emotional: Spikenard brings calm, a sense of centeredness, emotional balance, and most importantly, hope and compassion. Particularly useful where there is deep sadness.

Mental: Just like Metatron, Spikenard brings mental courage, strength, determination and fortitude. It also helps with insomnia where mental and emotional conundrums keep waking you up.

Relationships: Metatron is the Physical Archangel in Chief. He's one of the three 'Big Boys' as I call them. The other two being Melkizadek and Sandolphon. Once you experience his energies for the first time you will never forget them. His energies are very tangible, there is a 'thump' when his energies connect. He's not to be messed with and I say that in a very positive way! His energies are very 'external' to our physical bodies. He is out there around us to protect us and to bring in the support troops. He also has a sense of humour and knows no fear.

He is our connection to the Divine Male Universal energies as well as connecting us to our Earth Star Chakra. Imagine him as being the Commander in Chief of the military arm of the Angelic realm. He rallies the troops around you. His word is LAW!

Spikenard supports this energy by providing a sense of hope. Spikenard will comfort and support people who take on the worries of the world and tend to forget about their own lives. Spikenard helps you to communicate your emotions, feelings and thoughts, with love in a very clear and diplomatic way. Spikenard allows you to move forwards and away from any relationship that does no longer resonate with you. It is also useful for those in abusive or bullying relationships.

Together, they bring detached compassion to a difficult relationship by setting your boundaries, drawing a line in the sand, as it were.

Physical:

Muscular/Skeletal Systems: It helps relax muscles and reduce inflammation and has pain killing properties.

Circulatory System: For the heart is calms tachycardia and arrhythmia. It can reduce hemorrhoids and varicose veins. It reputedly helps anemia by aiding the body to absorb iron.

Lymphatic/Immune Systems: It is a support to the immune system in the presence of microbes, bacteria and viruses. It is said to be a natural antibiotic.

Nervous System: Has been used successfully in helping neuralgia.

Endocrine System: It can help male infertility, and menopausal problems in women. It can be a useful oil in birthing. It is an emmenagogue thus helps scanty periods and irregular periods.

Respiratory System: Because of its antimicrobial properties it can help all sorts of respiratory infections and allegedly asthma.

Digestive System: Said to expel parasites in the digestive tract. It helps calm spasms and aids normal functioning of the digestive processes. Supports the liver. Can shift constipation.

Excretory/Urinary System: A good diuretic.

Integumentary/Skin System: Spikenard is a powerful anti-fungal and a useful aid to serious skin conditions such as dermatitis, psoriasis, athlete's foot and fungal nail. Often used in mature skin products. It reputedly helps stimulate hair growth. Because of its antibacterial, antifungal properties it is a natural deodorizer. An excellent antiseptic.

Dreams and Aspirations: Spikenard will help bring your Dreams and Aspirations into the now.

Question: **Do you keep giving in to others when you know you shouldn't?**

Answer: **Use Spikenard to connect to Metatron's courageous spirit which abides within you.**

When you use Spikenard and call on Metatron's energies, you will certainly feel it if you have done so with the right intent. If you are needing protection from any negative situation or protection from outside influences so that you can have peace and space to focus on what you want in your life, they will come like a huge impregnable wall between you and whatever is interfering with your focus.

Notes:

Frankincense – Archangel Zadkiel

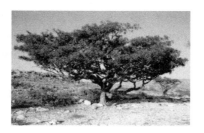

Botanical name: Boswellia carterii
Plant part: Resin
Country of origin: Africa. Almost all carterii comes from Somalia/Somaliland
Note: Base
Extraction method: Steam extracted

Author's Note: Most of the world's supply comes from Somalia, Somaliland, Eritrea and Yemen, countries which have seen or still experiencing conflict in recent years, this has impacted their Frankincense production somewhat. It is claimed that the Oman produces the world's finest, and most expensive, Frankincense, this is because it is the Boswellia sacra (which has 4 grades/types), not carterii. Boswellia Serrata comes from India and has contraindications.

There are probably no other oils which do as much as Frankincense does, safely. You might think Lavender does for example, but Lavender is not a safe oil. Although Frankincense is an expensive oil in relation to other oils, this expense is relative because firstly it is what we call in Aromatherapy a base note oil; which means we use much less of it and we do not need to use it as often because it remains in our system that much longer. Secondly, Frankincense is one of the oils that never ever goes off. In fact, there is a specialist market for mature Frankincense, and its price reflects this as the oil matures, rather like laying down a bottle of good wine! I would recommend that anybody who uses essential oils, or want to get started should make Frankincense top of their list as its benefits are unrivalled, it is perfectly safe, and can be looked upon as an investment.

Also Note: there are many types of Frankincense and the most common used in Aromatherapy is the carterii variety and is the one I am writing about here.

There is much misinformation on the internet including claims that Frankincense will cure cancer. There is ABSOLUTELY NO EVIDENCE OF THIS. What we do know is that the Boswellic acid which is present in the resin is a huge anti-inflammatory and on its own has shown to have positive results in reducing tumor size in vitro tests. However, the Boswellic acid does not cross over in distillation and is not present in the Essential Oil. Recently some CO_2 extractions have shown small traces of the boswellic acid but needs further investigation.

Contraindications: No known contra-indications, although I would urge caution during pregnancy and not use it until the 3rd trimester.

Emotional: Frankincense is relaxing, sedative and calming, bringing stability, comfort and even joy to the emotions.

Mental: Being a transformational oil it can turn mental fear into courage, mental weakness and lethargy to fortitude, dissolution and apathy to acceptance, mental blocks into inspiration, erratic thoughts to mental stability, a racing mind to a sea of calm and confusion into clarity.

Relationships:

Zadkiel's energies teach you forgiveness of self and others. When you forgive you can walk on in grace, with tolerance and the ability to see the greater picture. By forgiving without judgement, you can walk apart, or above, or away from negative influences with grace, dignity and integrity. The opposite of love is fear, what Zadkiel's energies do is encourage us to walk through life with love in our hearts and make decisions based in love and not fear.

To do this you have to reach into the depths of your soul and as high as we possibly can to the source, hence the reason why Zadkiel works with Jophiel on our Crown Chakra but his main role is with our 8th/Soul Star/Higher Chakra. Our 8th chakra forms the 'Earth Star' chakra of our 'higher chakra's'. When you are unforgiving of past issues or incidents you cannot move forwards with your life. If we don't get and give forgiveness, grace, tolerance, non-judgement right from the start, all our other chakras will carry the negative energy of blame, anger, intolerance and judgement. It is so very important to get these right or everything else will be influenced with negative thought forms.

Frankincense untangles and unties you from your attachment to past issues, thus allowing you the freedom to move forwards with your life, and thus manifest your dreams and aspirations.
It gently helps 'newbies' begin their spiritual journeys.

Frankincense is an ancient oil (infused) with ancient wisdom as far as the resin goes. Harvesting the resin to be made into an Essential Oil has changed over the years. Originally the Frankincense tears were harvested when they naturally occurred on the bark. Now, sadly, the practice is to slash the bark thus forcing the beautiful tree to 'bleed'. Being old enough to remember the difference in Frankincense that was allowed to naturally 'bleed' all those years ago, compared to Frankincense being forced to bleed, makes my heart sad. The difference is incredible! My belief is that with naturally occurring tears (takes around 30 years) you have the complete maturity and ancient wisdom of this tree. When the tears have been forced, it is more like dealing with a teenager.

Remember, Frankincense never goes off, so if you find an old bottle, +20 years old, of Frankincense somewhere, grab it with both hands!

Together, Frankincense in this case allows us to release the past as we know, however its purpose with Zadkiel is to make sure we remain our true selves. Frankincense is also a great protector and purifier of negative energies, an aspect of its vibration that is often overlooked. The key words with Frankincense are compassion, inner peace, tolerance and of course love. See how it sits beautifully with Zadkiel's energies? Together they are all about 'letting go of that which no longer serves us' or doesn't match our 'life plan'.

Physical: Because of the high triterpenoid chemistry of Frankincense, in order of efficacy it is antimicrobic, antibacterial then antiviral. What are terpenes and triterpenes? They are anti-inflammatory, analgesic, antipyretic, hepatoprotective, cardio tonics, and have sedative and toning effects on the whole physical body. Frankincense is often thought of being anti-viral, but in fact, is a highly efficacious and far better antibacterial, something I feel that needs to be remembered.

Muscular/Skeletal Systems: It will ease muscular aches and pains, arthritis and rheumatism through its effect on our breathing it allows more oxygen to reach these areas to relieve muscular tension, to carry away lactic acid build up in the muscles and joints. Relaxing, anti-inflammatory and analgesic for muscular aches and pains. Eases arthritic and rheumatic pain.

Circulatory System: It is warming to the circulatory system A tonic to the heart and circulatory system. Can calm palpitations and arrythmia.

Lymphatic/Immune System: It fortifies the immune system. It is antibacterial, antibiotic, antiseptic, antioxidant and helps cell regeneration. Fortifies the immune system overall. Staphylococcal and streptococcus infections are bacterial infections and Frankincense is excellent in treating both. Triterpenes have natural antibiotic constituents. There is evidence that Frankincense has been successful in treating scrofula which is tuberculosis of the lymph glands. TB is a bacterial infection and doesn't just affect the respiratory system.

Nervous System: A sedative and tonic to the whole nervous system. From my clinical experience, I would suggest a blend of Frankincense and Rosewood in cases of age onset epilepsy where there has been a history of abuse/bullying/victim of narcissism and their ilk.

Endocrine System: To the reproductive system, Frankincense has an affinity with the uterus and womb. It will relieve uterine haemorrhages, heavy periods and is a tonic to the uterus and excellent for prolapse. Of great benefit during labour, not just by easing the pain of contractions, but its calming effect on the mind and breathing. It will also help with post-natal depression.

Respiratory System: Clears congestion in the head and sinuses. Moving to the throat it soothes tickly coughs, laryngitis, sore throats and tonsillitis. To the chest, here we can see its connection with the mind. It relaxes and expands the lungs making breathing much easier, especially for asthmatics and people who have any type of breathing problems: bronchitis, pneumonia, COPD, and especially helps the panicky state one can get into when we can't breathe properly. By expanding the lungs, it loosens mucus and congestion and removes it out of the system. Probably best known for helping bacterial bronchitis and bacterial pneumonia in particular. Frankincense and Thyme linalool/white combined together are particularly effective on bacterial pneumonia. Remembering the contraindications to Thyme, the only one I would worry about is epilepsy. I used this combo on my grandmother's pillow when she had 20% chance of pulling through double bacterial pneumonia. In less than 2 weeks she was back in the resident's lounge. Although I don't suggest the use of Frankincense while pleurisy is still active, I would not hesitate to use it in recovery to help the healing process.

Digestive System: Moving to the stomach it will ease indigestion, dyspepsia, wind and belching. It has a particular affinity with the liver as it is a tonic and hepatoprotective. Triterpenes have also been shown to be promising in the prevention of diabetic complications.

Excretory/Urinary Systems: For the urinary system, it will ease kidney problems, remembering any type of kidney problems must be checked out thoroughly. Excellent in the treatment of cystitis, particularly when combined with Bergamot. Nephritis is a particularly painful bacterial infection of the kidneys. Frankincense combined with Sandalwood will greatly help the symptoms alongside the antibiotics you will in no doubt need to be taking. A gentle but effective diuretic.

Integumentary/Skin System: Its effect on the skin is second to none. Its healing, regenerative, softening and preservative effects are well known since Egyptian times. Mature and ageing skin is rejuvenated and wrinkles will be smoothed out. It will balance oily conditions. Its antiseptic properties help with all types of skin infections including wounds, sores, ulcers and carbuncles and all kinds of inflammation. It is rejuvenating for older, mature or sun damaged skin. Astringent properties balance oily and combination skins.

Dreams and Aspirations – Meditation, introspection, grounding. Links you to your higher self.

Question: What is the negative block you are hanging on to that is stopping you from manifesting your dreams and aspirations?

Answer: Forgiveness of self or others, which prevents you from following your life's purpose.

What can I say? When we pray, we are asking a question. When we meditate, we are listening for the answer. To hear that answer we must connect out-with ourselves or to our higher-self, as it is often referred to. Frankincense has an ancient history in meditative practices and religious ceremonies. It was recognised for it's introspective, calming and even enlightening qualities. Because of this combination of qualities, it allows space for us to forgive ourselves and others for actions of the past which have caused discomfort, disharmony and even anguish and free's us to move forwards.

Notes:

Elemi – Archangel Jophiel

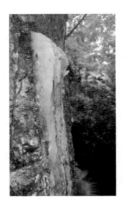

Botanical name: Canarium luzonicum/vulgare
Plant part: Resin
Country of origin: China
Note: Middle
Extraction method: Steam distillation

Author's Note: There are reports of Elemi being used for religious rites and for burning, from the 7th century so it is "Chinese incense". In the 16th century, Magellan introduced it in Europe and the Middle East for its fragrant and medicinal properties. Almost all now comes from the Philippines.
Use Elemi in very small quantities. Not just because Elemi will become the dominant odour, but used in smaller quantities it seems to enhance and 'turbo charge' as I call it, the efficacy of the other EO's in the blend.
Elemi is often referred to as "poor man's Frankincense" in the Aromatherapy world.
PLEASE NOTE FROM THE PHOTO's BELOW: In the Philippines Elemi goes by the name Pili. However, buyer beware, the distillers in the Philippines are now distilling Canarium ovatum, but this is from the Elemi seed/fruit NOT the resin. There will be a big difference chemically. So, I am choosing to use the name Elemi for the resin extraction and Pili for the seed/fruit extraction.

More information on Pili (Canarium ovatum) at this link:
(Appendix 9.)

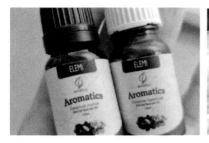 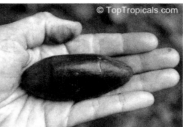

Contraindications: Possible irritant to sensitive skins.

Emotional: Elemi essential oil controls excessive emotions, dissipates fears, allows for clearer communication and helps restore confidence. It brings joy, peace and a feeling of general wellbeing. Brings balance and excellent for anxiety.

Mental: Elemi is an excellent anti-depressive, try combining it with Neroli and a citrus oil. It increases attention span and concentration, but contrarily it can also be very sedating to the mind and body when that 'state' of being will be of more benefit. This does not necessarily define Elemi as an adaptogen oil, but it is interesting that Elemi seems to 'know' what would be of best benefit to the individual. Is this the elusive 'secret' of Elemi that has eluded me for decades? More about this below.

Relationships – Compassion.

Jophiel takes us even closer to source, God, our soul or our Higher Self. He awakens our sleeping self to wisdom with imagination and inspiration. Once awakened we feel a new connection to something far greater than just our physical being. This brings joy and excitement to our lives. Although Jophiel is normally associated with our Crown Chakra ('I Know'), he also works with our Solar Plexus, the 'I Will'. Both of which, given Jophiel's directives make sense.

You see, the two phrases associated with him are 'Beauty of God' and 'I know'. So, when Jophiel's 'inspiration' hits us, through our Crown Chakra we suddenly 'know'. The reason why we trust this 'inspiration'? Because Jophiel is also associated with our Solar Plexus, the 'I Will'. It hits us in our gut, our gut instinct. It is so strong we then present it as 'I Will'. He certainly lets you know when he is around. Now you know to thank Jophiel every time you get 'divine inspiration' to follow your 'gut instinct'.

Jophiel is said to be the Angel of Paradise. There are two Paradises, the one heavenly and the other earthly. The earthly one we know as Eden. He is the first Archangel mentioned in the Bible, he sent Adam and Eve from Eden. Many, think of this as a banishment because they ate the apple of knowledge. In actual fact they were freed by Jophiel so they could experience life fully. The rest is history!

Jophiel is also the Archangel we should be calling on during exams, he will bring in that inspiration when you are stuck on that one darned question you know the answer to but have gone 'blank'.

Typically, Jophiel works in very subtle ways. Let's be honest, how many of us realise that those little 'sparks' we get come from him? It's a mystery.... Or is it a 'secret'?

Elemi not only helps us to trust our 'gut instinct', but also allows us to express this instinct through the 'I Will'. Elemi calms us down gently. It activates our intuition our 'gut instinct'. It enhances our psychic abilities and brings us that "aha!" moment. The 'secret' becomes manifest! Can you see why Elemi is Jophiel's oil?

Elemi is another oil that helps us accept changes, release blocks and move on. It is very much a **"be careful what you wish for"** oil, I mean this in all seriousness! It balances our physical, emotional, mental and spiritual selves.

Physical: Elemi is not called 'poor man's Frankincense' for nothing, the healing properties for both are very similar.

Muscular/Skeletal Systems: For back pain in particular, Elemi is an analgesic and antispasmodic. Try combining it with Marjoram, as it too has an affinity with lower back pain, with a dash of Plai. Otherwise, a great oil for general muscular aches and pains and helps arthritic and rheumatic conditions.

Circulatory System: Useful oil to add to a blend for varicose and thread veins. Generally warming and a tonic to the system.

Lymphatic/Immune Systems: Supports the Lymphatic system generally, but particularly at the start of an infection.

Nervous System: Sedating and calming for the nervous system.

Endocrine System: Effective on uterine and breast infections and also a uterine tonic.

Respiratory System: Like its counterpart Frankincense, Elemi has a rebuilding, repairing and strengthening effect on the respiratory system. It is an expectorant, helping to remove mucous and catarrh. It also helps to expand the lungs, but not to the same extent as Frankincense. Because of this action, Elemi is a boon to people who suffer from chronic bronchitis and asthma. It eases bouts of coughing. Elemi, like Frankincense, is recommended for sinus infections.

Digestive System: Helps to regulate digestive processes and return homeostasis to the digestive system generally. So, it might be worth adding that 1-2 drops into any type of digestive issue blend you are making. Particularly useful for diarrhoea, enterospasms and amoebic dysentery.

Excretory/Urinary Systems: Supportive, clearing and a tonic to the system.

Integumentary/Skin System: It is a powerful antibacterial and antiseptic, has anti-inflammatory properties and is regenerating for the skin, helping scar formation. Elemi can be used to treat numerous skin conditions including: allergic rashes, fungal growths, chapped skin, ulcers, sores, abscesses and particularly cuts and wounds that have become infected. Elemi also has a reputation for being effective in the treatment of gangrene, not that we would ever come across this in practice! Helps to stem excessive perspiration, but I would suggest the underlying cause needs to be investigated, but it would make a useful addition to a deodorising blend of oils such as Rosewood and Patchouli. Because it has a drying effect on the skin, it will be useful for oily skin and hair.

Dreams and Aspirations – Grounding, meditation, inspiring, manifesting.

> Question: **Don't know what you really want, but you know it's out there?**
> Answer: **Jophiel and Elemi guide you to your life path. They help you get to the answers that you previously did not understand.**

Jophiel awakens your sleeping self to wisdom with imagination and inspiration. Once awakened you will feel a new connection to something far greater than just your physical being. This in turn brings joy and excitement and therefore a 'drive' to manifest your dreams into reality.

Elemi balances your spiritual and physical lives thus bringing a positive surge of energies so that you can birth your dreams into reality.

Notes:

Guaiacwood – Archangel Gabriel

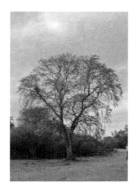

Botanical name: Guaiacum officinale/Guaiacum sanctum/Bulnesia sarmienti
Plant part: Wood/shavings/Resin
Country of origin: South American tropics, most coming from Paraguay these days.
Note: Base
Extraction method: Steam distillation

Author's Note: I know, steam distilled from wood, so why is it in this section that covers resins, grasses and exotics? Well, to put it simply, the oil is extracted from the resin which does exude from the tree, but they also fire up the wood to collect the resin that then leaks from the wood. According to Wanda Sellar, it is the Bulnesia sarmienti that gives off the most oil/gum by this method. The resulting 'oil' is so thick it is like a soft resin consistency at room temperature and needs warming up before you can use it. It behaves more like a resin than it does a wood oil.

Contraindications: No known contra-indications.

Emotional: If you enjoy a smokier smelling oil, then Guaiacwood is for you. It can be deeply relaxing where needs be, so be careful when you use it. Otherwise, it is soothing and balancing to the emotions.

Mental: Mentally it can bring inspiration, direction, determination and clarity.

Relationships:

We often say intuition is more a feminine trait, our third eye is associated with our intuition of things in our physical world. So, it is of no surprise that Gabriel connects us to our 'feminine side', our intuitive side. Gabriel opens us to messages from our Guardian Angel and Personal Angels. On a biblical note, it was Gabriel that announced the birth of John the Baptist and at the annunciation told Mary she would give birth to Jesus. For women, Gabriel helps us to communicate with our unborn child. He also helps with women's menstrual cycles and allegedly chooses which souls will be born. I have my doubts about the last aspect as it would remove free will and choice of the soul being incarnated. He is also said to be with your baby for the 9 months of gestation and when baby is born, he gently presses just below the baby's nose to make them forget 'heaven's secrets' thus leaving the little cleft above the top lip. I rather like that idea.

Gabriel's message to humanity is the importance of loving one another and encouraging unity. He brings transformation, change, mercy and forgiveness. As Michael is symbolised by the sword, Gabriel is symbolised by a trumpet and trumpet Lilly's. He is also associated with the moon, more feminine energy. His presence can be sometimes be seen as a streak of silver light, just like a moon beam. I cannot help but think Kuan Yin is a manifestation on earth of Gabriel.

If you have not seen the film Constantine starring Keanu Reeves and Tilda Swinton playing a very androgenous Gabriel it is well worth a watch. In the final scenes Gabriel is seen wearing hospital ID bracelets. They are labelled Awakening, Sorrow, Rage, Passion, Love, Joy, and Melancholy, totally sum up Gabriel's energies.

Guaiacwood with its cleansing properties helps you to find your purpose in life, and strengthens your will and resolve to manifest it, with clarity, integrity and determination.

Together they bring a sense of peace and loving security. If you feel you have lost direction, that there is simply too much going on, they will bring you 'back on track'.

Physical:

Skeletal/Muscular Systems: Asthenia, weakness in the limbs mainly after a viral infection such as Epstein-Barr. Helps rheumatoid arthritis.

Circulatory System: Being a sudorific (increases temperature) it helps to expel toxins aka viruses, bacteria, from our body. It can also decrease temperature in the presence of feverish colds, where it is a bacterial infection as bacteria do not survive well in colder temperatures.

Lymphatic/Immune Systems: It reduces swelling in lymph nodes, so might well be useful for Glandular Fever and Epstein-Barr virus generally and what can be the resulting CFS, Chronic Fatigue Syndrome. A support to the overtaxed Lymphatic System where there is oedema.

Nervous System: A lovely demulcent to the nervous system I would specifically add the word soothing here.

Endocrine System: Helps with the lack of vaginal secretions. Has a reputation as an aphrodisiac. Helps painful periods and menopausal problems.

Respiratory System: Tonsillitis, sore throats and general chest infections all respond well to Guaiacwood.

Digestive System: A good remedy for gout, whether treated directly on the digestive system or where the gout manifests in joints such as the big toe. A good laxative for constipation.

Excretory/Urinary Systems: A diuretic in the presence of oedema. It is antiseptic to bladder and genito-urinary infections. Reputedly breaks down bladder stones, but this should not be attempted without a full medical diagnosis. Syphilis is on the rise again worldwide, so might be worth noting this oil as it has a proven track record in helping.

Integumentary/Skin Systems: A great adjunct to a blend of oils for mature skin. Helps all types of skin diseases.

Dreams and Aspirations:

Question: You've got the bigger picture, but that 'little something' is eluding you?
Answer: Guaiacwood and Gabriel will bring clear messages, signs, symbology to you about that missing 'something'.

Guaiacwood and Gabriel bring guidance, vision, inspiration and even prophecy to you when you have strayed or are confused about your 'life path'. With Guaiacwood's help, Gabriel can come to you in your dreams, but don't expect an Angel, with visions and inspiration and sometimes prophecy! Their combined energies are also purifying, removing toxins, negative thought forms, feelings and energies from you and your environment, which block and restrict your progress.

Notes:

Benzoin – Archangel Michael

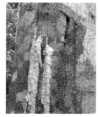
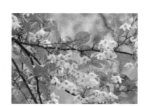
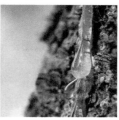

Styrax benzoin   *Flowers from both trees*   *Styrax tonkinensis*

Benzoin Sumatra   *Benzoin Siam*

White gum   *Golden gum*

Aromatherapy   *Perfumery/Incense*

Botanical name: Styrax benzoin
Plant part: Resin
Country of origin: Sumatra, Indonesia
Note: Base
Extraction method: Solvent extracted, an Absolute oil

Author's Note: Common names for the tree include Gum Benjamin. In older texts it is most likely to be referred to as Gum Benjamin.

In perfumery, Benzoin is used as a fixative, slowing the dispersion and evaporation of other essential oils and fragrance materials into the air. So, no reason why not to use it to extend the shelf life of your blends if they are for skin ailments, beauty products (particularly mature skin) or supportive fragrances for emotional/mental wellbeing. In fact, I would highly recommend it. **Be very aware which Benzoin you are purchasing.** There are two types of Benzoin resins: **Benzoin Sumatra** and **Benzoin Siam,** both are Styrax. Both varieties, like Frankincense, are known as pathogenic resins, meaning the resin protects the plant from insects and pathogens. The gums (they become known as a resin when they harden on contact with the air), exudes from the tree when it is damaged either deliberately or by nature, or naturally due to older age.

Benzoin Sumatra is obtained from Styrax benzoin, which is the one commonly used and written about in Aromatherapy, and is grown on the island of Sumatra.
Benzoin Siam is obtained from Styrax tonkinensis found across Thailand, Laos, Cambodia, and Vietnam and used in incense making and perfumery.
(See photo's above)

Contraindications: Not to be used if pregnant, breast feeding or on babies and children. Not to be used if undergoing treatment for a hormonal/oestrogen cancer. Possible skin irritant to a few.

Emotional By helping you cut emotional ties from the past, Benzoin brings calm, tranquility, peace, inner-joy, comfort and happiness. It can be very sedating if there is emotional stress.

Mental Benzoin is a wonderful oil for both emotional and mental sadness, loneliness, depression, constant worries, feelings of abandonment and then the mind justifies that feeling which, in turn, brings mental and emotional exhaustion. In their place, Benzoin brings mental (and emotional) balance, steadfastness, determination, focus, clarity, positivity and sense of belonging or secure and happy with your own company. It can massively reduce mental fear. A perfect combination with Vetiver at times of sudden trauma accompanied with a fear of a repeat.

Relationships:

Michael Ah, Archangel Michael, probably the most well-known of them all. Almost always depicted carrying a shield and a sword. Ready to defend and protect, to cut away 'ties that bind' and people/things that 'no longer serve your higher good' which you have mentally, emotionally or etherically with past or present issues. This is symbolic of protection, courage, strength and integrity.

When he is not doing battle on your behalf, Michael is a very easy-going Angel. Love being the driving force behind anything any of the Archangels and Angels do, Michael is no different. He teaches you to love yourself. By his own actions he encourages you to be courageous and stand your ground. He also teaches patience; winning battles doesn't mean you will win the war. He motivates you to accomplish all of life's tasks. He is the Peaceful Warrior. This is what he does to protect you 'externally', but what does he do to help you 'internally'?

Associated with our Throat Chakra, Michael helps us to remain balanced and steadfast to our principles, integrity and highest good for all and by doing so protects us from 'evil' or negativity. Our throat chakra is where we take in information and where we 'regurgitate' that information through communication whether that be through words written or spoken.

Benzoin immediately wraps you in a safe, warm and cozy blanket of protection and brings a smile to your face as you close your eyes and look up to the warming rays of the sun. It lets you know it is perfectly OK to be you. It removes those masks we don to different people and situations. It has a kindness and gentility which is under-pined with indomitable courage and strength.

Together Helps you move forwards with confidence and integrity, all the while offering feelings of protection.

Physical:

Muscular/Skeletal Systems: A gentle and effective analgesic and anti-inflammatory for general aches and pains as well as arthritis.

Circulatory System: Benzoin is a cordial for the heart, a tonic for the heart, and gently warms the circulation where there is coldness due to lack of circulation.

Lymphatic/Immune System: Helps swelling and inflammation of the joints associated with arthritis.

Nervous System: It is fabulously calming to the nervous system.

Endocrine System: A useful remedy for female problems such as leucorrhea and premature ejaculation for men. A well-known and effective sensual aphrodisiac.

Respiratory System: Benzoin is an excellent expectorant and tonic to the lungs and helps bronchitis, asthma, coughs, colds, laryngitis and sore throats, helps to expel catarrh. Like Myrrh, Benzoin is useful to help treat mouth ulcers.

Digestive System: It is calming on the stomach, eases flatulence. It strengthens the pancreas and said to control blood sugars, thus might help Type 2 diabetics by aiding digestion.

Excretory/Urinary Systems: More than just helps with urinary tract infections such as cystitis. It is also an effective diuretic.

Integumentary/Skin System: Benzoin is an excellent antiseptic on all kinds of skin abrasions, wounds, bedsores, rashes, chaffs, cracks, chapped, ulcers, eczema, red/inflamed, irritating, itchy skin, psoriasis and acne. A fabulous moisturizer for dry skin, by making it more elastic. Helps scar formation. Try it combined with Immortelle. Said to help particularly with frostbite/chilblains and other types of burns also respond well. It is a natural deodorizer.

Dreams and Aspirations:

Question: **Do you know what is blocking you, but you don't know how to cut the ties?**

Answer: **Benzoin and Michael can bring clear communication so you speak your truth with diplomacy, integrity, kindness and grace.**

Michael is associated with your throat chakra, he helps you to verbalise your dreams and aspirations in a clear, diplomatic, concise, assertive and even dramatic way – when required!

Benzoin will help dissolve any frustrating or negative thoughts that prevent you from manifesting your dreams and aspirations. It will help you focus your mind, not only for prayers and meditation, but to see clearly the resolution to manifest your dreams. As such, Benzoin helps to buffer and protect you from any 'self-sabotaging' thoughts and ideas that would prevent a positive thought process.

Notes:

Palmarosa – Archangel Raphael

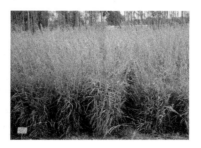

Botanical name: Cymbopogon martini
Plant part: Blades of the grass
Country of origin: India
Note: Middle
Extraction method: Steam distillation

Contraindications: No known contra-indications.

Emotional: Palmarosa brings emotional feelings of security, contentment, certainty, stability and is wonderfully uplifting to our emotions.

Mental: It is refreshing on our mind bringing clarity, focus, enthusiasm and decisiveness through wisdom and mental calm.

Relationships: Loyalty and security.

Raphael is the Archangel of healing. Raphael alongside Chemuel helps our heart chakra. Where Chemuel assists in our expression of unconditional love, Raphael helps with the healing of our love of self and others. Raphael brings healing, wholeness and unity to our heart. As Chemuel carries pink light for the heart and orange light for the sacral chakra, Raphael exudes both pink and green light associated with our heart chakra. Green is for healing; pink is for energising and anchoring.

Palmarosa gives you emotional stability and security in yourself.

Palmarosa allows us to express our mind and thoughts through our heart, to be mindful of our words, actions and deeds. It allows space for our love to grow until we know and act without any restrictions on expressing our love to all. Palmarosa protects our aura but at the same time projecting our heart feelings to others through our kind words.

Palmarosa is an oil that allows us to 'let go'. We all too often try to hide our insecurities because of past hurts. We can become almost 'obsessive' in holding on to past situations with people because the thought of 'letting them go' and stepping into an unknown future without them, is too terrifying to contemplate. Palmarosa helps us to embrace change, let go and move on and do so with kind words.

Together they clear your mind and focuses you on the emotional issues that need to be resolved or healed.

Physical: A huge antiviral, antibacterial and antifungal essential oil.

Muscular/Skeletal Systems: It is an analgesic (pain relieving) to stiff and tired joints.

Circulatory System: Calming and a tonic to the cardio-vascular system generally. Helps to reduce fever in the presence of a viral or bacterial infection.

Lymphatic/Immune System: A gentle but effective support to our immune system, particularly after an illness where our Lymphatic system is still working hard removing the dead debris of infection and any medication we might have taken.

Nervous System: Calming to an emotionally frayed nervous system.

Endocrine System: Palmarosa can balance the thyroid gland, but please seek the advice of a qualified Aromatherapist to help with this. Helps treat candida, in this case thrush in the vagina. Very useful for PMT/PMS and other accompanying menstruation problems. Strengthens the uterus.

Respiratory System: Helps fight fungal (think candida) and bacterial infections of the respiratory system, think bacterial pneumonia. Helps sinusitis and otitis.

Digestive System: A recognized tonic for the digestive system, and strengthens peristalsis i.e., the contractions of the digestive tract to help move things along the digestive system. Helps stop diarrhea and dyspepsia. A useful adjunct to a blend to help those with anorexia. Helps balance candida albicans in the gut as well as fight off bacterial and viral infections in the gut.

Excretory/Urinary Systems: Fights inflammation and infections of the urethra and bladder.

Integumentary/Skin System: Again, treats candida of the skin including fungal nail. Wonderfully hydrating to dry skin and balances excess sebum production in oily skins. It strengthens cell reproduction of the skin and hair. Helps dry and wet eczema. Reduces scarring and acne.

A little note on Candida. As you can see above Candida appears in many of our bodies systems. Candida usually appears in the gut, but can also be a fungal infection caused by a type of yeast (Candida albicans), even on the skin. Palmarosa is well worth a try against this fungal imbalance.

Dreams and Aspirations – manifestation

Question: **Are your dreams and aspirations being controlled by emotional fear?**

Answer: **Palmarosa and Raphael bring clarity and focus with healing to the emotional fear which is holding you back.**

Raphael's energies will heal any emotional issues you might have with manifesting your dreams, besides being the healing angel on all other levels too.

Palmarosa gives you emotional stability and security. It clears your mind and focuses you on the emotional issues that need to be resolved or healed, so that manifesting your dreams can come from a place of strength and most importantly wisdom. To do this, Palmarosa also helps you to 'think outside the box' for creative solutions. You'll know if that 'outside the box' solution is correct as it will make you smile and your heart sing. Unless you are emotionally secure, content and certain about what you want to bring into your physical world, it won't happen because it just won't have the right energy behind it.

Notes:

Vetiver – Archangel Uriel

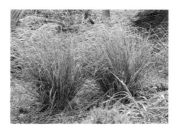

Botanical name: Vetiveria zizanioides
Plant part: Roots
Country of origin: India
Note: Base
Extraction method: Steam distilled

Author's Note: In India it is known as "the oil of tranquillity".

Contraindications: No known contra-indications.

Emotional: In the presence of grief, trauma and even obsession, Vetiver brings peace, tranquility, calm and serenity to our emotions. It is warming and embracing for our emotions and restores equilibrium both emotionally and mentally.

Mental: Mentally, Vetiver brings clarity, positivity, strength and wisdom. A huge help for insomnia, mental, emotional and physical exhaustion. Almost immediately will calm states of hysteria and repression.

Relationships:

Uriel's energies bring peace and tranquility, and the ability for you to receive as well as to give. His energies bring stability and 'self-knowing'. He helps us work on and understand and transmute negative aspects of ourselves and others so peace, tranquility and serenity can abide within us. When you have worked on, understood and transformed any negativity you become 'self-knowing' and truly connected to the 'I will', which is the essence of your Solar Plexus Chakra with which Uriel is connected to. When your Solar Plexus Chakra is clear and functioning in this balanced way, you can truly manifest who and what you are all about.

When we walk with Archangel Uriel, we walk in love, grace, peace and strength of character. He helps us connect with our creativity, our deepest insights into life, transform our worst nightmare into a gift and make our choices based in and with love. He helps us recognize the 'Buddha' within us and step back from judgement to recognize the same in others. When we can bring all these aspects together, we attract more of the same to us as others feel that energy in their etheric field and respond in kind.

Vetiver has a very strong association with your Solar Plexus. When you have a nervous 'butterfly tummy' just inhale the earthy fragrance of Vetiver and you will feel its physical impact on this area. I call it the Valium of the Essential Oils. Not only have I personally experienced its profound calming effect on states of panic, I have also seen it 'bring down' somebody who had experienced such a horrendous trauma he was close to being sectioned, in less than 15 minutes of inhaling this precious oil. Vetiver is also the only oil that can clear, balance and synchronize all your other chakras in one fell swoop. An amazing cleanser and protector both of your physical self and your aura, it brings in positive and grounding energies that promote strength and a deep sense of belonging and self-esteem.

Together they bring feelings of calm, tranquility, serenity, protection, focus, integrity, self-esteem, and a sense of honor and belonging to any given situation.

Physical: Excellent all-round tonic when it comes to physical exhaustion due to underlying emotional and mental stresses.

Muscular/Skeletal Systems: Warming for muscular aches, pains, cramps and spasms.

Circulatory System: It is said to aid in the production of healthy red cells in the blood. Because of this it helps to transport oxygen to all systems of the body. Strengthens and supports the circulation. Calming in cases of tachycardia and arrythmia. Useful in the treatment of coronaritis, which is inflammation of the coronary arteries.

Lymphatic/Immune System: Has a good record for helping rheumatic, osteoarthritic and arthritic conditions due to its anti-inflammatory properties. It supports and strengthens the Immune System.

Nervous System: A first 'go-to' oil in the presence of panic, extreme anxiety and hysteria. It has a direct impact on the Vagus Nerve and therefore our adrenals. I call it the Valium of Essential Oils.

Endocrine System: Well-known to have an aphrodisiac effect on many. Helps with menopausal and post-natal depression.

Respiratory System: Again, because of Vetiver's pronounced effect on calming the emotional, mental and nervous system 'hysteria' it also calms the breathing.

Digestive System: Helps overcome anorexia and bulimia. Used to treat intestinal parasites. Supports the liver and pancreas. Quietens a very nervous and anxious tummy.

Excretory/Urinary System:

Integumentary/Skin System: Antiseptic and healing for scars, acne, urticaria, skin parasites and indicated, like Patchouli, for mature skin.

Dreams and Aspirations:

Question: **Are you your own worst enemy? Are you constantly self-sabotaging?**

Answer: Vetiver and Uriel will connect you to your inner child and allow you to see yourself for the fearless person you truly are.

Vetiver and Archangel Uriel are known for their ability and deep commitment to finding unusual creative solutions to any problem. They do this by teaching us to see life and the World through eyes of love. It goes almost without saying that Uriel is the Archangel of 'transformation'. He brings peace, grace, insights and discernment. Bringing all these aspects to the table, he teaches us to understand, learn and experience the difference between listening to the limiting beliefs of our minds and thoughts which are based on past experiences, to following our 'gut instinct' and bring forth love in all our daily experiences.

Vetiver assists Uriel by connecting our past to the present. It teaches us to learn from our past experiences and shows us how to use the present to heal the past. You could say it mutates our past memories and experiences into present day wisdom and maturity.

Notes:

Galangal – Archangel Chemuel

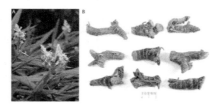

Botanical name: Alpina officinarum
Plant part: Root
Country of origin: The oldest reports about its use and existence
are from southern China and Java
Note: Middle
Extraction method: Steam distilled

Author's Note: *King's College, London, researched this oil and in its root form and found that its anti-oxidant and enzyme activation properties could possibly act against cancer. Their study concluded that "isolated chemical from the Galangal root killed cancer cells and protected healthy cells"
Galangal is a close relative of Ginger, Turmeric, Plai and Hydacheium and is sometimes goes by the name Galingale or False Ginger.

Contraindications: No known contraindications.

Emotional: An excellent oil for emotional fatigue. The kind of fatigue that gets you irate and even angry. It brings calm first and then emotional balance.

Mental: Once the emotions are settled, Galangal brings mental stability, direction, concentration, and focus. It goes without saying it also therefore alleviates mental fatigue.

Relationships:

Chemuel's energies are of pure unconditional love in all its forms. He helps you with all aspects of your relationships with partners, children, relatives, friends and colleagues. But most importantly his energies show you how to love yourself first – warts and all! Because, unless you can love yourself first, you cannot possibly truly and unconditionally love anybody else or recognise and accept genuine love from others.

Chemuel is associated with two of our Chakra's. Primarily our Sacral and secondary our heart Chakra.

Galangal connects you to your divine self or your higher self. This 'divine self' allows you to love and more importantly to trust yourself so that you can express who you truly are and explore hidden depths of your psyche and persona without fear or self-imposing restrictions. The phrase 'free love' from the 1960's comes to mind, where you can free your love to embrace who and what you are and accept who and what others are.

Together they bring courage, confidence and self-esteem.

Physical

Muscular/Skeletal Systems: Eases fatigue, stiffness in joints and muscles. Helps both rheumatoid arthritis and arthritis.

Circulatory System: Stimulates blood circulation.

Lymphatic/Immune System: It helps flush out free radicals. Stimulates the body to produce its own 'antibiotic'. It has good antiviral and antimicrobial properties. *King's College, London, researched this oil in its root form and found that its anti-oxidant and enzyme activation properties could possibly act against cancer. Their study concluded that "isolated chemical from the Galangal root killed cancer cells and protected healthy cells".*

Nervous System: Generally calming to the whole nervous system due to its effects on our emotions and mind.

Endocrine System: A known aphrodisiac.

Respiratory System: Sinus congestion and general stuffiness in the head. Helps at the first signs of bronchitis, catarrh, cough, colds and flu. Because of its calming influence it also helps in cases of asthma and where there has been shock/trauma which affects the breathing

Digestive System: An excellent oil for the digestive system which is often overlooked when it comes to Galangal. It helps constipation, loss of appetite, dyspepsia, flatulence, colic, travel sickness, nausea, vomiting and laxative. It also helps digestion of intestinal fats in the gut and liver and in turn supports the Gall Bladder. It has also had some success, particularly in its natural form in treating cholera.

Excretory/Urinary Systems:

Integumentary/Skin System: Quite similar to Frankincense in its actions on the skin. Wounds, inflammation e.g., rosacea, boils, cuts, acne and abscesses all respond well. It is also useful in a blend for mature and wrinkled skin. It is used to treat all types of skin infections, particularly Tinea versicolor is a common fungal infection of the skin. The infection interferes with the normal melanin of the skin, resulting in small, discolored patches. These patches may be lighter or darker in color than the surrounding skin and most commonly affect the trunk and shoulders.

Dreams and Aspirations

Question: **Have you forgotten how to love yourself first and foremost?**

Answer: **The answer is in the question.**

Galangal and Chemuel help you realise that you must love yourself first and foremost before you can give and receive love from others totally unconditionally.

Notes:

Patchouli — Archangel Sandolphon

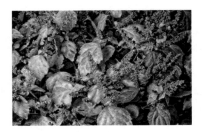

Botanical name: Pogostemon cablin
Plant part: Leaves
Country of origin: China and Northern India.
Note: Base
Extraction method: Steam distilled leaves, are lightly fermented before extraction making it an oleoresin.

Author's Note: First recorded use was in 5th AD in China and Northern India. HOWEVER, Pogostemon cablin appears to be native to the Philippines. It is believed that the plant now known as Patchouli was in fact different from the plants grown by the ancients in China and India. One possible candidate for the "original" Patchouli is a plant from the genus Microtoena (mints) that has a similar scent. Pogostemon heyneanus, described as early as 1690, and native to India, is one likely candidate.

Patchouli, strictly speaking is an herb, a member of the Lamiaceae family, just like the mints, and should belong in the Physical section of oils. However, with its well-recognised calming and grounding aroma and its popularity in the '60's where it gained an unshakeable reputation as a bit of a hippy oil, it has long been regarded and thought of as an Essential Oil used in meditative practices and as such sits in this section better in my view. It just doesn't behave like an herb!

You might read that Patchouli is sedating in low dose and stimulating in high. I would suggest, and from personal experience, that Patchouli being an adaptogen oil would mean it depends on the time of day as the opposite is true, i.e., one drop in the morning is stimulating and several drops in the evening is sedating.

Contraindications: Not strictly a contraindication but may cause loss/decrease in appetite in some people.

Emotional: Patchouli's sedating and calming properties bring emotional balance and feelings of grounding. Patchouli moves you from sadness to joy, where have we heard that before? It also re-instates emotional self-worth and confidence in yourself.

Mental: If you refer back to what I said about Patchouli being an adaptogen oil, it comes as no surprise that it is relaxing and invigorating, both mentally and physically. It sharpens the mind, combating lethargy, acts as a lovely antidepressant bringing mental astuteness, clarity and objectivity.

Relationships: Sandolphon is one of the three, what I have earlier called the 'Big Boys'. He is the Connector, the Archangel who oversees all the other Archangels and he is the great Angel Prince who oversees the Seraphim who, if you are religious, are the sphere next to creation, source or God. He therefore reputedly has the ability to soar well above or higher than the other Archangels can. Think of him in a lift that goes up and down through the spheres. He picks up and collects the relevant assistance you need from whichever sphere and brings the help or tools you need.

Having said this his energies keeps both your feet on the ground. He draws up the earthly energies of the Elementals or fairy/devic forces up to you and at the same time brings energies down from beyond the angelic realm. He works on both our Base/Root and Earth Star Chakras, alongside his buddy Metatron, and alongside Melkizadek to bring in the relevant resources you need from the etheric realms. So, you might feel his/her energies as a fleeting presence as he acknowledges what you are requiring and then zips off to fetch the 'right remedy'. Now that 'remedy' might not in fact be another Angelic being or Elemental, it might very well be a physical manifestation of the answer you need. Rather like finding your car keys..." but I had already looked there". Never forget the Angelic realm have a sense of humour!

Patchouli helps to ground your energies if you have become flighty or too detached from physical reality. It will relax your mind if it is over active and analytical which in turn can stop you from realizing the simple solutions and resolutions which are right in front of your nose very often. It reinforces our resolve and motivation to take action. Although a very 'grounding' oil it also awakens our subconscious and brings our thoughts, ideas and visions into the present. It allows us to see the 'bigger picture' by stepping aside and away rather than being embroiled and not seeing the wood for the trees.

As mentioned, it will give us flashes and insights to the Elemental and Devic realm. Difficult to believe that such an earthy and grounding oil can do this, but it can.

Together Patchouli and Sandolphon are all about rapport, not just with other people, but more importantly with yourself first.

Physical:

Skeletal/Muscular Systems: Patchouli is warming (febrifuge) and an anti-inflammatory to sore, aching and tired muscles.

Circulatory System: Can help reduce blood congestion and strengthen the veins as in hemorrhoids and varicose veins. It can also help calm an emotionally racing and palpating heart. Helps alleviate headaches brought on by reduction of blood flow.

Lymphatic/Immune System: It has strong antiviral/bacterial/fungal/parasitic properties, something often overlooked with Patchouli traditionally. It is an effective diuretic removing excess fluid from the tissue and can help break down cellulite. It helps to arrest heavy sweating, but the reason must always be investigated medically.

Nervous System: Strengthens nervous system over all. Its mild analgesic properties also help numb nervine pain and headaches.

Endocrine System: A very well-known and apparently effective aphrodisiac. It also, allegedly increases circulation in cases of erectile dysfunction. For women it is useful for vaginal infections such as vaginitis. I suspect it would be excellent in cases of PMT/PMS and emotional mood swings in menopause and has been reported to be effective for menopausal sweats, although not my first 'go-to' oil in this particular case.

Respiratory System: With all its antiviral/antibacterial/antifungal and antiparasitic properties it helps all types of respiratory infections including mouth infections.

Digestive System: Patchouli stabilizes either constipation or diarrhea. It can help weight loss if on a diet, but may also cause loss of appetite to some. It has been used successfully in the treatment of bulimia and anorexia. As mentioned earlier, Patchouli is an adaptogen oil and will help return things to homeostasis. Its antiemetic properties, helps to stop vomiting and feelings of nausea.

Excretory/Urinary Systems: It is a well-known diuretic thus helps in cases of water retention. Bladder and urethra inflammation such as cystitis can be helped.

Integumentary/Skin System: Being antiseptic it is useful on all types of fungal infections on the skin, including fungal nail. Being a cicatrisant it is excellent for tightening loose skin after weight loss for example, but this also applies to older and more mature skin where by it can reduce fine lines and tighten looser skin lying over reduced muscle mass. It has the ability to regenerate tissue, in other words it helps regrow skin cells and form healthy scar tissue. Often included in skin preparations to heal rough and/or cracked skin and helps with dry, itchy conditions such as dandruff, eczema and dermatitis. Being antifungal and antibacterial it is a natural deodorant. Also often used in preparations to help reduce cellulite. It repels fleas, lice, moths, mosquitoes and other insects.

Dreams and Aspirations:

Question: **Do you laugh off your dreams and aspirations because you think they are just a 'pipe dream'?**
Answer: **Patchouli and Sandolphon bring you the 'tools' to get the job done.**

A respected oil in meditative practices as it connects us to our consciousness and encourages you to listen to your own soul for truth and guidance. The answers always reside within us, Patchouli helps us connect to our own inner and ancient wisdom.

Notes:

10.

SAFETY AND BLENDING

Safety

There are some very simple safety guidelines that you must follow when using Essential Oils.

- NEVER EVER ingest EO's unless under the strictest guidelines from a Clinical Aromatherapist (UK), an Aromatherapist who has studied Aromatic Medicine (other countries), or a licensed MD who has a certification in Aromatherapy (USA), who have studied the ingestion of EO's.

- Always dilute your Essential Oils in a carrier oil or cream, unless otherwise instructed by your qualified Aromatherapist or Essential Oil Practitioner.

- If you are in **any way** unsure about which or how to use an Essential Oil, please contact an Aromatherapist.

- NEVER follow social media, online blends or recipes, or those in books, unless they also give you the contraindications to use.

- NEVER diffuse/vaporise EO's in public places or in your home unless the oil has absolutely NO contraindications and is safe for not only the adults who will come into contact, but children and pets too.

- Unless under the instruction of an Aromatherapist, NEVER keep using the same EO or blend of EO's because "I like the smell". You are in danger of sensitisation from which there is no known cure, and the ramifications to your overall wellbeing could be very serious.

- When buying pre-blended 'aromatherapy' products, read the small print. It might contain oils that are not suitable for you, contain preservatives, and long-term use can cause sensitisation. ALWAYS rotate your EO's and products containing EO's.

- EO's have a 'shelf life' like anything else. Oxidization is the main culprit. Once oxidised EO's are classified as hazardous in the industry, that includes just smelling them.

- Finally, ALWAYS get your EO's from a reputable supplier, that supplies oils to Aromatherapists, or ask your therapist if you can buy from them personally.

Blending

When blending your Essential Oils together you can add them individually to a base product such as a carrier oil (keeping in mind if you have a nut allergy) a cream, soap, in your bath or a diffuser/burner.

Adults

In a bath add a maximum combination of 7 drops of your chosen oils. In a carrier or base product add a MAXIMUM of half the milliliters, i.e. 30ml bottle equals 15 drops, 50ml bottle equals 25 drops. For daily products such as a shampoo, halve the dosage again, so 30ml equals 7 drops.

In a diffuser or ceramic burner, no more than 5 drops and only have it lit for approximately 30 minutes, one-hour tops.

Children

The dosage of Essential Oils and which can be used at each stage of development is best left to the guidance and advice of a qualified therapist. NEVER use ANY EO on a baby or child of any age without consulting a qualified Aromatherapist. You could seriously harm your child. There are very strict guidelines, dosage and application for children and babies. ALWAYS treat your EO's as 'medicines'. Keep them away from children.

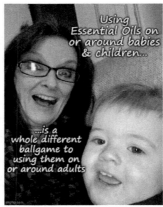

Me, with my grandson, photo taken by his mummy.

Special Needs children and adults.

This again is a specialist area. Please consult a qualified practitioner.

Elderly

Follow the guidelines as set out for adults, but halve the dosage again.

Appendix

1. "Repellence Effects of Essential Oils of Myrtle (Myrtus communis), Marigold (Calendula officinalis) Compared with DEET against Anopheles stephensi on Human Volunteers," Iran J Arthropod Borne Dis. 12/31/2011, PMID: 22808414.
2. "Review of Pharmacological Effects of Myrtus communis L. and its Active Constituents," Phytother Res. 2/4/2014, PMID: 24497171.
3. "Efficacy of myrtle oil against Salmonella Typhimurium on fresh produce," Int J Food Microbiol. 3/31/2009, PMID: 19217679.
4. "Hypoglycaemic effects of myrtle oil in normal and alloxan-diabetic rabbits," J Ethnopharmacology. August 2004, PMID: 15234770.
5. "In vitro and in vivo antimalarial evaluations of myrtle extract, a plant traditionally used for treatment of parasitic disorders," Biomed Res Int., 12/23/2013, PMID: 24455686.
6. "The efficacy of a paste containing Myrtus communis (Myrtle) in the management of recurrent aphthous stomatitis: a randomized controlled trial," Clin Oral Investig., February 2010, PMID: 19306024.
7. "First Case Report: Treatment of the Facial Warts by Using Myrtus communis L. Topically on the Other Part of the Body," Iran Red Crescent Med J. February 2014, PMID: 24719732.
8. https://www.kjpr.kr/articles/xml/GKad/
9. http://www.stuartxchange.org/Pili#:~:text=Both%20Canariu m%20luzonicum%20and%20C,and%20Canarium%20luzonicu m%20(sahing).

Index

Angelica – Courage of your convictions –133

Basil – Words have power/Integrity –138

Benzoin – Archangel Michael – 209

Bergamot – Spring –35

Black Pepper – Fire –53

Cardamon – Appetite for life –141

Cedarwood – Buddha/Dalai Lama – 99

Chamomile – The Now – 63

Clary-Sage – Perspective/Teacher – 144

Cypress – Peter Ustinov/Stephen Fry – 102

Dill – Smile – 148

Elemi – Archangel Jophiel – 200

Eucalyptus – Bruce Lee/Steven Segal – 106

Fennel – Fortitude – 152

Frankincense – Archangel Zadkiel – 193

Galangal – Archangel Chemuel – 221

Geranium – Balance – 65

Ginger – Courage – 156

Grapefruit – Water – 56

Guaiacwood – Archangel Gabriel – 205

Hyacinth – Journey away – 68

Immortelle – Journey within – 71

Jasmine – Acceptance – 75

Juniper – Eleanor Roosevelt – 109

Lavender – Calm - 78

Lemon – Air - 48

Lime – Earth - 51

Mandarin – Summer - 39

Marjoram – Perseverance/Badgering - 160

May Chang – A little bit of everything - 59

Melissa – Boundaries - 82

Myrrh Archangel Melkizadek - 187

Myrtle – Jesus/Christ energy - 112

Neroli – Bringer of light - 87

Niaouli – Mother Theresa - 118

Palmarosa – Archangel Raphael - 213

Patchouli – Archangel Sandolphon - 224

Peppermint – Focus - 164

Petitgrain – John Lennon - 121

Rose – Serene centeredness - 90

Rosemary – Memory - 167

Rosewood – Princess Diana - 123

Sage – Wise one/Wisdom - 171

Sandalwood – Ghandi - 126

Spearmint – Lighten up - 175

Spikenard – Archangel Metatron - 190

Sweet Orange – Autumn - 42

Tagetes – Divine masculine - 92

Tangerine – Winter - 45

Tea-Tree – Ellen MacArthur - 129

Thyme – Decisiveness - 178

Vetiver – Archangel Uriel - 217

Yarrow – Harmony – 182
Ylang-Ylang – Divine Feminine – 95

ABOUT THE AUTHOR

I am now what is colloquially termed as a Vintage Aromatherapist, having been qualified as a Clinical Aromatherapist for over 30 years and a teacher for over 25.

I am blessed with three beautiful grown-up children, and now two wonderful grandchildren.

Besides taking care of my clients, I also have a small and select number of students every year. I believe in quality over quantity and as Essential Oils and, what can only be termed as magical properties as they never cease to amaze me, have served me so well for most of my adult life, I honour them and respect them and the art and therefore want to maintain and pass on a legacy to future practitioners.

I am currently training past students to become teachers themselves, and thus safeguard what is a precious gift of Mother Nature to us. This is my legacy.

You can contact me via my website www.thenaturalapproach.biz

Printed in Great Britain
by Amazon

22110776R00136

Cosy Winter

A SEASONAL GUIDE

Melanie Steele

Follow me on Instagram @melaniesteeleauthor

Book design by Melanie Steele
Cover design by Melanie Steele

First Edition : August 2024

"Spend time close to home in awe of the simple treasures that make up your life. "

Dr Wayne Dyer

INTRODUCTION

I love that quote by Wayne Dyer. I'm very much a simple treasures kind of girl. Give me a book, a blanket and a hot chocolate and I'm the happiest girl in the world! I'm also one for staying close to home, especially in Winter. When the days are short, the sky is grey and the orange filled hues of autumn give way to drizzly days- my hibernation mode is activated.

That's not to say there isn't beauty in Winter. The crisp cold air, the tiny blanket of snow we sometimes get here in the U.K (that quickly becomes grey sludge) and days when the low winter sun shines bright- those are beautiful. A few years ago myself and my husband had a wonderful winter walk around a local National Trust property. It had snowed the day before, and it was proper snow- not the aforementioned thin blanket. The greenery was sparkling in the sun, and there was a fun trail with big frames that you could use to take photos! *That* is a Winter day out I can get behind.

For the most part, you and I are probably going to be staying home a lot this Winter. Largely through choice, but for readers in North America possibly through being snowed in! Either way, Cosy Winter is here to give you ideas and inspiration for enjoying this chilly season.

This book will be focused on the time after Halloween, which is where I ended my previous book *Cosy Autumn*. So if you're looking for ideas for earlier in the season, go check it out! (Us self published authors have to shamelessly plug our work, we don't have marketing teams to do it for us)

CHAPTER ONE

Winter Self Care

Winter is a difficult time for many people. The lack of daylight hours (A shout out here to our Nordic friends who experience twenty plus hours of darkness a day in Winter, yet manage to thrive!) the dwindling temperatures, the summer memories of being outside having fun are starting to dwindle... its no wonder we don't feel our best. We may be excited for Christmas, which has already been shoved in our faces by retailers for months by this point- but it is still a couple of months away.

What we really need to do now, is to prioritise self care.

The concept of self care has been a hot topic for years now. Sadly, like many things which become popular it gets twisted into an opportunity to sell us stuff. How many adverts have you seen online trying to sell you the latest self care item? Always with testimonials that the item changed that persons life. I'm sceptical of most everything online, particularly products that are expensive and supposedly life changing "must haves" that are replaced in a week by another advert for something else promising the same! The rise of TikTok shop, shopping directly through Instagram and other outlets have caused us to be inundated with products for self care- but they are only offering the retail friendly version of it.

So what is self care, really?

Self care is about doing the things that make us feel good, improve our health and help us to be our best selves- or some way on the way to that. However- self care is also about doing things we *don't* feel like doing, but are necessary to keep us healthy and well. That's the part they don't mention on social media- because it's not very sell-able, is it? Those things however are often more vital than anything else. You can't put a price on staying well both mentally, and physically.

Self Care that you don't always feel like doing, but probably should:

- Taking medication, vitamins or other supplements that work for you.
- Moving your body. I'm 100% guilty of not doing this as often as I should.
- Journaling to work through difficult emotions
- Saying "No" when you need to- set those boundaries!

These are definitely the less popular forms of self care in terms on what is shared online, but I think they should get far more credit. Things like journaling to work through difficult emotions will pay off long term so much more than just having a nice bath. Now there's nothing wrong with having a nice hot bath, and maybe that would be the perfect thing to do after that session- but doing the internal work is not to be missed.

Hard stuff done, let's move on to the fun stuff!

As I mentioned- self care has become a hot trend and it can be super tempting to buy the latest, greatest, most expensive things you see online. If that's what you want to do, and you feel that its something that really will work for you- do it.

However, if that's not really in your budget or you want to make simpler, more sustainable choices why not try some of these ideas?

Self Care that doesn't break the bank

- Making your favourite hot drink, grabbing a book and blanket and reading uninterrupted
- A hot bubble bath with candles

- A winter skin care routine
- Gentle movement like Pilates/Yoga/Stretching- there are plenty of videos on Youtube you can follow.
- Gratitude journaling- acknowledging what you are grateful for is great for your mental health.
- Giving yourself a manicure/pedicure.
- Preparing your favourite meal or snack.
- Enjoying a cosy movie.

If you're guilty of thinking "Ooooh that's a great idea, I'll definitely do that!" then remembering that thought a week later and realising you didn't do it- grab your planner, diary, notes app- whatever you use, and schedule it in *now*. Make self care a priority- it deserves to be on your schedule just as much as medical appointments, work meetings and other commitments.

IDEA TO TRY: SOOTHING OATMEAL MILK BATH

Ingredients

- 2 Tbsp Rolled Oats
- 2 Tbsp Baking Soda
- ½ Cup Powdered Milk (Can be Coconut milk for Vegan)
- ½ Cup Sea Salt
- ¼ Cup Epsom Salt

Grind the oats either in a food processor, blender or by hand with a mortar and pestle. Pour into a bowl and add the powdered milk and both salts. Stir to break up any clumps.

Store in an airtight container.

To use: Put 2 Tbsp of the mixture into running bathwater, then use your hand to make sure its fully dissolved.

"Winter is a season of recovery and preparation"

Paul Theroux

CHAPTER TWO

Notes From The Nordics

I'm a huge fan of all things Nordic lifestyle, and in the run up to writing this book I've been reading about three ideas from our Nordic neighbours that will definitely make for a cosy winter- Hygge (Danish), Lagom (Swedish) and Sisu (Finnish)

Let's explore how each of these concepts can help us embrace Winter. After all, our Nordic neighbours can experience up to twenty hours of darkness a day, so they know a thing or two about surviving, and thriving in Winter.

Hygge (Hoo-gah)

The concept of Hygge has surged in popularity across Europe and North America in the past few years. There are dozens of books on the market after the bestseller *The Little Book Of Hygge*, by Meik Wiking came out in 2016. However, the popularity of this idea has inevitably been swallowed up by consumerism, and to many its now just scented candles and blankets. There's so much more to it though!

Hygge is difficult to translate into English. To start with- It's both a noun and an adjective meaning you can both *be hygge*, and *have hygge*. It's about experiencing a mindful moment, typically at home, where you feel cosy, content and peaceful. The word itself dates back to around the year 1800, but various definitions can be traced back to Old Norse where a similar word was defined as "protected from the outside world". Yes, it can involve the aforementioned scented candles and blankets, but its also walking through a forest on a crisp winter morning, enjoying a Cinnamon bun with a friend, turning off harsh lighting in favour of soft twinkling lights, and of course candlelight.

Familiehygge is the Danish take on Friday family night where Danes spend quality time with family (and/or friends) after a busy week of work and other activities. I love the idea of a night dedicated to spending time with those we love, whilst simultaneously experiencing hygge.

Here are some ideas you can try for your own *familiehygge*.

- Cook a favourite comfort meal that will be enjoyed by everyone. You can serve it family style (where everyone helps themselves) to maximise the hygge feel.

- Serve the meal by candlelight to make it feel more intimate, and to differentiate it from having dinner on other nights of the week.

- Take time to have a really good conversation beyond "How was your day/week?" This is a time to build relationships and deepen them. To see how everyone is really doing- who needs support, who is doing really well but isn't being 'seen', and to see how everyone can come together in the next week to make it even better.

- I feel dessert is a must have for such a night. Even if you don't indulge on any other night, something sweet and tasty is bound to have everyone feeling hygge.

- After food it's time for quality time. Everyone should put their devices away, and no electronics should be part of this time. Think board games, storytelling or something creative that everyone can enjoy.

Lagom (Lawww-gum)

Another one that's tricky to translate directly into English, but generally speaking Lagom could be referred to as meaning "Not too much, not too little" It's about balance in all things- which is no surprise given that equality is a big deal in Sweden.

An example of Lagom would be *Lördagsgodis*, or "Sweets Saturday". In Sweden, sweets are typically only eaten on Saturday. Swedes eat the most candy per person in the world- 17kg (37 lbs) per person, per year! But only on Saturdays do they indulge their sweet tooth. This for Swedes is Lagom.

So how can Lagom help you have a Cosy Winter?

- Creating a work life balance
- Spending more time with friends and family
- Getting outdoors
- Enjoying occasional sweet treats
- Avoiding excess Christmas spending

One of the key tenets of Lagom is to own less, and keep it simple. Decluttering your home is a great way to bring some Lagom into your life this Winter. Do you need 3 can openers? 10 sweaters? Socks with holes in them? (Unless you plan to darn them- and you will *actually* do that!) There are a million books and blogs on decluttering out there so I won't bore you by repeating what has been said on the subject but if by chance these books and blogs have escaped you, go check them out for advice and practical tips.

Sisu (See-su)

Sisu was a brand new concept to me. I'd read about Hygge and Lagom previously, but when I stumbled across a book by Katja Panzar entitled *"The Finnish Way: Finding Courage, Wellness and Happiness Through the Power of Sisu"* I was intrigued. In Finnish Sisu is derived from the word for guts *(Gross yes, but bare with me here)* Whilst it's always been around, It's popularity as a concept was largely cemented when Finland became Independent from Russia in 1917. Sisu was seen as the "glue" that held everyone together as they worked to create a new society.

It's another concept that's difficult to translate (Are you noticing a theme here?) but it could be seen as a sort of mental toughness and resilience that helps Finns to thrive in what most would consider a harsh climate. It's what makes them get up and go for a walk in the forest in sub zero temperatures. It's what keeps them going through 50 days of darkness (in the North of the country)

Sisu then is less about the cozy vibes of Hygge, and more about the state of mind that allows Finns to thrive in long, dark winters.

Sauna is an *essential* part of Sisu for Finns. It's not solely about Sauna, but it definitely features! Finns will happily swim in freezing water safe in the knowledge they will go to the Sauna after. If you're not up for an icy swim, you can still definitely enjoy Sauna- but please consult medical advice as Sauna is not suitable for everybody.

On a deeper level, having Sisu is also what transforms perceived failures into events, not identity. Now, you might be thinking "whoah, thats a bit deep for this book!" but bare with me. There are many times in life when it feels like we are on an uphill battle with no end in sight. In the cold dark days of Winter, such battles can feel extra tough. But what if we reframed those events using the power of Sisu?

For example:

Starting a business even though no one around you has any idea about entrepreneurship leaving you to figure it out alone, and you do. Thats Sisu.

When you're running a race you've trained hard for but feel like you won't quite make it- you do it anyway. That's Sisu.

When you're balancing caring responsibilities with leading a big project at work and you nail it- thats Sisu!

How can Sisu help you make the most of Winter?

- Getting outside when it's dark and cold, when you'd rather be in bed.
- Signing up to volunteer cleaning up your local woodland even when its grey and drizzling out.
- Helping elderly neighbours weather proof their home, or shopping for their groceries, when the outside temperature has plummeted.
- Deciding to undertake a new venture such as a new job, going self employed, or moving to a new place where you don't know anybody.

Doing hard things makes us feel accomplished. I'm not suggesting you go out of your way to find difficult challenges to overcome, but a little Sisu this winter might help you discover courage and resilience you never knew you had!

RECOMMENDED READING

If the concepts of *Hygge*, *Lagom* and *Sisu* have got you intrigued, check out these books to learn more.

The Little Book of Hygge: The Danish Way to Live Well- Meik Wiking

Lagom: The Swedish Art of Balanced Living- Linnea Dunne

The Finnish Way: Finding Courage, Wellness and Happiness Through the Power of Sisu- Katja Panzar

The Little Book of Fika: The Uplifting Daily Ritual of the Swedish Coffee Break- Lynda Balslev

Nordic Lifestyle- Susanna Heiskanen

CHAPTER THREE

Winter Writing

The irony of this chapter is that I am writing this book in July! If you blog or write then you know you are typically writing content out of season, so that it's ready to go when the time comes. Nonetheless, it feels a little strange!

In my previous book, Cosy Autumn, I had a whole chapter devoted to journaling. I really felt as though this book ought to have that as well, because there is no better time to self reflect when you're indoors, feeling cosy and not having enough *Sisu* to get outside.

Journaling is hugely beneficial- it allows you to get all of your thoughts out of your head, and on to paper. It can also help you arrange those thoughts in a way that makes sense, and to see any patterns that are forming. This is especially helpful for identifying where your thoughts may be tricking you, as it gives you an opportunity to both reflect and change them.

As always, these are just suggestions. Sometimes it can be beneficial just to free write without any idea of where its going!

Journal Prompts

Write about your favourite winter memory. Describe the details of the moment, who you were with, and why it stands out as a special time in your life.

Think of a winter tradition you and your family follow each year. Describe what you do and why it's important to you.

Reflect on a snowy day from your childhood. What did you do and how did it make you feel?

Describe your ideal winter day. What activities would you do, who would you spend it with, and where would you go?

Write about a time when you felt the winter holiday spirit the most. What happened and why was it so memorable?

Reflect on the changes in nature during winter. What differences do you notice in the trees, animals, and weather?

Describe a winter sunrise or sunset. What colors do you see and how does it make you feel?

Reflect on the sound of snow crunching under your boots. What other sounds do you associate with winter?

Write about the wildlife you see in winter. How do animals adapt to the cold and what have you observed?

Describe your favorite way to stay warm and cozy during winter. What makes it special and why do you love it?

Think about a winter book or movie that brings you comfort. What is it about and why do you enjoy it?

Write about your favorite winter clothing. What do you love to wear and how does it make you feel?

Reflect on a time you spent a cozy day indoors. What did you do and how did it make you feel?

Describe your perfect winter evening at home. What activities would you do to relax and enjoy the night?

Write about a favourite winter scent like pine, cinnamon, or peppermint. What does it remind you of and why do you love it?

Reflect on the warmth of a winter fire. Describe how it feels to sit by the fire and enjoy its glow.

Think of a time you made a warm winter drink. What did you make and why was it comforting?

Write about a personal goal you have for the winter season. How do you plan to achieve it and why is it important?

Reflect on the past year and what you've learned. What were your biggest challenges and triumphs?

Describe how winter inspires you to grow and change. What aspects of the season encourage you to reflect and set new goals?

Think about a time you felt particularly strong during winter. What did you overcome and how did you do it?

Write about a book or article you read in winter that inspired you. What was it about and why did it resonate with you?

Reflect on a winter habit or routine you'd like to develop. How can it benefit your life and well-being?

Describe how you stay motivated during the colder months. What strategies do you use to keep your spirits high?

Write about your favorite winter holiday. What do you celebrate and what do you love most about it?

Reflect on the joy of giving during the holidays. What acts of kindness have you done or received?

CHAPTER FOUR

Winter Baking

If you've read any of my books- you know that my love of baking runs deep. In a book about being cosy in Winter, I had even more of an excuse to share my favourite recipes.

These are all brand new for this book. If you want more, I have a whole chapter in Cosy Autumn- which also includes a recipe for the quintessential baked good of the Autumn/Winter season- Cinnamon Buns. There are also recipes in *The Magic of Home*.

This time I've been inspired by my Nordic reading, and we are kicking off with a spicy twist on the traditional cinnamon bun recipe.

Swedish Cinnamon Buns (*Kanelbullar*)

For the buns

3 Cups (400g) plain flour
¼ Cup (50g) granulated sugar
1 teaspoon freshly ground cardamom
2 ¼ teaspoons (7g) instant yeast
1 cup (240 ml) warmed milk, no warmer than 120°F/48°C
¼ cup (½ stick/56 g) unsalted butter, melted and slightly cooled
½ teaspoon salt

For the filling

⅓ cup (⅔ stick/75g) unsalted butter, at room temperature

⅓ cup (65g) light brown sugar
1 tablespoon ground cinnamon

To Finish

Pearl Sugar

Method

Place flour, sugar, cardamom, and yeast in the bowl of a standing mixer and mix until combined. Attach the dough hook to the mixer. Add milk and melted butter to the flour mixture and mix on low speed until dough comes together, 2-3 minutes. Add salt and continue mixing for another 8 minutes on low-medium speed until dough is soft and pulls away from the sides of the bowl.

Alternative methods

No stand mixer? You can use the dough setting on your breadmaker, or knead by hand. You'll want to knead for at least 10 minutes if doing it by hand.

Place dough in a large bowl brushed with oil, and toss to coat (the oil will keep the dough from drying out). Cover with plastic wrap and let sit in a warm place or on the counter for 1-2 hours, or until doubled in size. Keep in mind that rising will be slower in cold weather.

To make the filling: In a small bowl, combine soft butter, sugar, and cinnamon until you have a smooth paste.

Shaping the dough

On a lightly floured surface or non-stick silicone baking mat, roll dough out into 35x35cm (14×14-inch) square. Spread butter-sugar mixture onto entire surface, making a very thin layer. Fold dough into thirds like a business letter, then roll again into a rough 35x20cm (14×8-inch) rectangle.

Facing the long edge, cut dough into roughly ½-inch/2cm wide and 8-inch/20cm long strips. Twist each strip several times, slightly stretching it as you do so. Grab one end of the twisted strip and coil the dough around your hand twice, then over the top. Coil dough again and tuck the loose end in at the bottom.

Arrange buns on a baking sheet lined with parchment paper (if they're too crowded, use 2 sheets), keeping as much space between them as possible. Cover and let rest for 45-60 minutes or until doubled in size.

Meanwhile, set the oven rack to the middle position and preheat oven to 350°F/180°C/Gas 4.

Sprinkle with pearl sugar, and bake for 15-20 minutes until golden brown.

Allow buns to cool on the baking sheet for 5 minutes, then transfer to a wire rack to cool completely.

Buns are best the same day they are made, but can be frozen for up to 2 months and reheated in the oven before serving.

Shortbread

Super simple to make, and delicious. Shortbread is a traditional biscuit (cookie) here in the UK. In the run up to Christmas the supermarkets are filled with pretty tins of it ready to be gifted to family and friends, but why not make your own?

Ingredients

125g/4oz unsalted butter, softened
55g/2oz caster sugar, plus extra to finish
180g/6oz plain flour

Method

Preheat the oven to 375°F/190°C/Gas 5.

Beat the butter and the sugar together until smooth.

Stir in the flour to get a smooth paste.

Turn on to a work surface and gently roll out until the paste is 1cm/½in thick.

Cut into shortbread rounds or fingers and place onto a baking tray. Sprinkle with caster sugar and chill in the fridge for 20 minutes.

Bake in the oven for 15–20 minutes, or until pale golden-brown. Set aside to cool on a wire rack.

Snickerdoodles

Snickerdoodles don't really exist here in the U.K, but I had some when I did a Semester in the States and loved them!

115g unsalted butter
130g granulated sugar
1 tsp vanilla extract
1 tsp apple cider vinegar
185g plain flour (all purpose)
1 tsp cream of tartar
1 tsp bicarbonate of soda
1 ¼ tsp cinnamon
¼ tsp salt
1 tbsp milk

For rolling

3 tbsp granulated sugar
1 tsp cinnamon

Add the butter and sugar to an electric mixer and cream them together. Add in the vanilla and apple cider vinegar and mix in.

Add in the flour, cream of tartar, baking soda, cinnamon and salt and mix in by hand (don't use the electric mixer for this part) until it forms a crumbly dough.

Then add in the milk so that it forms into a 'proper' cookie dough

Preheat the oven to 375°F/190°C/Gas 5.

Roll the cookie dough into balls and then roll the balls in the cinnamon and sugar mixture and place them onto a parchment lined baking tray. You can sprinkle more of the cinnamon sugar mixture on top of the balls before they go in the oven.

Bake for 10 minutes.

Remove from the oven and let the cookies firm up and cool down directly on the tray.

CHAPTER FIVE

Winter Comfort Food

Winter is synonymous with comfort food. If I'm being honest, all seasons for me are synonymous with comfort food! I'm just not a salad person.

Despite the cold, many fruits and vegetables are in season during these months. Eating seasonal fruit and vegetables is a great way to save money, and enjoy this produce at its best. Whilst we can eat many of these items year round thanks to global shipping-nothing beats eating locally grown!

What's in Season in Winter?

For readers outside the UK- please check your local information as it may differ.

- Apples
- Bananas
- Clementines
- Cranberries
- Dates
- Pears
- Pomegranate

- Beetroot
- Brussel Sprouts
- Cabbage
- Celeriac
- Celery

- Kale
- Leeks
- Parsnips
- Pumpkin
- Swede
- Turnips

My personal favourites from this list are Dates, Brussels (Yup, I'm a Brussel lover!) Kale and Parsnips. How about you?

Now we know what's in season, let's dive into some delicious comfort food recipes that make the most of this delicious produce.

Maple Roasted Parsnips

A perfect side dish for a Sunday roast.

500g parsnips
1-2 tbsp maple syrup
1 tbsp oil
Black pepper

Method

Peel and chop your parsnips into even size pieces.
Place the oil in a roasting dish. Preheat oven to 200°C/400°F/Gas 6 then place in the oven to heat the oil.
Meanwhile- Par boil the parsnips for 5 minutes.
Drain, then remove the roasting dish from the oven and place parsnips in.
Pour over the maple syrup, using a silicone or pastry brush to ensure they are fully coated. Grind fresh black pepper on top, then return to the oven.

Bake for 30-40 minutes.

Air Fryer Brussel Sprouts

450g Brussel Sprouts, peeled and cut in half
2 tbsp oil

2 Garlic cloves OR 2tsp Lazy Garlic
1 tbsp Balsamic Vinegar
1 tsp Lime juice
½ tsp Soy sauce

Preheat air fryer to 200°C/400°F for 5 minutes.
Place Brussel sprouts in a bowl, and add all ingredients to marinade them. Give them a good stir so they are evenly coated.

Once preheat is done, place in the air fryer basket making sure they are in an even layer.

Cook at 200c for 8 minutes, then shake. Cook for another 8 minutes.

Serve!

Tip- I love these as a side with Vegan Mac 'n' Cheese. My favourite recipe is from Veganomicon by Isa Chandra Moskowitz.

Leek and Potato Puffs

1kg floury potatoes (e.g Maris Piper)
2 leeks
2 tbsp oil

75g peas, defrosted
1 tbsp lemon or lime juice
1 tbsp curry powder
500g sheet of puff pastry
2 tbsp milk
1 tbsp sesame seeds

Preheat oven to 170°C/340°F/Gas 3 ½

Place leeks and potatoes in a roasting tin with oil.

Roast for 30-40 minutes.

Once cooled place the leeks and potatoes in a bowl and lightly mash. Add in the peas, lemon or lime juice and curry powder and mix.

Cut the pastry sheet into 6 even size rectangles. Roll out each rectangle so it's more of a square- this will help with folding!

Place 1-2 tbsp of filling in the centre of the square. Fold over one corner so you have a triangle shape. Use a pastry brush to put some milk on the edges to help seal them, then use a fork to crimp the edges.

Repeat for all the pastry squares, then sprinkle with sesame seeds.

Bake for 30-35 minutes until golden and puffed up.

These will keep In the fridge for up to 3 days. Enjoy hot or cold.

Sticky Sausage Potato Traybake

Serves 2-3 but if you add more potatoes and veg you could stretch it to 4

1 bag of frozen crispy potatoes (Also known as Parmentier Potatoes)
1 tbsp oil
2 medium carrots, peeled and diced into 2.5cm/1inch pieces
1 red onion sliced into wedges
3 garlic cloves crushed, or a heaped teaspoon of lazy garlic/garlic paste
6-8 plant based sausages
4 tbsp red onion chutney
2 tsp golden syrup (corn syrup)
1 tsp dried thyme or few sprigs of fresh
Sea salt and black pepper
Onion gravy

Preheat the oven to 200°C/400°F/Gas 6

Put the oil in a roasting dish and put it in the oven to heat up.

Once hot, add the carrots, onion and garlic. Roast for 15minutes.

Remove from the oven and add the sausages. Roast for 20minutes.

Meanwhile, preheat air fryer for 5 minutes to 200°C/400°F.

Add in around ½ the bag of crispy potatoes and cook for 15 minutes, shaking halfway through.

When sausages and potatoes are done- add potatoes to the roasting dish along with the chutney, syrup and thyme giving it a good mix.

Pop back in the oven for 5-10minutes to let it caramelise.

Make up the gravy. Once everything is cooked serve it up, pour over the gravy and enjoy!

Note- I cook the crispy potatoes separately as I find they are much crispier that way. You could add them to the roasting dish with everything else if you prefer. Alternatively, you can peel and dice any potatoes you have and use those. Par boil for five minutes, then add in to the roasting tray with the carrots, onions and garlic.

The Ultimate Lentil Loaf

I love serving this for Sunday roast. It freezes and defrosts perfectly.

3/4 cup lentils, brown or green, dry
2 cups vegetable stock
1 red onion
1 carrot
1 celery stalk
3 cloves garlic
1 cup fine oats (or quick-cooking)
1/2 cup pecan nuts, chopped
2 tbsp flax seeds, ground
2 tbsp soy sauce
1 tbsp parsley, fresh
1 tsp thyme, dried
pinch of salt

black pepper to taste

Wash the lentils under running water, then add them to a pot along with the vegetable stock. Bring to a boil, then reduce the heat and cook on low for about 30 minutes, until the lentils are cooked and fork-tender. Drain and cool.

Chop the vegetables. Heat a spoon of oil in a pan, add chopped vegetables, and saute while stirring occasionally, until the vegetables are softened, about 10 minutes. Then let them cool and add them to a food processor.

To the food processor now also add cooked lentils, oats, chopped pecan nuts, ground flax seeds, soy sauce, fresh chopped parsley, dried thyme, a pinch of salt and black pepper to taste.

Pulse the ingredients until the mixture starts to stick together. Don't overmix it, you don't want a pate, but to have some whole veggie and lentil pieces in the mixture.

Heat the oven to 180°C / 350°F. Line a loaf tin with parchment paper, then transfer the mixture to the pan, shaping it into a loaf and pressing it together.

Bake for about 30 minutes.

Once baked, remove from the oven, and leave to cool for a couple of minutes. This will help the lentil loaf hold its shape. Then lift it out of the pan with the baking paper and serve warm.

CHAPTER SIX

Winter Home

It's hygge time! *(I can't help but hear this in the 'It's moprhin time!' from the 1990s show Power Rangers- I'm showing my age here)*

Getting my home ready for cooler weather has already begun by the time Winter rolls around. By October the fluffy blankets are out on the sofa, the Autumn/Winter scent candles are out on the coffee table and my cosy socks are now front and centre in my sock drawer.

Of course- the main addition to your home in Winter is decorations for the festive season. Whether it's Christmas, Hannukah, Diwali or Winter Solstice- there's lots of celebrations going on!

In our home we celebrate Winter Solstice and Christmas. You can read more on how we decorate for festivities in the next chapter.

Our home is never more a sanctuary than it is in Winter. We relish the warmth and security it provides from the outside elements. We delight in the smells of freshly made Cinnamon buns, delicious stews and other seasonal foods. It may be raining (most likely here in the U.K) or snowing outside but it doesn't matter because we are inside- protected, safe and cosy.

To garner even more of those feelings, there are a few things you can do to up the comfort and cosy level in your home.

First up- blankets everywhere! The sofa, armchair, bed- everywhere where you might sit and curl up to read a book or watch TV. Blankets make everything better.

Hot drink station- readers of Cosy Autumn know all about my hot chocolate bar, but you can also expand this to a hot drink station. Think pretty glass jars of tea, coffee and hot chocolate on a neglected counter space, and fun add ins like candy canes, cinnamon sugar dust, chocolate chips, sprinkles and more! Of course, you'll want to display your favourite mugs here too. Don't forget tea spoons.

Natural décor such as an evergreen wreath, mistletoe, pebbles from the beach and wood slices are perfect for that in-between time before Christmas. They help bring the outside in- so you can still enjoy nature by looking at these beautiful items, without braving the outside weather.

Soft and cosy loungewear- there are so many cute sets of matching loungewear available these days. I bought a thinner set to wear on the plane when we went to Cyprus earlier this year. It was 3am in the morning when we set off for the airport and it wasn't super warm given it was early May. It provided just the right amount of warmth, was super comfortable to sit in- and it looked cute too! I opted for a neutral colour, but you can go as colourful as you want! You can get more fleecy fabric type sets for Winter.

Practical Winter Tips

If you have a boiler- get it serviced. Ideally you'd do this before Winter in case there is a problem that needs fixing before you need the central heating. I'd also recommend an insulation jacket for your hot water tank if applicable.

If you have a Chimney and you use it- get it cleaned!

If you live somewhere where pipes can freeze and burst (North American friends in colder climates!) make sure you undertake necessary preparations.

Insulation. We (Ok my Husband) insulated our loft (Attic) last year and it has made such a difference to our home in the colder months. We bought ours from B&Q- but any DIY retailer should have it. If you have in ceiling lights like we do, please make sure you purchase the appropriate covering for those before laying down insulation or they will become a fire risk.

Draught excluders for doors can keep cold air out, and they come in lots of designs so you can find one that suits your décor.

Thermal curtains- we have these up year round as they do double duty in keeping rooms cool in Summer, and warm in Winter.

Wash your windows! I know this seems more of a Summer job, but with reduced daylight in Winter you'll want to make sure your windows are sparkling so all that light can get through.

IDEA TO TRY:
STOVETOP POTPURRI

Ingredients

- 2-3 Oranges, sliced
- 2 Apples, sliced
- 250g Fresh Cranberries
- 3 Sprigs Rosemary
- 3 Cinnamon Sticks
- 1 Tbsp Cloves
- 2 Whole Nutmeg Seeds
- 3 Star Anise
- A Few Drops Essential Oil- Pine, Orange, Cinnamon (optional)

Add all ingredients to a large pot and cover with water. Bring to a boil, then reduce heat to a simmer. Leave to simmer as long as you'd like, remembering to top up with water as and when required.

"Winter is the time for comfort, for good food and warmth, for the touch of a friendly hand and for a talk beside the fire: it is the time for home."

Edith Sitwell

CHAPTER SEVEN

Winter Festivities

By this point, Christmas has been in our face for *months*. Home retailers like T.K Maxx (T.J Maxx in the US) Home Sense, The Range, Home Bargains and B&M's have had their Christmas stock front and centre since before the temperature plummeted. More upscale retailers like John Lewis, House of Fraser- even M&S have put out their Christmas Adverts on T.V filled with beautiful homes (and people) having the most perfect Christmas you can imagine with every present under the tree wrapped to perfection, a spread to rival a restaurant and of course- that *feeling*. The one that makes you feel, if only for a second, that you too can have this perfect Christmas if you *just* buy everything in the advert. Like all the decorations and presents In the world can offset difficult relatives, cooking disasters and frantic last minute gift wrapping!

Winter Solstice

Before we dive into all things Christmas, we have Winter Solstice.

It typically happens around the 21st December, and it's the shortest day of the year, with the longest night. This is for the northern hemisphere, with the seasons being reversed in the southern hemisphere.

For some, it is seen as the middle of winter- for others, it's the start. The further North you are in the world means you are likely to see it more as the start, as this is when the days are over twenty hours of darkness in some places.

Solstice has been celebrated in some form or another since prehistory. It marked the symbolic death and rebirth of the sun- the promise that days would grow longer again, the land would flourish and new life would begin.

Here in the UK- the neolithic monument Stonehenge was built to perfectly align with the Solstice- both Winter and Summer, and draws huge crowds every year (More so in Summer) It's amazing that thousands of years after it was built, people are still making a pilgrimage of sorts to see the sun align perfectly with the Heel stone.

How to celebrate the Winter Solstice

Watch it! Whether it's from your window or an outdoor space, it's a pretty majestic sight to behold. You might like to spend some time reflecting on the past year, or coming up with new goals to bring to fruition for the Summer Solstice.

Buy or make an evergreen wreath for your door. Evergreens are symbolic of safety and success, a perfect sentiment for Winter.

Burn a Yule Log. If you're lucky enough to have a fireplace, or an outside wood burner this is a fantastic tradition to uphold. Burning a Yule log was seen as a way rid the home of bad energy. Surround the log with pinecones, cinnamon sticks and mistletoe then allow it to burn down.

Declutter- The Solstice marks the beginning of the Sun's return, so its a perfect time to declutter the old to make space for the new.

<u>Solstice Recipe- Yule Log</u>

For those of us unable to burn a Yule Log, or for anyone who likes chocolate- this is the perfect excuse to make a Yule Log! Whilst these have become more synonymous with Christmas, you can still enjoy it in the few days before. This is a vegan recipe- other recipes are available online if you'd prefer a more traditional version.

For the sponge:

120g self raising flour
25g cocoa powder
100g caster sugar
1 tsp baking powder
10g cornflour
1/2tsp bicarbonate of soda
75ml oat milk
½ tsp vinegar (white or apple cider)
½ tsp salt
110ml aquafaba (the liquid from a tin of chickpeas)
50ml vegetable oil
1 tsp vanilla extract

For the filling:

2 tbsp icing sugar
200ml plant based double cream (Elmlea/Flora make this in the U.K)
1 tsp vanilla extract

For the ganache

250g silken tofu
150g dark chocolate, broken into pieces
2 tsbp maple syrup

Heat the oven to 180C/160C fan/Gas 4 and line a swiss roll tin (approx. 32cm x 22cm) with baking parchment.

First, make the ganache by combining the silken tofu and dark chocolate in a medium saucepan over a low heat, stirring until the chocolate has melted – it will look lumpy at this stage but don't worry. Add the maple syrup, vanilla extract and a pinch of salt, stir to combine and take off the heat. Use an electric whisk to transform the mixture into a silky smooth ganache, about 2-3 mins. Transfer to a piping bag and put in the fridge to cool.

To make the sponge, sift all the dry ingredients (flour, cocoa powder, caster sugar, baking powder, cornflour, bicarbonate of soda and ½ tsp salt) together in a mixing bowl. In a small jug, combine the oat milk and vinegar to create a vegan buttermilk. Set aside.

In a separate mixing bowl, whisk the aquafaba until the liquid has transformed to soft peaks – be patient as this can take up to 5 mins. It's best to use an electric handheld whisk or freestanding mixer.

Add the vegetable oil and vanilla extract to the jug of oat milk and vinegar. Pour the wet ingredients into the bowl of dry ingredients and use large metal spoon to combine until you have a thick batter. Stir a third of the whipped aquafaba into the batter. Once the batter has loosened slightly, tip the chocolate batter into the bowl with the remaining aquafaba and fold through until combined, being careful not to knock too much air from the mixture. Pour this into the prepared baking tin, level out with a spatula, and bake for 20-22 mins.

Christmas

Decorating

We put our Christmas decorations up on the first weekend of December. I know some people don't decorate until Christmas Eve to preserve the "wonder" of it all, or those who decorate as early as November! To each their own, but 1 month of decorations if just right for me.

We keep our decorating very light. For one, we are two adults so Christmas is always a low key sort of affair. Two- more decorations equals more dusting and clean up. As the saying goes- don't make a rod for your own back i.e. don't give yourself more work than is necessary!

Real vs. Fake

Ah- the timeless tree debate! There are *very* strong feelings around this and I'm going to say straight away that we have a fake tree. I have never had a real Christmas tree, and I don't feel like I've lost out on anything. My Husband however, who grew up at the opposite end of the country, *always* had a real tree.

Real trees are expensive (and were not very common when I was growing up- everyone I knew had a fake tree) and of course- they shed. There are products out there that claim to reduce this but the truth of the matter is if you buy a real tree, you accept that your floor will be covered with pine needles. Real trees have certainly become more popular in the U.K over time. There are a few places you can purchase them- and most of the time you are renting the tree. You'll buy it, take it home, then bring it back to be re-planted. This is a more eco friendly way to have a real tree for sure.

Cards vs. No Cards

The rule in our house is that if someone sends us a card, we will reciprocate. Other than that we don't send cards. We have had the same multipack of variety cards for about three years now because we send so few! Our lack of card sending is based on two things. One- the price of stamps is crazy. Two- it's not environmentally friendly. The cards we send are made of recycled card, but recycling should be the last resort In terms of being green with the first being refuse, then reduce.

Now of course if you are in a situation where your Great Aunt Brenda will lose her mind if you don't send a card then go ahead and do it. It's (probably) not worth the stress to refuse. Or if you're just really passionate about sending cards and that lights you up- do it. I'm not going to judge anyone for sending cards, I'm just here sharing what works for us.

<u>Gifting</u>

I think the buying and receiving of gifts is one of *the* most polarising debates of Christmas. That's before you even dig into how to react to a gift you don't want, and the complexities of re-gifting.

For us, we have a very specific set up. On Christmas Eve we do a grown up version of Christmas Eve boxes inspired by the Icelandic tradition of *Jólabókaflóðið* which loosely translates as "Book Flood. Icelanders buy new book releases in the months leading up to Christmas, and gift them to family and friends to be enjoyed on Christmas Eve. Reading often extends into the night, and is normally accompanied by chocolate in one form or another.

So, in our boxes we include a book. To make sure we get one we absolutely want we share 5 books off of our respective Amazon wishlists and let the other pick which one to get. My Husband and I have different tastes, so this takes the guesswork out! We also include things like chocolate, sweets and other small trinkets we know the other will like.

The reason we love this is that it extends the gift giving. When you are just 2 adults and you are only buying gifts for one another there probably isn't a ton of gifts to open on the big day (Or maybe there is in your house, but we aren't big on spending loads at Christmas) so this way we get presents both days. We have an approximate budget for Christmas presents for each other so there is no awkward "you spent more on me than I did on you" or vica versa.

To regift, or not regift

This is not something I've ever had to do- but my thoughts are if you receive a gift that you don't like or have no use for- why not regift it to someone who will love it? Make sure you stick a note on to say who gave it to you to avoid any disasters! Alternatively you could donate it.

IDEA TO TRY: HOMEMADE GIFTWRAP

You will need:

- A roll of brown (kraft) paper
- A Christmas themed stamp
- Inkpad

Most wrapping paper isn't recyclable (The test is this- if you can scrunch it and it stays scrunched, that's recyclable. If not, throw it away)

This is a fun idea I tried last year, so I'm sharing it with you.

1. Unroll the paper as much as you can- a big table helps!
2. Grab your stamp and put it in your ink pad. Don't roll it around or you'll get ink on areas of the stamp you don't want, and it will affect the printing.
3. Ideally come up with a pattern before you get stamping. You could do simple lines, alternating the stamp design if you bought more than one stamp- or any other sort of pattern.
4. Get stamping! Go slowly, remembering to ink the stamp each time.
5. Allow the ink to fully dry on the paper before cutting it for gift wrapping.

To take the rustic element further- wrap your packages with string (Hello The Sound of Music!) or pretty ribbon.

Christmas Food

My favourite bit of Christmas- food! I think as you get older it's less about presents, and more about the food and atmosphere. Note- we are vegetarians so I can't help you with cooking a Turkey (The traditional Christmas meat here in the U.K) or the like, but there are tons of helpful guides and videos online that can help you avoid the dreaded dry turkey.

I make the vast majority of Christmas food from scratch. Biscuits, cakes (including Christmas cake) the main course and the sides. I also make waffles for breakfast Christmas morning.

Things I do buy premade are

- Marks and Spencers chocolate Christmas biscuits (My Nan always brought these and my Christmas would feel wrong without them)
- Cranberry sauce (It's an ingredient in our main course)
- Gravy granules (So much easier than roasting tons of onions to make onion gravy)

Our main course is Gaz Oakley's Christmas Seitan Wellington. The great thing about it, other than the taste, is that you can make it up the day before- then cook it on Christmas Day! Whatever we don't eat we slice and freeze for later. The recipe is in available on his website.

Cooking Tips

Create a timeline of what needs to be cooked- starting with whatever takes the longest, and work your way back. That way you can see what needs to be cooked, and when.

For perfect roast potatoes- shake them in the pan once you've boiled and drained them. Roughing up the edges makes them crispy on the outside. Also, preheat the oil before you put them in.

To save time, buy Brussels pre peeled/trimmed! For other vegetables, prep them the night before. You will thank yourself.

If you are cooking a frozen Turkey (or other meat) please ensure you defrost it thoroughly before you cook it. This is so important for food safety!

IDEA TO TRY: CORNFLOUR DOUGH DECORATIONS

This is a spin on traditional salt dough. The cornflour and bicarbonate of soda make this sough bright white which looks beautiful against your tree.

You will need:

- 1 cup bicarbonate of soda
- ½ cup cornflour
- ¾ cup warm water

Place all ingredients in a medium sized saucepan and heat until it bubbles.

Stir it constantly until it starts to pull away from the sides of the pan.

Tip onto a surface liberally coated in cornflour and leave to cool.

Once cool, knead it until smooth- adding extra cornflour if too sticky.

Roll out your dough to around 1.5cm thickness, then use cutters to cut out decorations. Use a pencil or similar to make a hole in the top so you can hang them.

Leave to dry overnight, possibly longer depending on the temperature.

Hang them on the tree and admire your handiwork!

CHAPTER EIGHT

Winter Project

Winter is a perfect time to indulge in a personal project. With its long dark days making us feel less than great, having something to look forward to in the form of a personal project is a great way to stave off the Winter blues, and feel motivated to do something. Waking up with something to look forward to doing is a great way to start the day!

The question is of course, what are you going to do?

When it comes to picking a project, here are three things to keep in mind that can help you decide.

1. In the words of Marie Kondo, does it spark joy?
2. Will this project make me feel fulfilled, or accomplished?
3. Is this something I *want* to do, or feel I *should* do?

That last one is important. We so often get caught up in what we think we *should* do, we often ignore what we *want* to do. Now of course, some of those *shoulds* do need to get done- things like household tasks, and I'm not suggesting you forget all about those and only indulge in what you want to do. What I am saying is that you are *allowed* to make space to to undertake a project that you want to do- and I'd urge you to do so.

Feeling like you're on a treadmill with life- work, eat, sleep, chores, repeat is the fastest way to burn out. We all need to build in some time for play- even if it is just fifteen minutes.

My Winter project is of course writing. This ticks two boxes- it's fun, *and* it's a should- If I want to keep selling books! As I write this, my writing project is a little different from my past work as I'm planning on writing fiction. A big departure from my previous work, but one that most definitely sparks joy (and a little terror!)

So, what will your project be?

Here are some ideas to get you started:

- Knitting a blanket, scarf, jumper or other item that you've been putting off.
- Learning a new creative skill- like knitting, crochet or embroidery.
- Learning how to bake bread from scratch
- Decorating a space in your home that is in need of some love
- Writing that novel you've dreamt of, or even short stories or poetry
- Making it through your TBR (To be read) pile
- Turning a hobby into a business (ONLY if this sparks joy, you *do not* need to monetise your hobbies despite what the internet hustlers say)
- Volunteering your time with an organisation that is meaningful to you
- Learning a practical skill like canning (ideal if you garden!)
- Researching something that interests you but you haven't had time to dig into (Like a certain period of history for example)

To make a real go of this, schedule out the time you will work on it. Try to pick a time that you are unlikely (or less likely) to be disturbed, and when you feel more energised (morning gal here!) so you will feel more motivated to follow through.

Don't get upset if it doesn't always work out though. This if your project, *you set the rules*. If you need to break them, or something comes up- that's OK. This isn't homework, no one is going to tell you off for not finishing it!

I'd love to see your projects! Tag me @melaniesteeleauthor on Instagram.

CHAPTER NINE

Winter Books and Movies

As the nights draw in and the temperatures drop, who can resist curling up with a good film or book? I have a gorgeous purple armchair in my office that is the perfect spot for reading. There's always a blanket there ready to get cosy, and a footstool for extra comfort. Oh, don't forget about the cute upcycled side table where I put my hot drink and snack!

Hallmark Christmas Movies

Let me begin by making a plea- Hallmark please release your Christmas movies here in the U.K! We get some, but the new releases rarely make it over here, or if they do its quite some time after.

What we *do* have here is the channel Christmas Movies 24 which you can get if you have Sky/Virgin Media or similar. We don't have these services, or indeed an actual television (We have one *technically* but it is used exclusively as a computer screen) so sadly I don't get to indulge in these movies when they come out. I have to rely on Netflix and Amazon Prime for my cheesy Christmas movie fix!

My Favourite Christmas Movies

The Princess Switch 1,2 and 3
A Christmas Prince (and the sequels)
B&B Merry
Christmas Inheritance

Best Christmas, Ever!
Falling for Christmas
A Castle for Christmas
The Knight Before Christmas
Holiday in Handcuffs
A Very Merry Toy Store
The Muppet Christmas Carol

You'll notice that a lot of the *big* Christmas movies aren't on here- like Elf, Nightmare Before Christmas, Harry Potter, etc. My thoughts are that everyone knows about these, so you don't need a list!

<u>Winter Movies *(Where Christmas isn't the main focus)*</u>

Little Women
The Chronicles of Narnia: The Lion, The Witch and The Wardrobe
Love Actually
About a Boy
Miss Potter
The Holiday
Happy Feet

<u>Cosy Feels Books</u>

Now of course, you can ready *any book, any time*. But- if you want to read a book that feels cosy, here are some recommendations.

Lattes and Legends- Travis Baldree
Bookshops and Bonedust- Travis Baldree
The Spellshop- Sarah Beth Durst
Little Women- Louisa May Alcott
The Lion, The Witch and The Wardrobe- C.S Lewis.
Falling Inn Love (The whole series actually!) Erin Branscom
The Bookshop on the Corner- Jenny Colgan
The Little Board Game Cafe- Jennifer Page

Of course there are *plenty* more cosy books out there- this is just a list of suggestions to get you started.

CHAPTER TEN

Winter Days Out

Whilst we will probably spend the majority of our Winter days indoors, there are definitely some winter days out that can help break up the days and fortify our *sisu.*

Ice Skating

Whether this is outside on a frozen body of water (Please exercise extreme caution here, it may not be as frozen as you think) an outdoor rink set up for Winter, or an indoor rink- ice skating is a great way to get some exercise, and have fun!

Christmas Markets

Christmas markets are HUGE across Europe. Here in the U.K the biggest ones can be found in the following places:

- London
- Bath
- York
- Manchester
- Cardiff
- Edinburgh
- Belfast

These are the main Christmas markets- be sure to check out local information for smaller ones closer to you!

In Europe you'll definitely want to check out these locations for the best Christmas markets

- Hungary, Budapest- Advent Feast at the Basilica
- Metz, France
- Govone, Itlay
- Valkenburg, The Netherlands
- Brussels, Belgium
- Trier, Germany
- Vienna, Austria
- Dresden, Germany

Now of course there is bound to be a Christmas market near to you- even if it's a smaller, more local version. These are well worth checking out as they will typically be much quieter than those in big cities, and more likely to have local artisans showcasing their wares. Shopping local is *always* a good thing.

Steam Train/Heritage Railway

I can think of few things more romantic and cosy than a steam train ride on a cold winters day. Sitting in a beautiful train car bundled up in your cosiest layers and jacket looking out the window to frosty fields- heaven! There are numerous places to you can ride in a steam train here in the U.K with the most famous of course being the Jacobite Steam Train in Scotland, made famous by the Harry Potter movies. I'm not a Harry Potter fan, but this is very much on my wish list as a lover of all things steam trains!

Indoor Attractions

If you want a day out, but would like to remain warm and cosy than why not head to an indoor attraction?

You could try:

- Museums
- Aquarium
- Indoor Markets
- Castles/Other Historic Places of Interest
- Afternoon Tea

"No Winter lasts forever, no Spring skips it's turn"

Hal Borland

BONUS CHAPTER

Curating Your Perfect Winter Day

I hope you've been inspired by all the suggestions for having a wonderful Winter thus far. Now you're armed with ideas and inspiration, why not take a moment to make a mug of something hot, then sit down with a pen and paper to start coming up with ideas for a perfect Winter day?

To help you out, I've compiled a list of everything that's been mentioned so far and divided them into categories so you can easily pick and choose which ones you'd like to include.

Food and Drink

Set up a Hot Chocolate and/or Coffee bar
Make your favourite hot beverage and sip it slowly
Bake some Swedish Cinnamon rolls
Try one of the recipes from the Winter Food section
Shop for seasonal fruits and veggies

Heading Outside

Try your hand at Ice skating
A winter walk through local woods or forest
Visit a local historic monument
Head to a Christmas market

Self care

Have an at home spa day/morning or afternoon
Try some of the journal prompts from the writing chapter

Read a favourite book
Watch a favourite movie or show

Christmas

Have a fun day decorating the house (or more if you have a big space, or want to do it slowly)
Try making giftwrap and/or ornaments from the "Idea to try" section
Bake Christmas shortbread and put it in a lovely tin

Winter projects

Set aside a whole day (or a morning/afternoon/evening if you're pressed for time) to dedicate to your Winter project. Remember- it should be FUN!

Other ideas

Catch up with friends and family
Go to your favourite coffee shop with a good book
Check out your local library for books on your wishlist
Take photographs of nature in her winter glory
Volunteer your time with an organisation that matters to you

I hope these have inspired you- why not share your perfect Winter day with me at @melaniesteeleauthor on Instagram?

CONCLUSION

All good things must come to an end

It is my greatest wish that you have enjoyed this book, and that it has inspired you to have a great Winter season. Maybe if you're someone who is less keen on Winter, it has helped you reframe it as a season where there is still much to be enjoyed both indoors and out, and that with a little *sisu* you can make it through to Spring.

This will be my last non fiction book. I have loved writing this book, *Cosy Autumn* and *The Magic of Home* but it's time for pastures new. I am currently working on my first novel which will be a cosy fantasy, and I can't wait to share it with the world!

If you're interested in following my progress, come follow me on Instagram @melaniesteeleauthor.

As always, leaving a review on Amazon is a big help for us indie authors, and I would love if you would consider leaving one.

Printed in Great Britain
by Amazon

47439393R00036

THE B

BOY

A summary of my life through my eyes

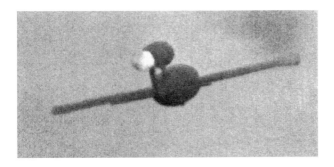

A V 1 Bomber seen from a chasing plane's
cockpit

TERRY FITZGERALD

PROLOGUE

I have listened to people telling me how lucky I was to be born when I was (1938) and how difficult it is to manage today. Life was apparently all coming up roses and life has never been the same since. Well I think that you should read this semi autobiography and see what some of life was really about and why you might think it was hard work and endeavour that produced today's life and that some of the same effort today can give you the same returns.
Shakespeare I understand noted the seven stages of life, this will have as many stages as I find relevant.

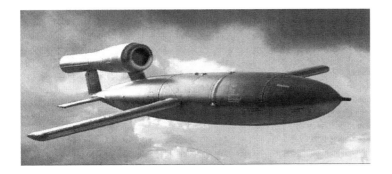

V 1 Bomber

CHAPTER ONE

Earliest memories

I was always the biggest bore that remembered all those things that no one else could even be expected to remember. You know we moved house from a basement flat to above a garage in Grosvenor Terrace. Mother, 'You cannot know that you were barely two'. Well here goes.

I started school during the war and was living in Lewin Road, Streatham. I went to school at St Andrews, Polworth Road.

My first day at school saw me led down a corridor passed various classrooms and a small kitchen to the last room which must have been separated from the rest of the school for some reasons as this was not equipped with a radiator but had a large independent fire in a stove with a long cast iron chimney. This was coal fired and had to be fed every hour or so. There was a guard all round it to keep us away. The room itself led onto the girls' playground. The boys' playground was at the other end of the building where we had come in. There were separate gates to each playground which allowed both sexes independent entry.

We met other children in the road on the way to the school walked in a crocodile accompanied by a parent as I recall but there was also an adult on the main road to ensure all the children crossed safely.

On the home trip I would call in at my fraternal aunt's house and on a good day pick a Bramley apple windfall to eat before dinner.

In the evenings neighbours used sometimes to come in and use our bath, as we were one of the few around with one, and they put money in our gas meter to cover the cost of running the boiler.

About once a week the dustcart came to clear our rubbish and this was a large cart pulled by two shire horses. Milk and bread also came by horse and cart.

The doctor was an occasional visitor as this cost money (minimum of half-a-crown) I think, and with dad at war (in England due to age and medical reasons) this was real money. With our luck both my brothers had scarlet fever, I think! Then my twin and I had mumps and measles before my twin had some other problem. This meant that the doctor was called as an emergency and very late in the evening. He prescribed M & B and gave him a tablet and said that he would be back the next day before morning surgery. The next morning the snow had fallen and the road was what looked like unpassable but to my surprise the doctor duly drove up in his old car with further drugs. He declared satisfaction with the progress and advised my mother how to proceed, as he was leaving my mother said she could not pay for both visits and the medication as all she had was at most the basic half-a-crown. The response was not to worry he could sort it later and would return soon to check on the patient. Our doctor luck continued when he advised that the twins should have their tonsils out and that he would arrange to do it himself in the Wilson Hospital. He was not only a GP but was the resident surgeon.

The day of the operation came and he met us at the hospital and said he would do the op and then meet afterwards and share an ice cream and jelly with us. All complete we returned home in a taxi. Who and how this was funded I will never know. Could this happen today!

We had a shelter put into the back garden and there was a communal shelter, which must have been for several hundreds of people, on the bottom of Streatham Common. I recall going in the one on the common and also remember when returning from school with a number of children when a rare German bomber flew over at a very low altitude. The parent in charge called for us to run for cover but one of the boys declared that the wind was in the wrong direction and we were not in trouble. Run for cover was the word but the boy was right and I amazingly watched the bomb doors come open and the spinning bombs came down with the wind taking them away from us to land, I think, on a common, causing little trouble.

One day a bomb landed nearby and we heard that a wall at the top of the road had collapsed onto a young lady who had later died. The war appeared to be coming closer.

For some reason that I did not know at the time my cousin was living with us. I discovered later that my aunt and uncle had split and that my cousin whilst in some form of care won a scholarship to a posh school at the top of Brixton Hill and

3

was assured that he would not be treated differently from other, privileged pupils. It turned out that when the LCC provided his full uniform and sports gear every article had a large label stitched in with a large council logo. My mother and father agreed this was not acceptable and arranged that he live with us and all the labels be removed.

Sundays were special occasions when we walked to the local Catholic Church where we passed a beggar and we boys gaily sang the then nursery rhyme,

Christmas is coming the goose is getting fat

Please put a penny in the blind man's hat

If you haven't a penny, a halfpenny will do

If you haven't a halfpenny GOD bless you.

On returning from church my cousin would have cleaned the flat and we, the boys, were then made to polish the table and sideboard until we could see the reflections of our faces

I seem to remember that Christmas (1943) was coming and we were, that is, the three boys would be expected to perform at the get together party. We did not like the idea of us each doing a special act and it was agreed that we could sing/dance to a new song 'coming in on a wing and a prayer' which finished with us down on one knee, big brother in front and twins behind and arms akimbo like a landing plane.

Six months passed and my brother's birthday came and went but before it was long passed the dreaded doodlebug was forecast. This duly came and the first we knew the Chimes garage at the top of the road had been hit.

On the 23rd June 1944 we were all in the shelter except for my cousin who remained in his bed in the house. The next doodlebug duly arrived and low and behold it stopped on the top of the poplar trees immediately behind our shelter. I was on the top bunk and as the engine stopped the silence was deafening.

The earth from the top of the shelter was shaken on to my head by the vibration of the engine then the engine stopped and all I could hear was the breaking of branches under the weight of the plane. A few moments, which felt like an eternity, later, the engine reignited and the doodlebug drifted on to the only empty house in the road and then exploded.

I, from my top bunk, was the first one out of the shelter and looked at the back of the house. Every window and window cill were piled one on the other with the house looking like an open dolls house you could see into every room. My first thoughts were that my cousin was in there somewhere. To my absolute relief as I ran down the garden my cousin came running towards me and we clutched each other then saw everybody funnelling to the centre of the garden.

What had happened to the neighbours! All the shelters nearer to the bomb than us were covered in debris and the adults immediately set to work clearing a space in order to get the occupants out.

The children were not allowed to get involved for some reason and at this time I found out that the boy up the road had been sheltering under the stairs but had managed to get out with only a large cut on the side of his face. He was about to be cared for by a neighbour when he remembered that he had not given my brother a birthday present he had promised him about a week before. He rushed into the house and retrieved his stamp album which he then passed to my brother as promised. I do not think I ever saw this boy again.

Many things seemed to happen but what I remember most are the large gash in the head board of my cousins bed settee and that it was overlain with the large French doors that had blown inwards and it seemed impossible that he had managed to get out unhurt, also the glass cabinet and all the bowls and glasses were shattered but on top of the piano were six unbroken eggs which I think we shared for breakfast next day.

Not too long after this it seemed we were being hurriedly prepared to leave and go to Streatham Common Station at the bottom of the road. It was a total surprise when a long goods train stopped and a guard opened one of the goods vans and helped us to climb aboard. The door was closed behind us and we found that there were some boxes to sit on and we shared our company with some dogs (greyhounds I think). We were on the train all day with the mother and son who had been staying with friends in the same house as us. I heard that they had a house near Manchester and had invited my mother with her three boys to come and live with them for as long as necessary.

The train eventually stopped at Crewe which made me laugh as this reminded me of the words to 'Oh Mr Porter' which said 'I wanted to go to London but they sent me on to Crewe'. We had to get off and run over a bridge to another platform and board another train. I know nothing about this train or how we got to our next destination as I think I was mostly asleep.

It must have been around midnight when we entered the house in Northenden near Wythenshawe where we were to stay until the end of the War. How all this was arranged and how accurate my memory is makes me wonder but I still think of it as miraculous and a credit to the ingenuity shown at many times in the Blitz.

CHAPTER TWO

Manchester

Where do I start as this period, in my mind, there is little or no chronology?

There was a field at the back of the garden that ran out on two sides to a railway line and it looked like an old sports ground as there was the remains of tennis courts within a wire fencing.

We visited and were enrolled at a school a couple of miles away which we were to travel to by bus. We would pay a halfpenny for the journey on the double-decker but the quicker route under a low bridge cost a penny. If we missed the morning bus we could catch the later single decker but this meant that we had to walk/run back after school.

We met a number of children who lived nearby and regularly saw a parrot in the window of a local house. There was another Terry in the road so I was given a specific nickname which eventually was only used by my elder brother when writing notes to me personally. We played mainly in the field at the back and someone in the family bought us an Atlanta kite. This kite was special as we had a set of parachutes and a releaser. This meant that we could send a parachute up the string of the kite from which it was released at the top. We then watched which way the wind took it and ran, sometimes for miles, in attempts to retrieve them for re-use. We had a high level of success. Unfortunately one day the unattended kite string rubbed against the gatepost and the whole thing disappeared forever into the distance.

We played a lot in both the street and the field and often came home together from the bus after school. The local shops were new to us as the greengrocer was also the wet fishmonger. We found the fish and chip shop and were introduced to a portion of mushy peas which were not to our taste really.

It did not seem long before I got what is still an unknown illness and we became acquainted with a local doctor. He was we all guessed to be a Hungarian, but whoever knows. He did not appear to understand why I ached so much and was very hot. He told my mother that I should be kept in bed but that I should not have any sheets and be covered only in extra blankets. I then got a severe pain in one arm and also felt quite shivery. My mother laid on the bed with me to comfort and keep me warm. The doctor decided to give some medicine and as he was going to make this up himself in his surgery (common in those days) he ask me what fruit flavour I would like it. Nearly two weeks passed and one day the doctor told me that the pain was moving and that it would pass round my body and the leave by the second arm. I did not really think he knew but was trying to keep my morale up. It turned out that he appeared to be right and as the pain moved round I felt a bit better. One morning, feeling somewhat brighter, I looked round the bedroom and saw a large bowl of fruit with a big bar of chocolate on top standing on the chest of drawers. Sweets were on ration and fruit a luxury. My mother told me that all the children in the road had given sweet coupons and pocket money in order to provide this treat with their wishes that I might soon be better. The desired result came in the next couple of weeks and I was soon up and about again. Such overwhelming kindness.

One day we looked out to the field and saw a number of soldiers or ARP (Dad's Army) who had commandeered the old tennis courts and were practicing throwing Hand Grenades They stayed for several hours throwing over the wire fence and other obstacles to gain height and distance. They never returned at a later date.

That Christmas Eve a doodle bug came over, immediately over our house, and as our next door neighbours were fairly old and did not know what the noise was my mother sent me to tell them that the plane would pass without harming us. I went to the front door and picked up a torch as it was pitch black. The ARP warden who had probably done nothing during the war was immediately out of his house and told me 'put that light out'. I replied that it was a V 1 and had no pilot to see the light and my mother rushed up behind me and shouted 'he does not know that, he does not come from London' and promptly clouted me round the ear for being rude.

We would always pop our heads into the local telephone boxes when we passed them and would press button 'B'. If users had not been connected and they had left without pressing this button their pennies would be returned to us. This money was sometimes used to buy six inch nails which we misused on the railway line. We would get through to the line and whilst waiting for a train to come would place the six inch nail on the rail with the point facing the expected train. The result was to produce a very sharp six inch dagger which we used as a toy. We also climbed tall trees. We would be out for hours but never seemed to be in trouble for it. Is this just rose coloured glasses? Anyway I was happy I am sure.

When the snow came that winter I recall standing near the window with my brothers as we sang 'Snow, Snow come down faster if you don't we'll tell your master'. Not long after we got up to go to school and the snow was deep enough to cover our ankle length wellies. We were delighted to have a day off until at about midday the sun melted the snow and we had to walk to school for the afternoon lessons. Would the teachers have been there today?

I being a natural left hander put my pencil into that hand. The teachers did not like this and tried tying my hand behind my back to help me write with the right hand but they soon gave up.

We were very much the average naughty kids and on the way home in the dark early evenings we would play 'Knock down Ginger' (knocking on doors and running away) and used twigs to release the air from car tyres. This apparently got out of hand and my mother decided that we must be reported to the police. We were then frog marched down to the local police station but it turned out to be our lucky day. It was a Thursday and it was the afternoon that the station closed and we were only taken back home and I think put to bed early.

We also made our own bows from branches of trees from the fields and arrows from golden rod stems.

Spring came and went and the rest of the year gave us the opportunity to have three bonfire nights (no fireworks as I remember) with baked potatoes etc. We spent many hours cutting trees and branches in preparation for these. V E Day, V J Day and Guy Fawkes night.

I do not recall when but by now the owner of the house and her son had moved up town and into a big house. We visited at times and saw there was a kitchen range with two ovens for cooking and making bread. Something way beyond our dreams. We were however allowed to rent our house until we could go back to London and in fact we were offered to buy it for what I understand was a good price. Unfortunately my father could only find work if he returned to his previous job in London and we arranged to return around Christmas

CHAPTER THREE

6 Nettlewood Road

Prior moving to Nettlewood Road we had to overcome a small trauma of discovering that the owner of the flat we had been bombed out in was not going, as we thought was the law, to rent it back to us.

My father was very angry and contacted the Local Council, his MP and his union as I understand and after what to me was a very short time but to my mother and father felt like an age the Local Council agreed to re-house us. We were allocated a requisitioned property in Streatham Vale. This would be available almost immediately but we had no belongings in London.

We were allowed access to the house and my two brothers and I were sent off to clean it up and as best we could prepare for the move. In the meantime we stayed at our fraternal aunt's and uncle's place back in Lewin Road. Our devilment came out again at this time and, I do not know how, but we tried our first cigarette. In those days they came as small packets of five and were in some shops sold singly. We also collected coal from the back of the goods yard where it was transferred from the goods trains to the delivery Lorries. Over time a lot of coal had fallen and was buried part way into the ground. This is what we 'scrumped'. This is the same goods yard where we first encountered container shipping. We had arranged for Pickford's Removals to bring what we had in Manchester to London; this was collected into a container on the back of a lorry and then taken to the local goods yard where it was transferred to a goods train. This wagon was sent to our local goods yard where it was then put on a lorry and brought round to us.

It was about my birthday when we at last moved in to this third house down the road which was the last house that had not been demolished by the bomb that had landed at the bottom of the road. The road next to us had also been destroyed to a great extent by the same bomb but in that road they had built the new prefabs and these were already occupied. Next to us from number eight onwards was a complete bombsite where we understood that they were soon to rebuild the houses as per the original designs. This is a small world as you will constantly hear in this narrative but in this case the couple who had lived in, I think No 14 had actually been living in the middle part of the house we were bombed out in in Lewin Road. We were to keep these people up to date as and when building started.

We started to settle in and got to know the neighbours at the back. This was easy as we all put our dustbins out in the alley behind our houses each week to be emptied. The dustmen, whose cart was pulled by two shire horses, walked through the alley with a very large bin over their shoulder and cleared our bins and carried the full large bin to the dustcart and then returned to where they had got to and repeated the process. This neighbour had an apple and a Victoria plum tree as well as a big Alsatian dog. When Pat was invited in to help himself to some plums he was given a rather nasty bite as the dog treated him as a stranger once he entered the garden.

There were, it seemed, a lot of children in the district and we learnt to play a game called drainhole football. This was played with a tennis ball and the idea was to kick the ball into the open gap in the kerbstone above the drain where it lodged and was declared a goal. The drains were not actually opposite each other but with teams of three or four we had great fun. Great fun that was until one of the two spinsters living in No 2 complained about the noise and told us we could not play on the road area outside their house. These same two had an orchard in their back garden and in order to stop us scrumping they tied all the branches back and put high wire fencing around.

The back garden became an allotment and a play area and believe it or not the home to our fridge. Well it was not a conventional fridge as these were definitely not on our shopping list or indeed were not yet available. Our fridge was a galvanised dustbin buried in the ground up to the lid and we made a couple shelves from orange boxes scrounged from the greengrocers. Milk and butter went lowest with eggs and cheese and meat, I think, nearer the top. We did not expect people to come into the garden and steal our provisions and similarly we, the kids, did not have keys to the house, but the key was left either under the mat or on a nearby window cill. Security was not considered in those days as we all trusted each other and helped each other out.

We re-joined the same primary school we attended when we lived in Lewin Road but now from Streatham Vale it was a much longer walk, over a mile at least.

One morning my brother fell over and cut his face and an employee of the head office of a big   jewellers took us into her building and got the company nurse to tend to the wound before we carried on to arrive at school on time. Questions were ask but there were no recriminations but thanks for the help and consideration.

I do not know how my mother coped with not knowing what time I would get home after school as I must have started my habit of meeting and talking to people at an early age.

Not far from the school near Streatham Station the trams changed from overhead electricity to underground. This was done by two men who maintained batteries and had very long hooked poles which they used to unhook the connecting rods from the overhead wires and anchor them to the tram then use a very large pair of pliers to run the new charged battery under the tram. This fascinated me and I would chat and then be allowed to help (unofficially, of course). This was only one of the regular delays on the journey home. Others were visiting the stables in Ambleside Avenue which later became notorious for the goings on at No 26, stopping at the cobblers at the back of the bus garage near where the sign-writers painted the adverts on the busses, talking to the lady and gent attending the public lavatories and then buying a stale bun in the bakers.

At school I think I enjoyed most of the days shared between learning and playing but two things stand out, first the daily milk ration which was third of a pint of milk in a bottle. I loved milk and without the teacher's knowing I would swap my empty with a full bottle that another pupil or pupils did not want, and secondly when I and another pupil had a problem with a particular teacher. Aiden and I had progressed with the mathematics to the extent that the school bought a special book just for the two of us. We were given the tests at the end of each chapter as homework. One day this Miss Ryan decided that each of us had made the same mistake. We were sent back on three occasions before she sent us to the headmistress for insubordination. This ended in our parents being summoned to the school to meet the head to clarify the situation which was deadlocked. On the day the head decided to summon the teacher to explain her problem. She said we would not re-do the particular sum in order to get the right answer. The head then asked her if she had completed the sum herself and she said no as she used the official answer book; at this point the head asked for the book and did the sum herself and came up with the same answer as Aiden and I had. She then chastised the teacher and apologised to our parents who were less than happy. This same teacher crossed my path a few years later which you will read about in the scouting section.

Out of school although only 8 or 9 I got a Saturday morning job with a greengrocer who drove round the local streets selling door to door. This was poorly paid and sometimes I did not finish until after three in the afternoon. I did however learn how important it was to think before you act. Whilst on the back of the lorry travelling from Streatham Common to Streatham Vale I purloined a Russet apple threw the core away on the driver side and the boss saw it fly past in his wing mirror. I got a telling off and a threat to dock some of my wages. I visited local shops and managed to get a job at a greengrocer/florist working from 7 to 1pm and gave the greengrocer notice. Mrs Stenning the owner of the florist told me I would earn half-a-crown but at the end of the first day she gave me a two shilling piece. I challenged her and she gave me the extra sixpence. Unfortunately after many months I was ill and when I returned the next week she told my job had been given to another boy. I told the boy my story but he suffered the same trick but did not argue. I moved on up the road and visited shop after shop in order to gain another job. I had luck at the top of the high street where a butcher ask me if I could ride an errand boy's bike. I said yes as confidently as I could and he ask his Cutter to fill the big basket at the front with as much as it would take and then ask me to ride down the road and back. This I managed somehow and he laughed and offered me 3 shillings if I got formal sign off from my college headmaster and then explained the law of working hours which he would proceed to break. I worked here until I left college and by then had increased my wage to ten shillings. I learnt a lot about life here and I think it helped me in my interviews for jobs at least two of which were successful. I joined Martins Bank Ltd direct from college. At the Butcher's I would start my day by cleaning the brass name outside the shop and then I might de-ice the fridge and then go on my rounds. I was conned out of ten shillings by one of our regular customers. When I got back to the shop I told Mr Wilson what had happened and he gave my cash to the cashier and I was sent down to clean all the copper piping on the motor that ran the fridge. About

45mins later he sent the apprentice down to say that I was right but that he had recovered the cost at the front of the shop and that I should treat it as a lesson. I was rarely off work but one week I fell off the errand boy's bike and did my knee up. By the time I got home I could hardly walk and virtually fell in through the front door. I finished up at the local hospital and was put on a stretcher on wheels next to a small table. The doctor inserted a tube in my knee and set a kidney shaped bowl on the table. He said he would aspirate the swelling and that if the kidney bowl started to fill up I was to call the nurse and have it replaced. Some hours later I was sent home and told that outpatient appointments had been made for me for Monday, Wednesday and Friday for the next three weeks. I was not allowed to put my foot down to walk on and was transported to and from the hospital for my appointments. The only good that came from this was that it was the Wimbledon fortnight and our next door neighbours had a small television and invited me in to watch with them.

The next year I started working on the Easter and Christmas periods. The apprentice taught me to truss the chickens at Easter but did it all wrong. The next day the manager checked my work, which fell apart, and he called the apprentice and asked him to truss a chicken, which he of course did wrongly. I was exonerated and the apprentice told to work overtime to recover the situation. There were six of us in the shop one Christmas when the manager ask the cashier to open the 'staff Christmas box' and split the proceeds. She counted the money and asked how she should share it out. The manager without hesitation said equally in six parts. The Cutter complained that I as only a Saturday Boy should have a lesser portion. The Cutter was adamant and so the manager said did he think it should be divided into only five and he of course agreed. The manger then said fine but he would be the one left out as we all worked together to provide the service which our customers were rewarding. The money was split six ways. There were many generous and business related things I learnt from Mr Wilson and when I left to start proper work he said if I did not get on with it and wanted a change he would always find me a job somewhere in the Company he worked for.

Note: From the first day I earned money my father insisted that I give one third of it to my mother. That meant that she started getting 10 pence and finished up with 3 shillings and 4 pence by the time I left school.

Not all of the time was taken up with going to school and working as play was a big part of life especially during the holidays. I particularly remember we went up to Streatham Common quite frequently and in the winter played football at the bottom end and also went up the top to the woods and climbed the trees by the rookery. In the summer we played cricket as long as we managed to get together a set of stumps and a bat and ball. We were given some ex MCC balls by an aunt who worked in the House of Lords and was given them by a member. When we were bored or there were only a few of us we might leave the common and go scrumping for apples in the grounds of the Convent, this was a challenge as we had to climb a high wall to get in and if we were spotted getting away before getting caught was not easy. One day I was the last down the tree and the scaffold pole we had used was displaced and fell on my head giving a nasty cut, but I still got away. Sometimes these sorties were reported to the school which was run by the nuns and they tried to find out who the little villains were, normally with no success.

Talking of scrumping we did not only go for fruit as there were a lot of allotments around and vegetables cost money so sometimes we took carrots etc. I think I mentioned earlier that our requisitioned house was the last one not knocked down by the bomb, well they started building next to us and this became an adventure playground. We would climb the scaffolding and run through the floors and then the lofts as the building progressed. This was particularly dangerous and I remember slipping at the first floor level but managed to hang on to a lower scaffold and continue on that level. The site was also another learning place where I watched the workmen use old scaffolds to make purpose size lintels by wiring reinforcement rods into the boxes and filling them with concrete. This was done last thing at night and they would then set and be tipped out for the template to be used again. When bricks were delivered we used to help unload the Lorries with one person on the back picking up three bricks and throwing these over the side for the next person to catch and then stack for later use. Later use was when I was allowed to fill a hod with 12 bricks and run up the ladder and deposit them near the bricklayer ready to be laid. We also hand prepared the pug (don't try to make too much at a time, it takes longer) and took this up the ladder in a hod to be tipped onto a square piece of wood near the bricklayer.

Somewhere along the way we came to look after two dogs for two years while a fraternal uncle worked on an engineering project in India. They were a dog and a bitch dachshund called Cobber and Dinah who were quite amazing animals as we taught them to beg and went out for long runs through the streets and over the many building sites where they should have fallen down footings and drain holes but never did. We also had a cat that delivered a dead or partially dead rat to our front doorstep each morning. These were we guessed being caught by the many fractures to the main sewer system. In order to go out early the cat used to come upstairs to one of the bedrooms and tap the face of one of the occupants with its paw to say 'let me out'. We lost the cat once for several weeks and then one day a door to door salesman stopped in the road and the cat popped out and ran over to me in the front garden. The salesman said he had no idea when the cat got into his car but had opened the boot on each stop but the cat stayed put until this time. Amazing! This cat also fell from the first floor window cill and I thought it would clearly be hurt, but no, it landed with all four paws on to the of the fence between us and our neighbour who is referenced again in the back of this narrative under 'it's a small world'

Our doctor lived a short walk round the corner from our house and we were regular visitors and we knew that he closed on a Thursday evening but unfortunately illness does not understand. One Thursday about June I had a severe headache apparently similar to one the previous year. My mother decided to prepare a hot poultice and placed it around my ear whilst singing 'up came the nurse with the red hot poultice, slapped it on and took no notice, oh said the patient that's too hot, oh said the nurse I'm sure it's not'. I seem to remember that my aunt and uncle from Canada were visiting at that time, anyway the poultice did not help and I got shooting pains from my temple up to the top of my head about every few minutes. This meant that I was walked to the doctor's house with a scarf around my head where the notice on the door told us where the partner was that night. This was a Dr Hutton Ash Kelly with a practice at the top of Greyhound Lane. We walked the mile to the Doctor's and waited to be seen. We had only been in his Surgery for a short time when he had hurried words with my mother and started to make phone calls. These seemed to go on for ever and get more frustrating but at last he told my mother that she had to take me to ETN Hospital in Greys Inn road in London. We walked the mile plus back home packed a suitcase and walked the almost half mile to Streatham Common Station boarded a train and somehow got to Holborn. Here we got a taxi to the hospital. On arrival we were apparently expected and nurses and a surgeon took us immediately to the operating theatre. Once there they administered Gas to put me out. The next thing that happened was all the lights went over the operating table. No panic, the doctor found a screwdriver and fuse wire and hey presto the lights came on. Again the next thing I remember is the doctor asking the nurse which ward I was going to and he would get a trolley. The nurse said I was to be taken to the Men's ward at the end of the corridor. The Doctor then took me in his arms and said that he would carry me there.

Next morning when I told the nurse my story she was distraught as she thought I might have been awake throughout the operation. During my stay the man in the bed next to mine taught me to play Chess, which was good and helped compensate for the fact that every four hours on the dot day and night I had an injection of Penicillin. My father worked in the road next to the hospital and visited, out of the blue, either before or after a shift. We had planned to go on our very first ever holiday two weeks after I had gone into hospital and they were not ready to discharge until they were convinced that my fraternal aunt was a qualified nurse and could care for me. The holiday was a great success.

My parents were regular churchgoers and I met a number of boys and girls after the service and we walked back to the various houses dropping off someone at each stop. The first stop was in Runnymede Crescent where my future wife lived (not interested at the time). I did however meet a close friend who was to share sport and holidays with me for many years. Chris Bruton, had a twin sister who was a good friend of Margaret's, gave us a painting as a wedding present many years later and we still have that in the family and still communicate with Margaret Bruton.

This friendship meant that I cycled from my house to his Council Estate regularly and on Thursday's in the winter we played pick up football on the green. We often met the Tooting and Mitcham side as they could not train at the own pitch and when they had finished formal practice they would often join us in a big pick up match which usually went on until it was too dark to continue.

When I was 11 a new scout group was opened in my old primary school which I joined and progressed to Troop Patrol

Leader. Whilst on various events including the St Georges Day Parade in Hyde Park in London I met a scout who lived up the road in Streatham Vale (more in a later chapter). I met the director of the Gang Show when it was moved to Battersea Town Hall and he was later to write some sketches for our groups Christmas Show and help us produce it. The scenery was painted by a friend of the group. Parents obtained reels of the destination boards from the local Bus Station which were stitched together before being painted. In the show I played several different parts and when the family came to see it they said that it was a success.

It was also at this time that I passed my eleven-plus and obtained a place at Clapham College. My elder brother was already there and my twin brother also joined me. Mick was not to find the grammar school to his liking and our parents arranged with the authorities for him to leave early and take up an apprenticeship in Printing Papermaking and Bookbinding in which he was to be very successful. I completed the course to GCE

My father worked part-time at the local newsagents and one day he said he was going to buy the weekly newspaper called Ice Hockey World on a sale or return basis. This meant that he would stand outside Streatham Ice Rink on a Wednesday night before the match to sell and again after if he had not sold out. Most weeks two or three of us boys used to go along to help and shout 'Ice Hockey World, don't forget your Ice hockey, Ice Hockey World' to which late in the season we would add the words 'and annual'. This must have been quite successful as we got the franchise to all of the London rinks and two of us boys would travel across London by tube from

Tooting to Harringay, Wembley or Earls Court. This only stopped when the league ceased and the rinks felt they made more profit from skating than they did from staging ice hockey matches.

Sunday afternoons in the summer often meant that I went out on a cycle ride with a friend who lived at the top of Streatham Common. We used to ride randomly in any direction for about anything from 15 to 25 miles and stop at a common or park for a little while and then ride home in time for tea. One year we had 13 pleasant Sundays in a row which nobody today seems to think possible. In the winter one year we had a friend of Pat's (Peter Bonthrone) visit on Sundays and sometimes his brother to play Monopoly, this could be one game carried over from one week to the next.

Going to school meant getting a train from the station to Balham and changing onto the tube to Clapham South and it was about 100 odd yards from there. Starting at the College meant taking or avoiding the induction ceremony administered by the elder boys, being introduced to your form master and then taken to the Physics and Chemistry Laboratories to be acquainted with the layout. We also had a geography room and Gym but all other lessons the teacher came to our form room. When the teacher came in we were expected to be quiet and to stand to attention by our desks until the teacher had settled and advised us to sit down. The teachers were strict and punishment could be administered on the spot, e.g. a chalk board rubber thrown at your head or a thwack across the hands with a monitor or by being sent to the Headmaster. Going to the Headmaster could result in the cane across the backside or a long wait outside his office, only to be dismissed to return next morning. Next morning you would either be caned or let off. I always liked school but will cover my time there in the next chapter.

CHAPTER FOUR

144 Topsham Road

We were rehoused to Topsham Road in Tooting I think in early 1952 but it could have been earlier. We did not exactly choose the location but the system for rehousing Council Tenants was to offer them a viewing of a premises and if you did not like it you would be offered a further viewing.

This could happen only three times and the belief was that the third viewing would always be the worst, so we took the second which was, in fact, very nice but not in a location of our choice.

I had saved up some money and decided to buy a Coronet Box camera which was in a sale in the photographic shop over the road. Later I went to evening classes to learn how to develop and print my own films and my cousin's husband helped me to make an enlarger which gave me lots of pleasure and satisfaction, as did tinting the prints to provide colour.

I was involved in athletics at school and as Tooting Bec track was within walking or running distance of the house I started to go on Tuesday and Thursday evenings and Sunday mornings. I joined a club and met some good athletes like Gordon Pirie who let us join in his training routines. I did middle distance running and the High Jump. My best height was 5 feet 3 and a half inches and I did a 2 minute timed half mile and my best mile was on grass at the Midland Bank Ground when I recorded 4 Minutes 43 Seconds. I was part of the college team in the Wandsworth school sports but my best results came after I left school, so more details later.

School went quite well and I was always in the top ten of a class of 32. This was despite the fact that I usually got single digit marks for Latin and French. I did well at all the maths and art but could not sing a note. Our class were in general very poor at chemistry and we stopped English literature in order to spend more time on English language.

In 1952 the king died and Princess Elizabeth acceded to the throne. For the coronation day my father obtained Press passes for the occasion and we were given a 'Reveille' each to pretend we were selling but to definitely not let it out of our hands. We walked along the front of the crowds in The Mall and saw the procession close up. Because there were such big crowds we found it easier to walk the five miles or so back home in the early evening.

When I completed the fourth year I was expected to have good results in the GCE's but things changed that year. Mick started his apprenticeship and started to earn money and Pat also was going out to work. My uncle Ted with the support of the Balham Church started a Youth Club who were destined to have meetings at our house and I got involved in helping to produce a club magazine, this involved me in cutting stencils for a Gestetner machine both by hand and with a very Old Royal Typewriter (very time consuming). These side attractions did not help me concentrate on my studies which went backwards rather than forwards. I did leave the scouts to give more time for study but it did not seem to be effective. Just about my sixteenth birthday I decided that I had to get a job arranged before the exam results were published. I originally wanted to become an apprentice architect but would have needed a pass in Technical Drawing and this was not taught and it was too late to do a crash course. I then felt that I would like to go into a Bank and wrote to each of the Big Five asking for an interview. The result was that it was fairly easy to get the interview but if you passed it the next step was to do some form of exam. Nat West made me sit a modern (for that time) aptitude test which took a good hour. Midland Bank asked me to attend for a full day to complete three exams each over about 90 minutes. Two in the morning and one after having lunched in the staff canteen. This was then to be marked, but to our horror, (there were about 20 odd attendees), we were advised that the 6 with best combined results would be offered a position and some of the others might be allowed to come back a couple of weeks later and try again on the same terms. I got an invite to try again. I was invited to take a Company medical at both of these companies but after well over a month as I had heard no more from them I applied to Martins Bank. Here I had an interview a test and a medical within three days. The following Saturday I received a formal job offer from both Martins and Nat West. Big problem. I wanted to go to Nat West because they had an excellent sports ground only three miles away in Norbury and a great record for supporting average to good athletes. I eventually settled for accepting the Martins Bank Offer as they had been so much more efficient. This proved to be a good decision and I was assigned to the Foreign Branch in the city of London in Gracechurch Street.

Starting out to work was quite daunting and you had to get to work on time and as the six new entrants each year had to run the post room this meant being in before the regular 9 o'clock start and staying on until the mail was all franked and taken to the Post Office , often nearer 6 o'clock. I soon enrolled into evening classes at the City of London College in order to pass the Institute of Bankers exams. This turned out to be three evenings a week from 7-9pm. The exams were divided into Part 1 and Part 2. Each part had five subjects but you were only allowed to take and pass three before going forward to the next stage. I stayed with Martins for 7 years before moving on to First National City Bank of New York and that year completed all of Part 1.

During my time at Martins I helped start a Table Tennis Club and we joined the Business League which had matches after work in local business premises and an Athletics Club who competed alongside the Big Banks at meetings, mainly at Motspur Park in Surrey. We also arranged three sided matches with other Banks and Clubs like Blackheath & Greenwich. There was a football team playing in the Banks League which was played on Saturday afternoons after work. I felt that I was lucky to have selected Martins Bank as they rotated their Staff for the first few years around the various departments and I learnt Foreign Exchange, which in those days covered checking import/export restrictions, Bank of England weekly and monthly returns (aggregate total of imports and exports handled split down by country and currency and commodity). I moved on to Cheque clearing in the mid-morning and early afternoon which was divided into large town clearing for all amounts of large denominations for taking to the Clearing House by 3.25pm for clearance the same day and an ordinary clearing which we picked up and balanced in the Clearing House at 8.30 the following morning. I moved on to the Bills department and learnt about the documents for Imports and Exports including what special needs the various Countries Embassies required with regard to Bills of Lading, Certified invoices etc. This experience stood me in good staid for moving to an American Bank when they started expanding in London.

The Youth Club went from strength to strength with Mick and Ted running the Committee and Pat as Captain of the football team. We purchased an Adana Printing press and apart from printing our own 'you have been selected to play' postcards we supplied them at a very small profit to other clubs in the League. We printed letterheads and Dance tickets and 8 x 5 flyers. We played our matches on Sunday afternoons and were able to get most of our best players who had been called up for National Service to get a 36 or 48 hour pass and they could return on the Sunday to report back to the coaches that departed from Wembley in the late evening. We won the league most years and many cups and in fact one year we won the league and all the cups. The prizes were presented at the Catholic Hall at the Oval and that was the first time I went home feeling ill on beer after we had filled the cups with Babycham and several pints of Bass or Red Barrel.

We had a Parents Day at the Club in Balham and spent all morning setting up equipment for the music, table tennis, judo and dancing in the evening. We stopped for a break and had a cup of tea in the church presbytery. When we went back to check all was ready we found that the expensive audio equipment that we had borrowed had been stolen. We managed to get some replacements and the event went off without further hitches. After this Pat and I got together and he suggested we ran a dance and make a profit to pay for the lost audio equipment. It was quite a large sum so I agreed to go to the Priest at the Church Hall in Clapham and try to get him to rent us the Hall at a peppercorn rent for the following Valentines weekend. To my surprise he helped out and Pat got a Band on the cheap with the sob story from a friend. This band played for us on a number of occasions later.

The dance itself was a great success after we printed posters and tickets and visited all the clubs around to tell them why they should come and support our cause.

An outcome of this was that I was to become a regular M.C. and organised dances for our own and some other clubs. We got very ambitious ourselves and rented the Streatham Baths and the Syd Phillips Band. We got the local pub to provide two bars at the venue with the agreement that if it was successful they would give us a donation. Pat kept all the accounts and we made a small profit. Later we ran further Dances at the Baths and got money up front from the pub as they had obviously done very well. I remember that we had Ronnie Scott before he went to the 51 Club and a modern jazz group called Tommy Whittle.

Staying with the Youth Club we entered the Wandsworth Youth Clubs sports and won the event at Battersea Park and I seemed as captain to run in every event, under and over eighteen Mile, 880 yards, high jump and relay. At this point we were neck and neck and only one event to go, the 3 mile. We only had one volunteer but even if he won we were not sure to win overall. I talked a member into running but he insisted I ran with him. We won the race and Mike and I came in side by side, both gaining further points to confirm our win. I remember finishing and trotting to where my family were on the side-lines and collapsing quite exhausted next to my father and his comment was that is how you should finish every race if you want to excel. On a different occasion I was running second part way into the last lap of a mile at Tooting Bec track and needing to accelerate but feeling somewhat lethargic when a man appeared through the trees at the back of the track and I heard 'Come on son'. Right! That was my father and I did win the race. At the Presentation (after my rupture) I felt an absolute fraud as I limped over to the Mayor using a walking stick to collect the trophy.

Parents were always very supportive and my mother used to come over to the common on various Sundays but I especially remember when all three boys played in the same team (a rare happening) both mum and dad gave us full support. I also recall being taken to hospital for stitches to one eye and later making a difficult save clearing the ball too quickly and realising I had hurt myself. This turned out to be the Rupture that when operated on kept me out of National Service. This was instrumental in my not pursuing athletics for greater success which could have been assisted by a spell in the forces.

The cousin I mentioned who lived with us until we were bombed out stayed in London to finish his exams and although we heard from him after we left Manchester and were given a bike from his sister we did not seem to meet. A quick aside, I taught myself to ride on that bike. I got up earlier one morning determined to ride, I set the bike up in the kerb and pushed off and cycled totally pleased with myself until I got to the bottom of the road when I found out I had no idea how to turn the corner. I carried on and hit the wire fence to the prefab and sailed over it into the garden. No real problems and low and behold I could now ride. I do not recall meeting my cousin until he started visiting my mother fairly regularly in Topsham Road. We were invited to his wedding to Pam which involved the usual family party and the party pieces. This was one of the first times I was introduced to 'Marching with the band', 'The old fashion razor', 'The pessimistic character with the crab apple face', 'The inside is quite new' and 'the coon song'. My father did this last number as he said he could not sing and then recited what is definitely taboo today.

This is how it went:

> Coon-Coon-Coon how I wish I were a different shade
>
> Coon-Coon-Coon how I wish my colour would fade
>
> How I wish I were a white man and not a Coon, Coon, COON!!!!!

Back to my cousin. When leaving the house he always ask my mother if there was anything he could do for her and she always said no I am alright. Then one day my dream came true and my mother said 'Oh yes, Terry is absolutely mad keen to learn to drive a car. Maybe you could teach him'.

We started lessons on my 17th birthday in February in a Morris Minor (split screen I think) and booked a driving test for mid-June. Unfortunately at the last minute we had to cancel as his car was run into at a crossroads. We arranged an early booking at the end of July when I was lucky enough to pass first time.

This led on to me wanting to buy a car and I obtained a Saturday and Sunday evening Potman's job in Camberwell where my uncle worked, This paid 10 shillings each night and I calculated that I saved by not going out on weekend evenings. This meant that about my 18th birthday I had 50 pounds to buy a car. I looked at a nice Austin Ruby Seven but when I went home on the test drive all the family laughed as I unwound out and towered above it. To my lasting regret I gave up on it and bought an Austin 1934 12/4. This was good car but several things used to go wrong and it was expensive to maintain. The Ruby would have been better and cheaper. After about 18 months and many trips to the coast and dances etc. I had to replenish my wardrobe. This meant selling the car for 35 pounds and buying socks, shirts and shoes. I had had lots of pleasure from this car but the most memorable times were the problems. We were coming back from Southend when all the lights went out and although I thought I had gone on in a straight line I was almost touching the outside of the dual carriageway. I arrived in Brighton and pulled up quickly at a pedestrian crossing and we lost all electrics; the battery under the seat had lost a lead. I took my family to Fontwell races and as was usual in those days a lot

39

of cars broke down on Bury Hill. Whilst we were waiting for the police to sort it out, a Rolls Royce driver left his seat and opened the boot and removed a hamper. This contained a bottle of champagne which he proceeded to open and share with the occupants of his and a car two or three places behind him. He also offered a glass to the policeman who politely refused.

When I was 18 my father said that I could join him at that lunchtime in the William IV pub over the road where he would buy me my first alcoholic drink. In those days for most boys this really was their first. He told me I would not like the Light and Bitter that he was drinking but a better introduction was to have a Mackeson Stout. It was not long before I was also drinking L & B and playing darts. We bought a dart board and my friend's father made an excellent proper cupboard and we fitted this above the fireplace in the front room. This was often used after committee meetings and also on Sunday afternoons after lunch. There were a lot of Sunday afternoons when the Drawing room had two Solo card schools going and maybe others playing darts. We might on other occasions play cribbage and maybe chess particularly with my mother. We converted the mahogany leaf to the dining table into a very efficient Shove-Halfpenny board which we kept in top order by polishing it regularly with French polish. Mum was an expert at this and the story goes that when she and dad were on holiday in Somerset they put down their sixpence by the board to play the previous winner. The gentleman mum played had been on the board all evening winning sixpences. When she beat him and further players she was told that he was the County champion and always earnt his beer money but not that night apparently.

Our involvement with the Youth Club football team meant that most Mondays my mother would wash eleven shirts and pairs of socks ready for the next week. Sometimes when the water was either iced up or not working on Tooting Bec Common the whole of the team would trudge back to our house and get most of the mud off both boots and body before using the bath in turn.

Pat became quite good at darts and managed to get into the pub team at Clapham Common. He played in an eight man team and I understood that he often had only three darts at the board in the first straight eight and if he did not get a 60 he was not sure to be picked the next week. One Friday I remember he asked if I would like to join him and visit the pub for a drink and a game of darts. We totalled up how much money we had between us and decided that we had the fare each way, enough for two beers each and two sixpences for playing pairs. This format was similar to when my mother played shove-halfpenny. In this pub there was a couple of older ladies who were renowned for winning and drinking halves of Guinness. We lost both of our games and were still early in the evening so Pat said we could have another try but if we lost would have to walk the three miles home as we would be using our return bus fares. He was good and I managed some scores on the sixteens and guess what, we stayed on the board for most of the evening and had an extra pint and a bus home.

A friend of the family and a school friend ran a bring-and-buy shop at Clapham Common, which I used to visit regularly. He started a new venture and sold purpose made golf clubs. This entailed him fixing the required head to the club and then measuring the shaft to fit the individual. When he had cut the shaft to size I had the job of gluing the leather grip to the top of the shaft. He did well for a while but I think it became easier to get this type of service from a sports equipment shop. Golf shops or Pro shops did not exist at that time.

The Streatham Church opened an over 18's club at the side of the Thrale Hotel where we met once a week. It started about 7pm and for about an hour we would play games and then go over the Pub for a quick pint. On return the club room was set up with music for dancing and we did this until about 10 or half past when we went home, either directly or if lucky via one of the girls houses for a coffee and then home. This club used to organise coach outings and I remember several times going to Climping Bay near Littlehampton. In those days there was no Car Park or Café on the beach and our coach dropped us off on the A259 and we walked past the Black Horse Pub down to the sea with instructions to meet the coach at a fixed time in the early evening. We always had a Priest and several adults in attendance to make sure the party stayed totally respectable. One weekend the Priest was away and he said that I could borrow his car and take a car load out for a day to the coast. We arrived at Pevensey Bay after nearly rolling the car when the person who said he knew the way called an extremely late left turn when we were only just in front of a heavy lorry and travelling at nearly 70mph. The day went well from then on.

My friend Adrian and I decided as we had not arranged a holiday that we would try and cycle round Holland, Belgium and some of France. We cycled to Liverpool Street Station on a Friday evening. Travelled to Harwich and slept on the overnight ferry to the Hook of Holland. Our plan from thereon was to cycle in the mornings. Stop for a snack lunch and sightsee in the afternoon before finding a Hostel for the night. We were members of the YHA and the Catholic equivalent. The other aim was to have a very nice meal each evening. In the YHA we had to be back before 10 o'clock but not until 11pm in the Catholic Hostels. We cycled to The Hague, Amsterdam, Rotterdam, Utrect, and Chaam in Holland. Our first serious problem came in Turnout when we tried to change Martins Bank Travellers Cheques in the local bank. The Cashier told us he could not cash Midland Bank Cheques as there was a problem with counterfeit cheques. We tried to explain that Martins and Midland were two different Banks and eventually after calling my London Office they agreed to cash some of our cheques. All seemed O K until about an hour later a lad came cycling past and accosted us. He was the Cashier from the Bank and he told us he had not completed the transactions with the full documentation and could we return to complete it. Although amazed we did as requested. This town did not seem to like us as when we tried to enter a good restaurant in the evening the Head Waiter, seeing us in Jeans and Jumpers and being foreign visitors he thought we might not have enough money and were not dressed appropriately. We had propped our bikes against his window and told him we liked his menu and showed him our cash. He reluctantly ushered us to a hidden corner table and then gave us first class service and a very good meal. No more problems passing through, Antwerp, Brussels and Ghent where we saw the early work on the new Basilica. We left Ghent in heavy rain and where they were building the new Motorways we took a wrong turn and actually finished up on the Motorway. A lorry driver put his head out of his cab window and yelled at us until we realised what we had done. We stopped at the next township and climbed over the barriers into the town/village. We had not been able to change money in Ghent so our first aim was to find a Bank. We ask the locals but communication was not easy. One resident then started shouting 'English, English' and several people appeared from their houses and they were over excited to meet us. By the time we stopped them enthusing we found out that the Bank had shut just a minute ago. We were then invited to have tea in one of the houses and were introduced to local pipe tobacco (which half killed Adrian), his racing pigeons and Belgium cake. This cake could be served at any meal and kept for several days as a cold delicacy which we struggled with and Adrian managed to feed his to the dog. We left late in the day with no Belgium money and a thought we might cycle as far as France as we had French Francs and English money. We got as far Dirksmuide and it was dark and we were very hungry. We entered a local pub and enquired for food and drink. The answer was first that they would not go near French Francs under any circumstances and could not cash pounds. We were downcast but the Owner told us not to leave and asked if Ham and eggs on two slices of bread would sound nice. We showed him the few coins we had in local money and he said O K. He asked the man in the corner if he could go to his bakery and bring over a small fresh loaf and we were given a meal that felt to us 'fit for a king' and for about one and sixpence we had that and a full pot of tea and were waved on our way. We arrived at Dunkirk Railway Station at about two thirty in the morning and received very different hospitality. No hotel answered their night bell so we flagged down a Police car for help and while my foot was still on his running board he told us 'What did we expect' and put his foot on the accelerator. We stayed in the waiting room at the station until the café opened at 6 0'clock. We travelled on to Gravelines and found a bed for a few hours before travelling to Calais and the ferry home. We cycled from Dover and having gone 440 miles got back 8 days later in time for a dance at the Youth Club.

Another time saw us holiday in Gorleston and while playing darts in the knockout tournament we came up against pair called Johnnie Bennett and Paddy Lightfoot who we discovered played in Paddy's brother's Jazz band. We struck up a good friendship back in London and we went to many gigs where they played and were about when they left Terry's band and joined the newly formed Kenny Ball Jazz Band. Our long weekends and often late Wednesday evenings started to take their toll and one Monday morning I realised that it was more important for me to arrive awake and ready for work if my future was to blossom so at that point I decided to stop going out so often and concentrate on my career.

Another pastime that we indulged in was dirt track racing. This was done on specially stripped down bikes with wide handlebars and no gearing and usually fixed wheel. It was based on speedway but although there were some purpose made tracks e.g. at the park in Morden, we prepared our own track in the disused bombed out site in Hackbridge. We joined a club at the Castle Pub in Tooting where on a Sunday morning they converted most of their car park into a track, and we competed in a local league. We did not use our regular bikes but collected old parts from the local dump to both make, repair and improve our models. This getting things from the dump was taken to quite an extreme when my cousin in Morden with a mate collected enough parts to build a small motorbike. He felt forced into this as his father would not buy him a new bike for his birthday. His father was so afraid that he would hurt himself on this contraption that he then went and bought him a new Triumph 250cc. He was mad keen on this but unfortunately he died a year later in an accident at a crossroads near Blackfriars Bridge.

My next big event was mine and my twin brother's 21st birthday. We booked a hall invited about 100 relatives and friends and arranged to provide our own food and music. The food was done by a cousin who was in the trade and the music came from borrowed turntables and speakers. On the day I hired a Van to collect all the food drink and other gear. The party was great as were all of those family parties in those days. At the end of the day I ran the van as a ferry service to take local guests home and just my luck I parked badly alongside Wandsworth Common and inadvertently turned the lights off. Yes at 1.30 in the morning a Police car pulled up next to us and ask us what was going on. Well they looked into the back and saw a couple of guests and various Shirts, socks etc. that were some of my birthday presents. We tried to explain we had not robbed the locals and that we were waiting for a chap to come back from saying goodnight to his girlfriend. After a little while when the lad came back we were cautioned to be more careful in future and sent on our way with a cheery goodnight and drive safe.

With the monies I had received as presents and by selling some Premium Bonds to my brother I gathered together enough money to buy a Lambretta Scooter which later I sold and bought a DKW 200 cc motorbike from a friend of Pat's who was emigrating to America.

I cannot be sure which year it was but my mother slipped a disc about early December and we took the door off one of the rooms and laid it on Pat's bed in the small bedroom as this was the only treatment known to us at the time. This was obviously not comfortable and also very boring so we as a family decided to rent a small television set and fix it up on the top of the wardrobe where she could see it. We continued renting televisions at Topsham Road until my mother died. Anyway, mum was not recovered by Christmas and it fell to me to cook the Christmas dinner while the rest of the family went over the pub. Having spent most of the time running up and down stairs for instructions the dinner was served about 3 o'clock as was usual. I had passed my first cooking lesson. I think there were 7-8 at the meal. I think that it was this year that I started to make a Christmas flower arrangement which I did for several years.

The months after my birthday started well with both of my brothers either engaged or to become engaged to be married. And then for some reason one Wednesday evening Pat and I went to a social evening at the new Youth Club at the Catholic Church in Norbury. When we returned home we found out that our father had come home from work feeling unwell and had experienced double vision and a doctor had been called. Not long after we got home he was taken to hospital and when we visited him he was numb down one side and could not speak to us. Using eyes and one hand he gave us his blessing and we left for the night. Things did not get better and he was transferred to the Atkinson Morley specialist hospital. By Saturday morning the doctors felt they had identified the problem and arranged for some form of surgery to be done at 1 o'clock but sadly at about 11 o'clock he died before anything else could be done. Pat took over and I used my new motor scooter to transport him to Insurance and Council offices and the Co-op funeral directors.

Later in the year at the same Youth Club in Norbury I danced with Margaret and escorted her home at the end of the evening. The rest is history as we have now been married over fifty years.

Both the weddings were planned and after a very short discussion we decided that they should go ahead as planned. The three girls got on very well and Margaret was a bridesmaid at both events. I proposed to Margaret before Christmas 1960 prior to both weddings.

As mentioned earlier I made a conscious effort to improve my lot in life and in April 1962 after several interviews I started a new job with First National City Bank of New York in Old Broad Street. I was lucky enough to be given several job offers but chose this one as there was to be no commitment to move and work abroad written into the contract. My new boss told me they did not need to put it into the contract as it would never be refused because of the obvious perks for the employee and his family. As it transpired I was more interested in bringing up my family in England and being with them it was many years before I even travelled abroad on company business.

I still played for Balham Youth Club on Sundays until I was to leave Topsham Road for my next stage in life. I also played for the College Old Boys on a Saturday and used my Motor Scooter to give lifts to other players. My most frequent passenger was a John McGowan who lived in Streatham Vale with his family which included his sister Cathy (a known pop singer) who co-incidentally was a good friend of Margaret's sister, Mary.

Margaret worked at Boot's Booklovers Library and enjoyed it very much until it was merged with W H Smith's Library and she was originally offered the Librarian's job at this point. What happened next was that the Smith's manager came to Boot's and brought his old librarian with him and turned out to be somewhat of a bullying type and none of the original boot's staff enjoyed the new regime and many left including Margaret after I got her an interview with Pratts (The John Lewis Store). This was not a great success but lasted until she gave birth to our first child, Christine, in June 1964.

We agreed that we would make our first home with my mother and proceeded to identify and buy furniture for when we moved in. The first item we found was the bed and then from Limelight Furniture Co a bedroom suite. We then found a dining room suite with gate leg table and cocktail cabinet for the front room. We had spotted this in a tally shop at the top of Brixton Hill and it seemed too expensive so we went to Croydon and found the same for a mere 50 odd guineas instead of the 63 in Brixton. This set me thinking and I went all over the suite until I found the maker's name and when I looked them up I found that their warehouse was in Hackney Road and that I could get there in my lunch break. This was the start of another success story. When I got there the place was in chaos and the owner explained that they were moving premises to a warehouse in the new town of Basildon in Essex. He told me that I could buy the suite with the best uncut moquette at £35 and have the choice of any in the factory at the time. The problem, of course was that he could not do business at that time and told me I should bring my prospective bride on the back of my motorcycle to see him in his new premises two weeks later. On arrival I introduced Margaret to this very nice Jewish proprietor. We picked out a suite and agreed the price which still seemed too good to be true but what next! He asked if we had found any other furniture and that if we had he would purchase it on our behalf and then pass it on to us with a 33% discount on the retail price. I told him we had already ordered the bed but only identified the rest. He said no worry he could arrange it all and would keep it in his warehouse until nearer the wedding which would give me time to decorate and lay carpets. He was as good as his word and when we had

50

settled with him he asked to ensure that if I had friends getting married I would put them in touch with him for a similar deal. I did this and several friends were very happy. Many years later he wrote with sincere apologies, that as times were hard, he could not continue my deal and was sorry but he would have to reduce my discount to a mere 25%.

Our wedding took place in June 1963 and this was arranged as was traditional then by the bride's father and took place in St Bartholomew's Church in Norbury with the reception in the Sussex Tavern just up the road. I hired one of the fairly new Mini's for a two week stay in Cornwall at the Bederuthen Steps Hotel in Newquay. This was the first time either of us had been away for a whole two weeks. We stopped on the Saturday of the wedding at a B & B Farm in Somerset on the way as the roads did not allow us to travel the whole journey without an overnight stop. We had a pub lunch in Exeter and looked around the Cathedral. The lunch was my favourite at the time; a full mixed grill which consisted of Steak, Chop, Kidney, Gammon Bacon, Sausage, Tomato, chips and veg and to this day I cannot recall a better mixed Grill. The first week was brilliant weather following the wedding day, which was the hottest day of that year. The highlight was our trip by plane from Penzance to the Silly Isles, the plane took about 13 passengers, a Pilot and a Stewardess and we were not allowed to sit together as everyone was weighed and seated appropriately to properly balance the load. The second week was a washout and in truth a waste of time and money. The highlight was probably the journey from Falmouth to the Hotel across Dartmoor as we had our heads out of the car window to identify the kerb or the middle of the road through the thick fog. We just made it in time for dinner. Our return was on the Summer Solstice and we visited Stonehenge where parking was easy with no crowds or tourist restrictions. Once inside the stones we found that the Druids were part way through some ceremony and they offered us what appeared to be unleven bread from a pewter plate, a lovely break in the long all day trip back to South London.

Before the baby arrived we enjoyed what we called ear-holing round the countryside on Sunday afternoons which involved finding a pub and sharing a drink and a packet of crisps. We also had the occasional treat of eating out after Margaret finished work on a Saturday. This consisted of going to the local café and having a main type meal before going home. We met friends and spent evenings playing music which was supplied by the guests and we shared cups of tea or coffee. Sundays usually consisted of a roast lunch cooked by my mother and assisted (in a learning capacity) by Margaret. This has held her in good stead throughout the rest of our marriage including excellent Christmas puddings and mince pies to die for. After our engagement I managed to find the time to decorate mum's house and make the front room into a cosy lounge where we were to spend many happy evenings. We continued when possible to go to as many dances as possible including trips to The Locano Streatham, The Orchid Ballroom Purley and various youth club venues. We managed to have several trips to the London Theatres seeing some of the big Musicals (Flower Drum Song, Starlight Express and My Fair Lady and at later dates included Evita, West Side Story, Most Happy Fella, Oliver, Fiddler on the Roof, and Miss Saigon and Cats.).

Our house was behind the sweet shop on the high and they were very well known for their coconut ice. This was made in the factory on the other side of the road to us and was carried past our side entrance to the shop. The lads who cut the blocks of coconut ice had to cut away the rough edges around the large blocks before they cut the smaller blocks and as they passed, if we were in the garden, they would pass the offcuts to us. Unfortunately the husband, Mr Crawford died and after this his wife was asked to sell the recipe to the known Company of Crawford and Crawford. Mrs Crawford refused and said she would rather destroy the recipe and true to her word when she sold the shop she did indeed destroy the recipe.

At around this time I became interested in collecting foreign coins and arranged to import some full sets and some 5 dollar coins from the new release of Bahamian coins that were being introduced with the change of currency from sterling to dollars. This was not a great success as when they arrived several of those people who had ordered the coins told me that they could not now afford them. I sold some and kept the rest (more later). I also bought new releases of English Crowns ensuring that I got four of each as it was our intention to have four children and they have one each on an appropriate occasion. Why we settled for five children will be made clear later.

After Christine was born it soon became apparent that living with my mother could not go on for too long and the search for our next home became a priority. We were very lucky as at this time the London County Council made an offer to all second generation family members who were willing to leave London and settle elsewhere to apply for a 100% mortgage. My brother Mick and I decided that this was an opportunity not to be missed although it was a 25 year fixed term fixed interest rate at well over bank rate. Pat has told me the rate was over 6% but I always thought it was more and Bank rate was only 4%. The crux of the matter was that I could borrow up to 4 and a half times my salary for under £17 per month. Mick found work and a house near Maidstone but this was not good for me as the time and cost of commuting into the City was too costly and exhaustive. One day however I found an advert for some new build semi-detached houses to be built in Milton Regis, just outside of Sittingbourne. They were a modern two up two down property a lounge and kitchen/diner on the ground floor and two bedrooms and a bathroom upstairs, no garage, an eight foot front garden and 26ft back garden on the long side. The total width of the land was about 24ft and the house from back to front less than 30ft. Pat had a car at this time and said he would come over from Thornton Heath and take me to view the site on the next weekend. The trip was very satisfactory until Pat got a speeding ticket on the way back as we were hurrying to ensure we were not late for lunch.

I started the ball rolling and signed up with the Council and on the dotted line with the builders. I did not have a penny in savings and decided to look for weekend or evening work. I am not too sure nowadays how I managed but I discovered that moving and getting started in the house would cost around £100 and that I would need a further £100 for the solicitor.

When the time drew close for completion I was still broke but had probably the best bit of good fortune ever in that I won £100 on the Church Sweepstake. When the solicitor needed paying a German colleague in the office heard of my plight and took pity on me and bought some of my coin collection for, guess what, £100!

Now our first real move and our own home!!

CHAPTER FIVE

22 Dobbie Close

Great expectations but then to the reality of moving house. Has one ever passed without at least one certain trauma, let me begin with our first. The removals van came to Topsham Road and loaded our belongings and we were then to proceed to Margaret's parent's to collect further items. The driver ask me for directions as he did not know the area and I proudly started directing him. What's this he said in horror when he saw the low bridge sign, I said I did not think it was very low and that his van would pass through it; the driver's mate got out to take a look and seemed to agree with me. Well sufficient to say we did get under the bridge but with barely 3 inches to spare and a considerable delay. We got on our way with Margaret, Christine and I sharing the cab with the removals men for the journey.

When the removals men saw our new property their first comment was that it was small and modern and that most of our furniture destined to go upstairs would not make it up the narrow wall staircase and then turn at the top. As usual these people knew what they were talking about but in our case they were also not without initiative. They found out that the builders were still on site and that a glazier was present. A polite request for help and the upstairs front window glass was removed and the removals then took place in what seemed no time. The glazier was recalled and replaced the window and said he was pleased he could help and would not take any money for a beer.

Shattered but happy to be settling in we eventually put Christine to bed and were able to make a cup of tea and sit side by side on our bed settee in the lounge.

Getting to work meant leaving the house at just after 7 and walking the mile and a bit to Sittingboune Station to catch the 7.25 to London.

I worked a five and a half day week in those days and decided to play football for the company team which meant we could meet up after work on the Saturday and travel together on the tube to Northolt for home games and make other arrangements for away games. I also trained with the Sittingbourne Colts team on our local recreation ground on Thursday evenings and did get one game with them in the winter we lived in Milton Regis. This was memorable as once again I was to finish up in hospital. I played left back on the day and just before half time our very athletic goalkeeper managed to pull the ball down from between the opposing forward's head and mine. Our heads collided and we were both in an ambulance on the way to the Isle of Sheppey hospital quite quickly. The doctor was a Pakistani and listening intently to a transistor radio to the proceedings in the war out there with particular regard to hearing about his family. He took a look at my eye and said he would have to stitch it up, apologised that he would keep his radio on but also said that he would do a much better job than the doctor who had stitched my other eye up. He was true to his word and I was back at the Eastleigh Prison Pitch in time to board the coach back home.

Early recollections of this time include when we bought a Baby Burco, for the uninitiated this was a simple boiler which you could put on the draining board and plug in to the power supply to allow you to boil nappies etc. in real boiling water and not carry on scrubbing and rubbing in a sink. This might seem strange but washing machines were a new innovation and far too expensive; it was to be several years before we hit these heights The actual immediate pleasure of buying this Baby Burco was the pleasure Christine had playing with the empty cardboard box in the garden, this gave us lots of fun.

One of the first things I and two neighbours decided to do was build a base each for future purchase of a garage. We arranged to have ballast and cement delivered on Easter Thursday for the weekend. All went well until we got up on the Friday morning to find that it was snowing and three bases in two days looked a very long shot. The snow stopped fairly early in the morning and we started to mix the concrete by hand and barrow it to the first pre-prepared base area. This base was for my next door neighbour and was for a double length garage 24ft x 8ft. The next two bases were only 16ft x 8ft and by late Saturday we had completed the job. Totally exhausted we felt we deserved a pint and gathering together the pennies we had between us we found we had enough for a pint each and a little bit extra. We bought the three pints and approached the fruit machine with the extra coins. Our lucky weekend, we got three of a kind and we felt that we must now have a further celebratory drink or two. My mother was visiting at that time and when I got home after eleven o'clock she asked me to throw my hat in first. I knew I should be in trouble but both she and Margaret accepted the explanation and I was sound asleep within a very short time.

Christine was becoming the usual difficult child and Margaret and I shared the night duties but I always did Saturday's as I did not have to get up for work early the next morning but we played the problems by ear and how we felt and our recent successes with coping with her persistent crying episodes. We got by and then also found out that we were expecting our next child.

My mother came over quite a lot and Margaret, at times, travelled by train to Tooting and walked with the pram to visit her parents in Norbury. We managed to buy a car (Austin 1954 Somerset) which gave us a chance to visit my brothers and have the odd Sunday afternoon trip. We also rented a Television but this meant that I had to manage on 10/- a week which included buying my newspaper, paying for my canteen two course lunch and my Saturday football match fee. On occasions the match fee was a few pence cheaper and I put this in the club fruit machine at Northholt and when I won I managed to afford a beer after the match. I did quite well as far as pay rises were concerned and felt quite lucky and decided to buy a garage. The cheapest 16 x 8 was an asbestos and wood one from the Co-op which I bought and assembled. I thought I had done a reasonable job but was surprised when in the early 2000's Tim rang me to ask which number Dobbie Close we had lived as he was working nearby. I identified the house for him and he said there was a rough looking shed in the back garden. On closer inspection this turned out to be the garage I had put up in the early 60's.

Going back to making money stretch out I was lucky to have Margaret as she managed very well and even with our next door neighbour went out pea and fruit picking. They would walk a mile or two to the other side of Sittingbourne either down Mill Lane or up to Snipes Hill pushing prams. I had to do my bit and I acquired an allotment which was nearly two miles away. This took a lot of hard work clearing stinging nettles etc. before planting. The greyhound cabbage and runner beans were a great success but the potatoes were riddled with worm. To our surprise Christine loved the cabbage and sometimes ate only this for a meal. She must have been fed well enough as we lived next to a recreation ground with a very high slide and in no time she was climbing to the top on her own and sliding down into my arms if I managed to get round from the bottom of the steps to the bottom of the slide quickly enough.

My friend Chris and his wife bought a house a few miles away in Rayleigh and it fell to me to cycle over to the new property and fit his new carpet before the next weekend hiring a van and collecting furniture from his house and driving through the Dartford tunnel to pick up more goods from her place north of the Thames. Another long but satisfying day particularly taking a van through the tunnel.

When the time neared for Karen to be born we had regular visits from the midwife and I explained how quickly Christine had been delivered in Weir Hospital who at 2.30 told us to go home and not bother to call for an update before 6 o'clock. At 5.30 we rang to be told that she had been born at about 3 o'clock. One morning Margaret woke about 6 am and asked me to walk to the phone box up the road and call the midwife. The Midwife duly came and said that the baby would come later in the day and that she would go to visit a patient in the next village and we could call her mother if we needed to get a message to her. True to form about, probably less than an hour later, Margaret said I should get an urgent message out. I went to the local telephone box and as I was trying to get through I spotted the midwife's car approaching. I ran out into the road and waved her down and in well under half an hour we had our baby girl in her mother's arms.

Our neighbours were a strength to our pleasure and progress at this point in our lives. I must mention our next door neighbours Seth and Rosemary whom we still exchange Christmas cards with. On the other side of the road Brian and Elaine Luckhurst had a similar property to ours and I trained with him as he played regularly in the winter with the Sittingbourne football team. He told me he played cricket for Kent in the summer and worked for a local removals firm in the winter to make ends meet. Little was I to know that when he scored a double century for Kent and could not sleep that night that he would become an England player. Sport did not pay a lot in those days and it has only been in recent years that footballers have been able to earn more than £50 per week. He may not remember me but I certainly remember him and his family.

With the new baby in mind and a need for more space we started to look for another house on the edge of the commuter belt. We visited a new build building site in Crowborough quite near Jarvis Brook railway station. There was very little to look at except mud, rock and one or two almost completed houses. The semi-detached we could possibly afford was at the bottom of the steep hill backing onto a brook and a copse (privately owned) and there was a footpath to the road by the station about a ten minute walk. We had already looked at the Beaver estate in Ashford and a very wet site in Buxted but these were very small whereas the Crowborough house had a third bedroom 10ft x 10ft. We decided to take a further look on the following weekend and it was a particularly wet and miserable day but as we departed the site on the road to Eridge we both admired the view and the district in general and Margaret said 'if we can like it on a day like this we must like it'. Our minds made up we started on our next house move which was going to prove anything but straight forward.

We were told that the build would be ready for early June and we managed to sell our house with this in mind. The place was not finished, or likely to be for at least six weeks, so we arranged to move in with my mother in Tooting for about a month prior to completion. In the first week in August we were still trying to arrange completion and I developed a severe permanent headache. We had arranged with my brother Mick to go on holiday with him, his two kids and our mother in early September. In true Terry style I made a pact that in no circumstances would I not go away. In short we agreed for completion during the week before the holiday and planned how we would cope. Never think you can plan anything where builders are concerned. Yes we did keep to the date but only after the Managing Director had agreed to some of my conditions.

Still suffering from my headache I leave Tooting with the car and roof rack jammed and I think I am feeling better. No such luck when I get out of the car to get petrol my head hits back with a vengeance.

CHAPTER SIX

70 Medway

When we arrived with our removals van the men saw that there was no path to the front door and that there were an army of painters trying to complete their work. The best we could get was to have the downstairs lounge and the garage filled with our belongings and (as per the Managing Director's instructions) be put up in the local pub on a half board basis. The work on the house was going to take at least a further week so on the Saturday our holiday plan came into force. Early in the morning I drove to Coxheath to pick up Mick, Jean and the children. I returned to Crowborough to add Margaret and our children to the car and the luggage. We travelled with little mishap to Selsey in West Sussex and there picked up my mother and added her and her luggage to the car to continue to the Pontin's Holiday Camp. You will spot here that I still had only my Austin Somerset and that it had nine occupants and luggage. Not a particular problem in those days as long as you were loaded safely and had good mirror vision all round. First and main memory of the holiday was the next morning when with the sun shining we set ourselves on the grass around the swimming pool. Christine saw a father dive off the board and his daughter jump up and down with glee. She basically demanded that I do this for her. With my head still painful I reluctantly agreed and walked slowly to the diving board. Well I completed what I classed as a swallow dive and disappeared under the water. When I broke the surface all I could see was Christine jumping up and down in obvious delight but the big bonus was that from that moment on my headache had left and I was relaxed for the first time in ages. A good holiday but now to the real world.

The house was not fully fit for occupation but we moved in and settled quite quickly considering the 20 or so problems we reported to the site manager a Mr Bulldock who had a limp which seemed to match his very up and down moods. To say the least he was not the most popular person about and when he sacked some of his brickies on a Friday morning they bricked over the chimneys of a pair of semi's which they boasted about in the pub but was not actually proven until after the buyers moved in (only one of his major problems).

We found several inches of water under our lounge floor and arranged for the Irish labourers to run earth drains down the garden to the brook at the back thinking this was a problem related to the way the house was sited on the hill. Days later it was discovered that the mains water inlet to a house two doors up was not properly connected and instead of going into the house it was releasing into the ground 24 hours a day. Once mended the base dried up.

At this time the Beeching Report came out that announced massive station closures and included in the list was Jarvis Brook. I supported a group of locals who rounded up support to stop the closure and we managed to get our point over on local television. We had tried to get the backing of our M P but he did not immediately get involved. We had a very positive meeting in the Assembly Halls in Tunbridge Wells and got what appeared to be an agreement to keep the line open as far as Buxted. At this point our M P turned up at our next meeting in Crowborough. Guess what he addressed it and said he was proud to support a winning cause. My question was why had not said this earlier and he replied that he had always been behind us. Anyway we kept our rail service unlike a lot of the rest of the country.

In my usual fashion I designed a garden on the back of an envelope and then got on with it. Outside the kitchen door I built a low walled vegetable patch and at the back of the house I laid a very large patio area with large paving slabs. We moved a lot of earth and built an eight or ten course wall half way down the garden split by an at least six foot wide gap with three ample steps for child safety. Later we cut down two fairly young silver birch from the land at the back and by burying them a good two feet in the ground and using 3 x 2 and some hooks made a grand swing although I say it myself. The rest of the garden was grassed over for a playing and sitting area.

The front garden came later as this fell over 3 feet from the pavement to the house. We thought it would be a good idea to have a tiered and stepped area down to the front door level and flatten out under the lounge window. This meant building a retaining wall about 3 foot high to support the pavement. My neighbour told me he could co-opt the dumper truck when the site was vacated and we then collected massive ironstone rocks from a seam part way up the hill. This provoked the building site manager to advise us that he would not allow us to take any more rock unless he provided it and charged as appropriate. We ignored him.

Digging out and levelling was a big task and Margaret insisted on doing her bit. I thought it was a good idea but as she was now again pregnant most of the neighbours thought I was nasty and could cause her significant health problems. It did not help a lot when I explained that I could not stop her if I tried and that anyway she was very capable of looking after herself and did not intend to do her baby any harm.

Margaret got on very well with the woman over the road and our children played with her boy and Margaret still corresponds with her. I got on with the chap two doors down and during the rail strikes I was able to give him a lift into London on a number of occasions. I used to meet a resident from up the top of the hill and one of the experiences we shared was the ability or not to get into local sport. My problem was that our road was planned as an extension to the road in Jarvis Brook by the same name. Our end of the road was in Crowborough but when I applied for membership of the local tennis club I was told that I could become only an Associate Member and play only on Wednesday evenings as Medway was in Jarvis Brook. No amount of documentation would persuade the committee that I qualified as a Crowboroughite. Needless to say I did not join the club but did later have the pleasure of playing against them. My neighbour tried to join the highly prestigious Beacon golf club and as his handicap was only nine he would not automatically get into their first men's team, there was not a vacancy for him. Some weeks later he told me he was going to play golf and when I asked which club he had joined he said he was in the local club. Well the club had not suddenly lost all of the best players but his wife's application for membership was accepted as her handicap was eleven they were willing to bite her fingers off to have her in their ladies team, and low and behold because she was a member he as her spouse was offered membership. This was my second brush with snobbishness in tennis but fortunately it did not put me off enjoying the game. Other neighbours had closer relationships and had what were known as key parties and this eventually led to broken marriages and new partnerships but with only the same people living in different houses (not a way of life I understood). Our house was surrounded by steep hills which meant that if I needed the car on a winter's morning then I had to park it up near the Post Office/Corner store in order to be sure of getting out. The hills were however a boon for Margaret when she started to learn to drive. She was a very good diver but very bad at taking exams, sadly after her first test she stopped lessons as she was by then very pregnant.

One of my abiding memories was one day we were stood at the front of the house when one of the neighbours came down the road and told us that her husband had just left to go and pick up their new car. We chatted for a while and Christine who was standing getting bored suddenly started jumping up and down shouting Tractor! Tractor! The next minute this brand new VW Beetle came trundling round the corner. I was supposed to be embarrassed but did not feel it.

It was about this time that Christine was due to start school and we arranged for her to attend a pre-school introduction in the summer holidays. This was one of the early signs of how obstinate she could be if she didn't want to do something. We got her to the hall on the green and she started to scream that she would not go in as this was not proper school and that was it not for her. She would not shut up until we took her away. Later, of course, we had to take her to proper school and this being a small school with only two classes the head teacher had heard about our earlier problems and came to meet us on the first morning. She made friends with Christine and arranged for her to ring the bell for assembly and all went well. She did really well that day and came home happy to be going to PROPER SCHOOL.

The golf playing wife was also the local midwife and attended Margaret throughout but the big surprise was that one day she came with a trainee who thought she had met Margaret before. Low and behold she had been a junior nurse at the hospital in Balham when Christine was born. She obviously did not remember the birth as the day before Margaret felt the baby would arrive she insisted that I be brought home from work as the baby was due. This cost me a day's holiday and left me to twiddle my thumbs the next morning. This turned into a useful exercise as I found some floorboards and skirting on the site and spent several hours making a wooden steam engine which was to be a kid's toy for many years to come. That afternoon although forewarned the midwife was caught out with the birth and basically panicked. I rushed upstairs to find out what was happening and helped her regain control and complete the delivery, for a little I thought she was going to strangle Robin with his own cord. This midwife however was expecting a baby when we left

Crowborough and we always wondered how her midwife coped with her.

We used to keep in touch with Pat and Mick and one day we agreed to have Mick's kids for an afternoon soon after Robin was born and late in the afternoon we went into the local café for tea. We were very conscious of the stares as we entered with five very young children.

For no particular reason that I can remember we agreed that it was time to move on and we looked for a detached house and found one being built privately above Crowborough town centre. We chose all the colours and bathroom and kitchen fittings. We had problems with our buyer and his mortgage which delayed proceedings and the old lady who was having the house built decided that I was no longer a suitable buyer and withdrew from the sale. This was, as it happened, a good thing as we found a more convenient and larger property in Lingfield. The Estate Agent in Lingfield was very resourceful and felt he could let me view a house that was on the market for over £9000 when I had told him that my approved mortgage was only £7500 and that getting more would be difficult. Having driven to Lingfield we did take a look at the house and did needless to say, like it. We continued our search with little avail and a couple weeks later the Estate Agent called me and suggested that I take another look at the £9000 property. I told him in no uncertain terms that I could not afford it but he convinced me that the sellers were desperate to sell and that if we liked it at this viewing he would talk to me about pricing an offer. He told me an offer only a little higher than my top figure would secure the buy. He turned out to be right and we bought for somewhere around £8000.

My mother was unable to understand why I was going to move as we had put so much work into creating a beautiful garden and met such nice neighbours. I think I just felt that as we had decided we could at this point not afford to have the fourth child we had planned it would be a good idea to find a place to make a future for our family. Margaret could stop trudging up the hill to get the family allowance from the local Post Office and pushing the pram with two kids on it into town and back which was further up the steep hill. I could also leave the car on my drive and know that I could start it and drive away without getting stuck on the hill. I could now keep the spade in the garden instead of the boot of the car. Christine would miss her school, we would miss local events, particularly the annual fireworks, but anyway the time had come to move on.

CHAPTER SEVEN

44 Saxby's Lane

This time we appear to have had better luck than on previous occasions and the move went well. We had a corner store a few hundred yards up the road and a good butcher with his own abattoir where he had at least one cow and several lambs delivered each week. A good baker and a supermarket and several pubs were just beyond the Library and the Church all within a five minute walk. We had a village hall with a working men's club with a stage and a badminton court which was used by the local club. I met some locals and we set up a tennis club in the grounds of the local school. This flourished and we joined the Weald League. Our best win from my point of view was when Crowborough visited us and we gave them a thumping. I also joined the Badminton Club and eventually got into their team (on occasions when they were one short) but I did get to play in a number of mixed matches against local villages.

I had two work colleagues living nearby in East Grinstead and we met at each other's houses for dinner parties and or family afternoons. We also got together on bonfire nights and shared snacks and fireworks in one of our gardens. It was much later that we started taking the children to organised events. I also remember that when we took down our conservatory we then made it into a greenhouse for one of these colleagues which we erected having laid a proper base to accommodate it.

One day we had a problem with a sudden leak on a radiator and I went in search of a plumber. The man lived round the corner and his wife rang him to see if he could help. He left the job he was doing and came to look at our problem. He had not been working long when Christine decided to 'help' him. This turned out alright as they seemed to get on well together. When I related this story to other people in the pub I was told he would never come again as he had a dislike for children. Well some time later when I decided to have the Garage pulled down and replace it with a two storey extension of a garage utility room and upstairs bedroom with an en suite I thought I would call on him for advice regarding local builders and fitters. He made an excellent recommendation and his two sons worked alongside the builder doing the electrics and tiling. He himself did the plumbing. I asked why if local gossip was true about him not liking children did he come and work where I had three of them. His reply was it was not children as such that he did not like but little interfering brats. He said my children were well behaved and a pleasure. We were to meet again when I designed a further extension and the same team built a large family room attached to the back of the house and extending across the lounge, kitchen and utility room.

I remember that one day I took it into my head that the original design of our house was obviously only three bedrooms and that the second bedroom had been converted into two small rooms. Margaret wondered what I was doing when I took a club hammer upstairs and started to knock down two walls and a door. She did not at the time complain that all the debris was landing on our nice carpet which I had failed to cover with dust sheets, however, she set too and by late afternoon we had made our two rooms back into one. The kids seemed delighted and this meant that Karen did not have to be encouraged to climb from one bedroom to the other via the outside wall. Although Margaret accepted the occasion she has often related the story in more recent years in both positive and some definitely critical ways. It was also about this time that I built a Wendy house out of some cheap plywood I acquired and I used an old wooden window frame for the door and window. I never felt this was used much after the spiders took residence but have been assured of late that I am mistaken. The garden did not get a makeover as it was a good play area and was bordered by some beautiful May blossom.

The three children went to the local schools up the road. In this area there were two schools before the move to a Comprehensive probably some miles away. We moved before this came to pass. One of the parents at the first school felt it would be a good idea to start a PTA and the Headmistress agreed to come and sit in on the platform at a discussion meeting. During this one parent asked if the PTA was formed and they wish to change the method of teaching arithmetic how would she respond. She clearly said I am the Head and what I want is what gets done. I said this meant that a PTA could have no effect on what went on in the school and she agreed. Needless to say the meeting agreed to inaugurate a PTA and make the building of an adventure playground a specific task. Over the next year this was done and then on the first day of term they told the children it would be open in the area adjacent to the playground. On that morning the Headmistress came out and said that her teachers could not supervise the children and that the parents were not insured to do so. True to her word the Head was in charge and the playground was still not open when we moved several years later.

We used to attend the local Catholic Church which seemed to suit our needs with a Sunday Children's Service; unfortunately they changed the priest at the same time as they converted to using local language services. This seemed a good idea for the kids but the change recommended new hymns that none of us knew, particularly the children. It appeared that we were allowed to use any hymns of choice but this priest decided this was not for him. The kids did not want to go to Church and Margaret had always gone to it for me and so when Christine joined the Church of England choir with her classmates we stopped going. We were not alone in finding the Priest unacceptable as when Margaret's mother came over for Christmas I used to accompany her to Midnight Mass. One year she asked could I take her to a different Church as she had not enjoyed the Service in the two previous years. I took her to Mass at the local Nunnery.

One day a car took our gatepost out of the ground and left the number plate and part of the bumper on the drive. We found the car abandoned down the road and tried to find the owners to get our repairs done. We did find where they lived but decided that for the amount of money involved it was not a good idea to enter the middle of the Council Estate in that part of Crawley.

After a particularly windy night we woke up one morning to find that a tall tree from the chicken farm next door had fallen across our garden with the top in our other next door neighbour's garden. That day I managed to borrow a two handled logging saw from a friend and each morning before work my neighbour and I met and cut one log length off. This went on for over two weeks. He had an open wood fire and later chopped and stored the smaller logs for drying out.

My association with hospitals reared its ugly head when I returned home from work latish one evening to see an ambulance with lights flashing parked outside the house. A very sobering effect and then I was asked to follow it to Redhill Hospital after Margaret was loaded on board. When we arrived at the hospital Christine said that the car was on fire. This was not totally true but the rear wheel was red hot and when we returned to the car later the break was ineffective. I rang the garage and he was great. He said if I could get insurance cover then he would leave a car at his garage for me to pick up and could use it to collect my mother from London and get the family home. I rang Pat and got insurance and drove the car very carefully to the garage. The owner of the Garage told me to call him when Margaret had recovered and then we would sort something out. Another case of meeting with a Gentleman. Does this happen today, one wonders. Margaret made a quick recovery as it turned out to be an allergy to penicillin.

Somewhere along the line when all three kids were at school we decided Margaret would like to have another baby and when I agreed I insisted that with such a gap it would be unfair to have only one and that we must try for two quite close together. The closeness was not totally successful but having five children was.

About this time I used to walk over London Bridge and they started to take it down stone by stone. They closed one side of the bridge to replace it and were then going to repeat the process on the other side. This was a mammoth task and we wondered why as each stone was removed it was carefully numbered. We then heard that a town in Texas had bought the bridge and were going to rebuild it in America. I think we were right when we assumed that they thought that they had bought Tower Bridge. The two projects were completed and London Bridge is now rebuilt in the USA and the New London Bridge is completed with underfoot heating to keep the snow clear. This was the early days of the modern day idea of underfloor heating. All the time the work went on building the bridge there was a man in a rowing boat keeping a lookout for anyone who may fall into the river. I guess a boring but necessary job.

When we had the first extension done our next door neighbour, who was a trainee architect, agreed to do my drawings for an agreed small sum of money, I got all the planning agreed and when the job was complete I offered to pay my dues. At this point he ask for a much larger sum and when I reminded him of our agreement he advised me that he had just qualified and was bound to charge me a percentage of the estimated enhanced value gained. It did not totally please me that Margaret got on very well with his wife and it seemed I must keep a good relationship.

The thought of paying this man for the drawings for the planned rear extension put me into thinking that a lot of the work had already been done and that maybe I could do these myself. I completed the drawings and obtained three sets of blue prints and sent them off to the Council for planning permission. A couple of weeks later I received a phone call from the head of planning who quizzed me about the extension and particularly the drawings. It was agreed that I would call into his office and discuss the matter. I was very aware that I could have made mistakes as I had based everything on my reading of the other plans. When this man discovered that I had prepared all of the documentation myself he seemed very impressed and treated me like a pupil. He pointed out minor errors which he said he could handle but then ask me how the wall of the side was not going to be blown over and fall into the garden. I pointed out the lintel over the door and he said yes but where was this fixed to the main building. I had not shown the wall tie on the drawings. Interview over he congratulated me on my efforts and seemed pleased that I had not had to pay and architect. The plans went through without a hitch.

Having done all these improvements what would I do next. MOVE.

This did happen but it was definitely not planned. We had all we needed in the way of convenience for bringing up a big family but my workplace had changed from the City/West End to Lewisham in SE London. This was not a work problem but travel became impossible. The train would be up to town via London Bridge and take endless time both going and coming. I decided to travel by car but the route was not straightforward. A couple of years later the road through Godstone/Oxted would be available but my journey was immediate. From the September through December I witnessed several severe accidents and as I was often a tired driver because of my long hours I felt I could not cope for much longer. I therefore planned to move nearer to my work. Margaret particularly did not want to move to town and I managed to find a place on the edge with immediate access to the countryside. I took Margaret to view the place by driving through total countryside until we were within less than a mile from the property. This was a success and we made the decision to put in an offer. In the long run there were many plusses and minuses. Plusses were local facilities for the kids including swimming and later job opportunities. Minuses were the loss of the family room and although the footprint was equal the facilities were not nearly as practical. The new property had an unheated swimming pool and the garden had massive potential. I will address this later in the next section.

Our move was to take place on Karen's birthday when Peter was only six days old. As he was our fifth child the doctor insisted Margaret was in hospital for the birth and she came home after 48 hours. This meant that within a day or two we were completing on our house purchase and the midwife told Margaret that it was too soon to move and we would have to delay the move. Needless to say we did move and all the family rallied round to ensure that all Margaret did was to sit around and look after her baby. I have mentioned that a car hit our gate well it was not uncommon for a car to go into the hedge as we were on a sharp bend. On the morning we were moving the school bus came towards the house and the kids were looking for our children to say goodbye when the coach driver misjudged his course and hit our removal van. Not too serious but hilarious to the kids.

We settled in very well except that Robin raced down the hill on his bike and fell off and split his nose and I finished up making the first of what was going to be virtually a season ticket to Bromley Hospital over the years to come.

MIDI-LOGUE ONE

Think of the foregoing as a list or catalogue of reflections on life in general that run in parallel throughout life and have been part of the learning and as a result of the learning.
`

So far I have described the process of building life for a future like climbing a staircase and now I have arrived at the landing.

From here on I will dwell on the various themes that run through life in parallel with each other. That is until I get to retirement. I suggest that as with me in life there will be repetition and a few too many words.

CHAPTER EIGHT

Projects

My first effort apart from garden design (there is still one to come) was the wooden steam engine and the project theme is going to be things for the children.

In Crowborough I built a swing and this idea was carried through to Lingfield where about the only out door plaything that I got involved in was building a Wendy House from an old window frame as already mentioned. The recreation ground was only across the road and provided for most of the children's needs. We did however provide two games indoors, particularly after we built the playroom on the back, and these were unreasonable amounts of Lego and Scalex which was later passed to the care of one of the boys and now apparently nowhere to be had. (sad!). Robin was ahead of the market and put headlights onto some of the cars and used them in the evenings after dark.

It was when we got to West Wickham that things got more ambitious as we bought into an unfinished swimming pool. By unfinished I mean it had a rough concrete lining which was rough on the skin and often encountered as the pool was only about 17ft x 11ft and five foot deep. I had already decided to rebuild the bathroom which was lined with marble so when my mate and I converted the bathroom into a stand-alone shower, a vast corner bath and stereo sinks we dumped all of the marble into the back garden. We moved in during the hottest year recorded since the war and the kids spent many hours messing around in the water. I bought a sizable summerhouse and put curtained cubicles in to make it into a proper changing room so that we could entertain guests. The next year came round very quickly and the kids realised that the water was not going to be as hot this spring and summer so I arranged to extend the central heating into a shed in the garden where we installed a heat exchanger and a pump and ran piping across the lawn to heat the pool. We also had people in to line the pool with mosaic tiles and to level and cap the surround. This done we cleaned up the patio area at the side of the pool and proceeded to cover the outside surrounds with the marble from the bathroom. This done we started to look at the rest of the garden and realised that the big sugar pine tree could support a rope which was duly attached. Next Karen, whilst hanging on to the rope, finished up going through the window into the pump shed. Out came my season ticket to Bromley Hospital and within a few hours we had agreed with the doctor that we would accept his recommendation that he graft the wound with skin taken from her thigh. We managed to get back home in time for a late Sunday lunch and I made it to the bowls club for the afternoon match.

The next thing was to design the garden for the first time. I contacted the local garden nursery which was owned by one of the bowling club members. I invited him over one evening and introduced him to my ideas of using York stone in most of the front garden and round the side of the house to a very large patio with a small side pond. I know that he had never had a Project this big and for many years was reminded of this by his son who often said so and also that he had never had another like it. This had cost a lot of money so when we felt it was a good idea to have a large garden pond we all got together and agreed this would be a family project. We drew the plans up and settled on a main pond with a cascade waterfall pumped by a pump hidden under it. We added a side pool which was to be fed from the bottom of the waterfall and provide a breeding pond.

The digging out started and we finished up with an at least 18inch deep pool which was pear shaped and 17ft x 10ft. Whilst building the water feature one of the large rocks was too heavy for me and it and I finished up on the already full pond. I was unable to get this out and it became a fixed feature of the final job. We added coloured lights in red, blue and green which were probably the only colours available in those days. We stocked it with Golden Orfe, Green and Golden Tench and Sucker Loach and I think, from time to time, as recommended by the Beckenham shop, various other species. At this time the children's play part of the garden was near the house and after a while I felt it wise to put a portable fence up to keep the younger ones protected from the pond and the pool. This was probably after Peter climbed up next to his mother who was sitting on the side of the pool and promptly fell straight in. Margaret followed in next to no time and realised that she was in a nice summer outfit but knew even if it had been designer she would still have done the same.

The next innovations were more of the winter type and took place indoors. First carrying on the fish theme we started with some cold water fish in a tank and soon added a warm water tank with heaters and filters which needless to say mum looked after but in this case both the children and she were very happy. We always had trouble keeping mum away from all the needs of the fish as she actually preferred this to regular housekeeping. It was around this time that we had other animals e.g. a rabbit and guinea pigs but I only really remember the budgie. The animals had to stay in the garden because of Margaret's asthma and we found that if we tried to have two budgies this also affected her.

We started to get into satellite TV and TV games to the extent that we were using all the available channels, which in those days was only five or six, to accommodate our perceived needs. The first game was very simplistic but also very up-to-date and it was basically on the lines of table tennis. I was encouraged to invest in all new technology as it came along but we still limited the time that was allowed for play unless it was me and Margaret.

I think it was about this time that I obtained some cheap plywood and set about building a doll's house which was a replica of the layout of the house in Crowborough on a scale of 1 inch to 1 foot. I managed to get an old transformer with switching and using fine wire and touch bulbs put in room lights. The windows were made of clear plastic on homemade frames and the furniture mostly made from the plywood offcuts. The kitchen was purpose bought and stair and room carpet came from real remains from our house carpets. Individual red tiles were cut from office red folders and stuck one by one onto the roof. The end product worked and was only passed on to another family when I was well into retirement.

We soon came up with the idea of building a model railway and true to form we decided on an 8ft x 4ft double 'O' gauge. I think Robin and I mainly sorted out the layout. I created the landscape with a fine chicken wire and a Polyfiller type plaster. Margaret and the kids sprinkled loads of coloured dust onto glue in order to create fields and pastures representing wheat, grass for the cows and yellow for rape etc. I cut out grey cardboard for the roads and pavements and painted white lines and curb stones. We assembled rows of shops and houses and made a roundabout. Of course we made a station and platform and bought a signal box. We made our own level crossing gate and later out of foam hardened with glue we made hedges and trees. On this layout we could run two trains at any one time which gave us many hours of fun.

Sometime later we repeated our model railway building and created a layout in 'N' gauge which was run on a four way controller. This was done to a higher standard than the first effort but probably did not come anywhere near Robin's exacting standards in his model making.

Staying on the indoor games I bought a 6ft x 3ft slate bed snooker table and Margaret proved to be more adept at this than was expected and it was not unusual for her to be overall winner at the end of a session. The table only just fitted into the room and one day when we thought it might be better in the back room and I allowed the children, in particular Robin, to arrange to dismantle it. This was very nearly another visit to the hospital but fortunately Robin managed just in time to get out of the way as he removed the last leg and the whole thing smashed to the floor. It was cracked and therefore only good for the dump. We manhandled it into the back of the car in got rid of it. We replaced the table and had the new one for many years.

It was not long before we decided to move the play area to the back of the garden and enjoy using the patio and pool and pond surrounds for pleasure. This came about as one of the fruit trees was falling over and the other looked on its last legs and we were able to pull them out of the ground and take them to the dump. With the space in front of the summerhouse cleared I then thought it would be a good idea to invest in a proper climbing frame. I know that this initially had quite a lot of use but later all I can remember is Robin creeping out in the evenings and doing what seemed like hundreds of chin-ups.

When Chris was sixteen I gave her a motorbike for her birthday and this of course then had to happen for all future sixteenth birthdays. Many neighbours and parents appeared to condemn me for this but as I and Margaret had enjoyed our scooter and bike I thought it was right to start the children off on a proper learning curve. It seems to have worked as we have had no serious accidents and still have five children. Tim and Karen fell in love with bikes and biking and it was Karen at only about 5ft high that invested in large heavy bikes but she seemed happy and competent. Tim also followed suit and as I did, he gave up soon after he was married. He has now however in mid-life bought an almost classic bike without all the electronics and gets out on it in the summer when possible. Robin progressed to a classic MG Midget but has now started to ride a moped to work which saves both time and money. Peter has a love affair with Hillman Imps and having spent some time using one to run around he then restored it and then sold it and bought a Hillman Imp Van in pretty poor condition and then restored that. It is running at this time. Going back to the original bikes the negative for me was that I seemed to be forever leaving home in the late evening and recovering the bike and rider after some fault had occurred. I remember one evening when Chris called for me to go to near Brixton to get her and as I was leaving home the phone rang and Karen was calling from the A2 near Rochester. In my usual optimistic way I got into the Peugeot Estate and felt that I could kill both birds with one stone. Well, I picked up Chris with her little bike and we then proceeded to look for the petrol station and find Karen. Karen's was a bigger and heavier bike and I was not going to be able to lift this without help. We were in luck and there were some young lads who I asked to give me a hand. The first lad said he could help lift the bike but how did I expect to get it into the back of the car as there was already one bike inside. I said don't worry I am good at this having had lots of practice. I was at that point actually pretty doubtful and was contemplating the need for a further trip. Not something I relished. The lads were pretty strong and sensible and in next to no time the bike was well into the boot and to all of our surprises I was also able to properly close the boot. Another bike mission complete but the repair was not simple and later that week saw Karen riding one of the boy's bikes and towing me on hers down to the Garage at Elmers End.

Before I stopped working in Data Processing Apple brought out what was probably the first 'portable' computer. I was given the use of this for some of my work and took it home on occasions. This was no easy task as it weighed nearly 40lbs. Robin was interested and we learnt from some manual about how to pick and put pixels. He thought that he would be able to recreate an arcade game and with a boat on the bottom of the screen and a plane above he wanted to gun down the boat. We soon found out that the speed or lack of it in the computer was no match for the chip that had been put in and arcade machine. In truth it took about three minutes to get one bullet from the plane to the boat. Our experiment was a total failure but an excellent learning medium.

When I left the IT area and started working normal hours I found that I had time on my hands in the evenings and as I have never watched seriously anything but sport on television I felt I should find something to fill the time. I thought that it would be a good idea to build a wooden model boat. I visited the model shop in Woolwich in one of my lunch hours and chatted with the manager. He asked if I had done any model making and when I said no he recommended that I start off small and progress to larger if I enjoyed the experience. I said that I would rather build a big boat that I could be proud of and proceeded to select the largest Billings boat in the shop. The 'Norske Love' was a72 cannon man of war and was a definite challenge. I learnt to bend strips of wood in hot water in the bath and found out how useful a pin pusher was. Three years later the boat was complete and Robin set about building an airtight cabinet to house it. We set this up on the stair head where in general it stayed until we moved on retirement to Findon Valley.

My efforts had inspired Robin and before he left school he had completed a model of the Danish paddle steamer. During Robin's school years he became very good at woodwork and for his GCE he built a compendium coffee table which we still have. He used the boat and photos of this to apply for an apprenticeship at Piper's who built models for the building industry. He got down to the last six from over fifty applicants but as only four were required and two sons of current workers were among the six he did not quite make it. He did not then just give up on woodwork and we designed a nest of coffee tables which he still has and is along with the rest of the family proud of.

Robin returned to boat building and started to model the Golden Hind. We travelled to Plymouth to see the full size replica in order that he could get the detail right and he was meticulous and covered interior benches in velvet and carved the lifeboat from a single piece of wood. He did go through a spell where he lost some interest but tells me that I somehow re-inspired him. He still displays this in a homemade cabinet on the wall in his apartment and visiting deliverymen and tradesmen always admire it.

Timothy did not usually ask for a lot but one day he said he would like an aviary in the garden and again not doing things by halves we bought a 6ft x 4ft shed and made the top half a roosting area and the bottom a place for storing seed etc. We then got a lot of three by two ex-council paving slabs. We buried these almost three feet into the ground so that the foxes would not be able to get to the birds when we had finished building. With posts also three foot into the ground we created the sides and roof all attached to the shed. The end product was 24ft across the back of the garden up to the shed and came away from the back fence on the left a full twelve feet. This extended about 18ft to a five foot by two foot six door which also attached to the shed. Not feeling this was enough we then used and old plastic pond and created a spot for the birds to drink and wash.

Then came the birds. We had two cockatiel which bred annually and two pairs of diamond doves which also produced one male and one female each year. We bred many foreign finch and other related birds. We had a pair of Chinese and a pair of English quail for the ground cover which never seemed to do anything.

Somewhere along the line Margaret got interested in doing embroidery. I think it came after I brought a cross stitch of a country girl back from Copenhagen for Karen. Anyway she did a number of these and I got to framing them and some still hang in our present apartment.

CHAPTER NINE

Sport

My over commitment for all my sport must have been overbearing on the rest of the family but it was my way of coping with home and work and keeping myself sane.

Football started with us kids playing drainhole football in the street when I was just eight. Winning became second nature to me and I never liked the idea of coming second or losing. We played cricket on Streatham Common in the evenings but my first real encounter with competition came when I went to Grammar School. We did PE classes twice a week and had sports on Wednesday afternoons. We played football in the playground before school and in the breaks and according to season we played cricket or football either in the paddock or on the common. We had all been assigned to one of four houses and these competed against each other at the end of each season. In the summer we took the little exposure to athletics in PE to a further step and after school either one of the teachers or the headmaster supervised and coached long jump, high jump, javelin shot putt and hurdles. I found that I was quite good at the high jump and practiced the Western Roll as my jump of choice. I liked running on the track and as we lived near Tooting Bec Track I joined a local club and trained on Tuesday and Thursday evenings and Sunday mornings. With the Bank and the youth club and school I participated in a number of knockout competitions and was in winning teams for the college in my age group in the

Wandsworth School sports, the Catholic Youth Club sports and Junior Banks. I was never quite good enough to represent the local club although at their annual sports day I won club credits in five events when I ran the Mile in four minutes and forty seconds and the Half Mile in exactly two minutes. My best mile was I think when I ran the same 4min 40sec but on grass at the Midland Bank Sports Ground at Elmers End in a three side event between Martins Bank, Blackheath Harriers and Midland Bank. It was not long after this that my cousin and I discussed the possibility of me devoting myself to trying to achieve the four minute mile. It did not take too long to understand that with no returns except personal prowess this work ratio to life style was inequitable and I thought that my social life would give me more pleasure.

Football was to take up a lot of my winter weekends as I played on Saturdays for the Clapham Old Boys and Sundays for Balham Youth Club. The friendly events were for the Old Boys as I played in a second or third eleven and the social side came high on the agenda. When I moved away from Tooting I got more involved with the Bank's team as it was easier and less expensive travel. Whilst I played in the team I was not selected for the five-a-side team when the Inter American Banks arranged a knockout tournament. As each bank was invited to enter two teams I, for some reason, was asked if I could find four employees to join me and make up a second five. I knew one player who played for his local team who was a good centre half and a little very quick winger who knew more staff than I did. This lad helped me select two more players and as I discovered later he had found a very good goalkeeper. The games were arranged for evenings over a two week period at the Chrystal Palace Sports Centre. We played two games on each evening and if I remember rightly there were two leagues and the top two in each league played off a semi-final and final. I think that both of our teams got to the semi but were not drawn against each other and they lost and we won. The final was well supported by many staff members and we finished up at full time drawing one all. A penalty kick out then. In those days you nominated one penalty taker and played as many times as it took for one team to miss if after the first five it was all square. Earlier in the tournament I had asked the centre half to take the penalties but he had refused and the team were unanimous that the captain take responsibility. My first penalty hit the post in the first round and came straight back and hit me in the face. I insisted that our centre half in future reminded me to aim at the back stanchion and not the inside of the post in future. This went well until the final when the occasion appeared too much and no one gave me any advice. Yes it did happen again. I hit the post with my first try and the ball hit me in the face. I told you we had a good goalkeeper, well we were 4-3 down and they had one shot left. A magnificent save to his left and we were back in the game. The rest of the game seemed endless but in the end I did not miss and they did. 15-13 winners. A night to be remembered particularly as the Leisure Centre bar had closed and we had to find a pub up the road before it closed.

Mostly the Saturday fixtures were uneventful but one with the Old Boys could have started the change to the offside rule as in a Cup Final our left winger scored directly from the by-line. On this occasion we had official linesmen and to our total horror he ruled our right winger, who was standing almost beside him on the line, offside and the goal was disallowed. We lost 1-0. Another reference to refereeing was when I was playing on the left wing and chased a ball down to near the corner flag. I got my foot round the ball and sent it into the penalty area where our centre forward headed into goal. The ref said that I had carried the ball over the goal line. The opposing goalkeeper searched out the referee in our half of the field where he had been all along and told him politely but firmly that it was a good goal and should stand. The referee still disagreed and again we lost 1-0 in a cup game.

The Sunday games were different as I played with what I felt were good players some of whom either played on the Saturday for Crystal Palace or Sutton United. They gave me the privilege of playing and then most of the time gave me nothing to do. I was however quite good at getting the ball downfield and to the feet of one of my players which often finished up as a quick goal. I was always determined but it was not until many years later that I was told by one of the players that he thought I was the bravest keeper he had played with. I wish he had told me earlier. This Balham Youth Club Team often won cups and leagues over the years and one year we swept the board and claimed all that year's trophies which were presented at a presentation evening in the Catholic Hall just behind the Oval Cricket Ground.

At this point you will have realised that I had been playing football most Saturdays and Sundays in the winter but in the Summer I enjoyed friendly tennis with friends over many hours. Having moved to West Wickham I must have realised that my footballing days were slowly coming to an end and I actually played my last proper game for the company Vets side on my 40th birthday. I refereed for a few years but found that the social life was changing and lunch time drinks after the match became more isolated by the captains not buying the ref a drink and constantly moaning.

I visited the local tennis club and felt the competition would not be strong enough and I did not feel I wanted to travel further afield. Getting old?? No never! So I visited the local bowls club one Sunday morning. I was with a friend and we got there about five to midday. My friend had a set of woods but I had only bowled a couple of times in my life. Once in a challenge at a hotel in Torquay when my boys were making fools of this chaps boys in the pool and he wanted to take it out on me and when I was alone in Central Park New York. In this instance I came across two bowls greens in the middle of the park and there were a few locals from the club playing a threesome. When I was at college in Clapham my uncle used to play bowls on the common greens and I learnt the basics of the game. For my sins I congratulated some of the shots with a shout of 'good wood'. One of the players came over and greeted me and guessed that I came from England or South Africa as these were the only places she knew that called the bowls, woods. She insisted I went inside to meet her playing partners and to see the clubhouse. I stayed and enjoyed the company and after about an hour one of the members said it was time for him to go home. I was then promptly invited to replace him in the threesome. I guess I did not do too badly as we played on for a further hour and then had a light refreshment. In that club it was a soft drink. That said we now asked how we should go about becoming members of this West Wickham B.C.

The typical bar lawyer was propping up the corner of the bar and he proceeded to advise us that it was exclusive and there was a waiting list. He twigged that we were new to the district and told us that we had to get two existing members to propose and second us and then after displaying our application on the notice board we would be offered trials to see if we could bowl without spoiling the green, and then it would be put before the committee. By this time it was well past the Sunday opening time for licensed premises so we asked if, as we had come out for a drink, it would be possible to buy one here. Well, said our expert, only club members can buy drinks at the bar. I at this point was losing patience and made to leave with quite a negative comment about this local club. Wait a minute said the barman he did not say you could not have a drink, only that you could not buy one. The air cleared and we stayed for a further three hours and true to their word they did not let us buy a drink. The outcome of this was that we were both later accepted as members at the next full committee meeting and my friend is still there and when I moved away after seventeen years they made me a life member.

This started a total over commitment to bowls for the next thirty odd years. I was accepted as a member of West Wickham B.C. just before Christmas but of course could not actually bowl until the next May when the season started. As it happened I was working in Lewisham and the local council opened a new indoor bowing club in the Leisure Centre over the precinct shops. The club opened in the February and I honed some of my skills at this venue.

Starting with the outdoor bowling I managed to get into the club league team and was advised that I should enter the county and district knockout tournaments. One of the senior members of the club told me that he thought I had promise and should leave the club and join a more prestigious one where I could play with better players on much better greens. This was probably true but I liked the club and it was convenient with a nice little bar which was usually well attended. In truth the club and the green improved over the years and I was pleased that I stayed. In order to gain a County Badge in Kent it was necessary to get to the area final, which was known as the second round in whites. Both this and the previous round were played on neutral greens. There were five tournaments for the men, the open singles, un-badged singles, pairs, triples and fours which were competed for each evening of the week. If you did really well in most of these you could be playing every evening plus two or three times at the weekend because the Club, District and sundry other representative knockouts overlapped the timetable. There could be eight rounds sometimes to get to the badged round and in our area which was the home to about three quarters of the county team it meant that however well you felt you played you always had a chance of playing a County or England player. I never did get my badge but was on five occasions the bridesmaid. Twice losing to the future England Champion, the County lead and once a County four. If I had gone to another club I may have been carried as a two in a four and obtained a badge but I have no

101

regrets. I managed to win, at one time or another all of the club knockouts and always enjoyed things like selected pairs where you might play with a complete rooky and make good headway or even win. I particularly remember when Kent needed a White Horse League representative four to play in Middlesex against them and Surrey in a three-way match. On the previous Wednesday I was asked if I could stand in and help out. On the Thursday I got a call asking could I find a further player and on the Friday it became 'can you bring a four'. I asked those at the bar if they could support me on the Sunday for an all-day competition and offered to do the driving. The outcome was, to the clear dismay of the Kent first four, we took the overall prize for best four and were part of winning for Kent County. I could be my usual boring bowling self and recall endlessly many, many, outstanding exciting games but these will remain in my memories.

I had made my mind up not to join most of the many committees in the outdoor club because of other commitments in the summer but at Lewisham Indoor I did serve many roles starting as Treasurer and later as Secretary, Captain and President. In one of these roles I attended a meeting after someone had suggested at the previous meeting we consider whether we could re-introduce the Presentation Dinner and Dance. When the item came up it appeared that the main problem that had stopped support for this event was that it never got round to the dancing until far too late in the evening. I said this was because they took donations for raffle prizes and as we had so many generous members it took all evening to complete. I also thought that the price was a defining factor and made the following

102

proposal. That we have only three very good prizes in the raffle and I suggested Crystal Glasses perhaps whisky, red wine and white wine sixes. That we fix a price of only £5 and publish the menu and timetable. The voice from the committee was that at five pounds this did not even cover the cost of the band and that we as a club had no funds to cover a loss. I being me put forward £200 to cover any shortfall which would be returned if I made a profit. I co-opted my brother to run a Tombola at the point of entry and got several of our ladies to walk round the tables just prior to coffee and sell raffle tickets. The evening was a great success even though my daughter Christine drew her own ticket to win the whisky glasses. End product I got my money back with a small profit to the club. The deal I did with the Leisure Centre manager for the cost of the room rental was on a sliding scale of the number of people that he was to cater for and as our attendance turned out to be full capacity this helped no end.

Indoor bowling was quite new in Kent although David Bryant's Club in Margate was one of the first in the Country. My business moved me back into London and at that time I found that by driving to Beckenham for the morning train I could get back in time for evening bowls at the Cyphers Club and even get home at a sensible time. I therefore applied for membership and was pleased to join them. This did not give me the opportunities that I had hoped for as my perception of supporting the club and the committees of supporting players was somewhat different. I spent a lot of happy hours at the club and represented them on various occasions particularly at weekends and was not unknown as one of the people at the bar even after my membership lapsed. I returned to Lewisham when my business returned me to the district and remained a member until I retired and moved away. My bowling involvements changed when I moved to Sussex and these experiences will appear in the retirement narrative.

CHAPTER TEN

Work

My work experience started when I was very young, about 10 years old, and I worked in a florist/greengrocer, for a man selling door to door fruit and veg and then for several years for a butcher. These were very different and very rewarding training for the real world. As you have already heard I learnt that people could be both nasty and kind, helpful and destructive and all mixes in between. I believe I was more prepared for the bigger business than the others I met starting out to work even the university graduates.

My first real, quote, job was at Martins Bank. I was fortunate, although I did not realise it at the time, to be assigned to their London Foreign Branch. In those days the Banks and similar organisations employed staff on an incremental salary scale. This ran from 16 years old to late twenties or early thirties. This still exists today in things like NHS and Local Government. My scale took you up to management level and if you had not been promoted by the time you reached the end of the scale you would not expect to get any more than a nominal cost of living increase. Pensions and family insurance were deducted as a percentage of your basic wage.

I understood this and was happy to aim for more money in my pocket than the manager figure at least two years before I attained that age. I could never compare or prove this goal as I moved on after seven years. Whilst at the Bank I worked my way through most of the jobs related to international banking but in the first two years also had to do the menial junior tasks. I used to start my day in the post room sorting mail and end the day addressing and stuffing and then franking and mailing. My day job moved round the departments and I learnt about Town and General Clearing, Foreign Exchange, in particular documentation for imports and exports and making returns to the Bank of England, Bills of Exchange, Bills of Lading and cashing of foreign cheques, drafts and letters of credit. I did a spell on the counter where we had a sub counter on the Dover Ferry and learnt about balancing outstanding travellers' cheques particularly for end of year returns. Our Accountant who was a barrier to anyone wishing to speak to the manager had been a conscientious objector and did not go to war but ran the office like a little Hitler. One day when a new girl started work in the typing pool the first letter she passed to this Accountant had the point of the pin showing. He tore the whole thing up and told her to redo it and present it with the head buried. The next letter had a few commas/full stops missing and these got the same treatment. That evening when I went to the Post Room for the evening duties she was in tears and had been told that she could not go home until the letter was completed satisfactorily. I finished up typing the letter with my two finger system and she managed to leave before six. She was not looking forward to the next day but to her credit she became well respected in the typing pool. I had my really bad experience with this man just before the Christmas after my father died. My mother woke that morning rather depressed and after sorting her out I made work for about a minute to nine. This would normally have been okay but on that day I was due to supervise the incoming post and run the Post Room. I entered the room to find the Accountant at my desk and he gave me a good dressing down. I flipped and told him that my mother had been reacting to my father's death and I had got in as soon as possible. He told me I had a job to do and had I not got brothers or sisters who could have handled the situation. I asked if he had a family and maybe a heart somewhere. I was about to go home when he exited the room. At this point all the post boys started clapping. The first day after Christmas I arrived to the signing in desk at two minutes to nine and found myself standing next to the Accountant who deliberately engaged me in conversation. At exactly nine o'clock he picked up the signing in book and told me to go with him to his desk and sign on in red as being late. This was probably when I made up my mind to look for work elsewhere in the Bank. I did however get involved with the social side of the Bank and organised an Athletics team and played table tennis and chess for them as well.

At this time with new markets emerging there was a need for a trainee foreign exchange dealer and I put my name forward for consideration. I was eventually told that the choice was to be between me and a chap called Barry. Barry was given the job and when I ask Personnel Department where I had failed I was told they could not split between us and they gave him the job based on his longer service with the Bank. When I pointed out that he was a relatively new arrival they disagreed. I had to point that he had been credited with two years based on the fact that he came straight to us from National Service which was their practice, they said they had not realised but could not alter their decision. I later applied to be considered for a senior job at the new branch that was to be opened in Streatham. The process seemed endless and when they announced the opening date I again enquired of the Personnel Department as to my situation. I was informed that I was the best candidate but that with all of my experience in the London Foreign I was too important and could not be released. I at this time decided that with an obstructive Accountant and a manipulated Personnel it was time to move and I started looking for other jobs in the City.

On April 2nd 1962 I started work in The First National City Bank of New York.

On day one I was taken to the department behind the counter on the ground floor and introduced to the Head and Deputy Head of the department. They were introduced as Les and Tom. They then said I would be working for Jim. This completely baffled me as I had only ever referred to my seniors as Mr this or Mr that. It took me a long time to adapt. The job was fairly easy to understand and the most important was to work within City deadlines to ensure every cheque etc. got to the right place by the right time. I worked alongside a lad called Frank who I got on well with and one day when I went to Hackney hospital to try and obtain some important medicine for my sister-in-law's boy I got severely delayed. I knew I would possibly be in trouble as hitting the next deadline would have been almost impossible. To my complete surprise my job was fully up to date as Frank had stepped in and taken over. We learnt more about each other after that day but unfortunately tragedy was ahead. I helped him organise buying wood for DIY in his bedroom after his parents split up and he felt he needed commitment. All seemed well but the next day he did not arrive at the office and we heard later in the day that he had died. Rumours were rife but I just felt very sad and helpless and I think the lads in the department then realised it was really no joke.

One morning soon after I got to work one of the staff tapped me on the shoulder and said 'I know you, you used to live in Nettlewood Road and went to 29TH Streatham Scout Group'. He was right and he had competed against me in local scouting events and when I was at the Gang Show in Battersea he was performing there. We have remained friends ever since that day.

In those days the City depended on a number of Money Brokers; we like others had a Money Desk and this was situated in the corner in front of the counters for Cash and Foreign Exchange. The Money Desk gentleman was always immaculately dressed in black jacket and stripped trousers and each day he had a standing order for a Red Carnation for his button hole. The Internal Audits and Bills Departments agreed one day that they would take the micky out of him and agreed that the next day they would all come in wearing a Red Carnation buttonhole. As I left home that day I spotted we had lots of Red Pinks in full bloom and picked about 20 of these and took them to the Office. The joke was appreciated but to all of our surprises a Photographer appeared from New York with the intention of taking a Group Photo of as many staff as possible in front of Tower Bridge for part of a worldwide advertising campaign. We were all offered 10 shillings overtime to go to the Tower of London and have our pictures taken. I was one of the first to arrive and this very American Photographer saw me in my Motor Cycle gear and asked me to keep it on, including the helmet for the shoot. I refused and then he saw our Money Desk man complete with Suit, Carnation, Bowler hat and rolled umbrella and exclaimed 'great man where did you get the gear'. I explained that this was his regular dress for the office and he shrugged. Later many others turned up still sporting their buttonholes. The final picture eventually appeared on the back page of the TIME magazine.

I moved from Cash One to Cash two and supervised Standing Orders, Direct Debits and various foreign payments and receipts but also had to cover for the Receiving Cashier for holidays and sickness. He was a definite hypochondriac and there was a whole drawer full of anything from Aspirin to plasters but particularly he had a bottle of TCP. This was kept for when we received notes and cheques from the Kuwait marketplace. These had to be counted and he did not want the foreign germs. We all stayed late when these arrived and shared the counting with some licking their fingers and others using a sponge and water. The Cashier used a sponge and neat TCP. Guess what he was the only one to get dermatitis. He also signed up for the new flu jab and for several years was always away for at least a week after it with Flu symptoms. Another job on the side was to carry gold bars from the open back of a lorry to the vault. This was quite a trek and two bars was about all you could manage for more than one journey but every time a new member of the staff started we arranged with the delivery man to give him three bars and it always worked, he would stagger into the vault and go back for more too proud to admit it was really too much for him. Pranks like this were commonplace in the office but we did have one practical joker who always went, in my opinion, too far. One of our managers nearly had a nervous breakdown because of his continual actions. I progressed to the Foreign Exchange Department and then to the bookkeeping area where I got involved in the statistics side. The Office was moved from Old Broad Street to Moorgate and about this time I was asked to run a small department of two or three to provide monthly breakdowns of the earnings from all the various trades and deposits with various interest and earnings cut by day, week, and month and to present these personally to some of the senior managers including the head of trading.

I was enjoying my work but at that time all of the staff were asked to take an IBM computer aptitude test. I finished in the top six clerical staff and was asked to join the others on an IBM sponsored training course on Computer Orientation and then on how to program in COBOL. This resulted in me joining an International team who were developing a Bookkeeping system which was to be implemented throughout Europe.

For this project I was to work in Paris for about 3 months from January to March 1969. This meant I shared an apartment with another employee in Port de Saint Cloud. I travelled by Metro to the office in the Champs Elysees and ate out in evenings either in the vicinity of the office or near the apartment. The restaurant in Port de St Cloud was privately owned and we ate there a lot and I learnt about good French wine but particularly I discovered I was quite partial to St Emillion. I sometimes worked nights to test programs and in the time when I had my car I was returning to the flat at about 3.00am when I stopped on a totally clear road at a traffic light. Half asleep waiting for the lights to change I was suddenly fully awake when two policemen with white gloves a side arm each and a kind of sten gun tapped with the butt of one of the guns on my driver's window and demanded 'identitie si vous plais'. I had never realised how quickly you could produce a passport from a back pocket. Very, very, scary. This kind of thing happened again at Le Tourquet airport and I produced a few coins from the depths of my pocket even though I only had less than the maximum I was allowed to take out of the country.

I was assigned a boss and had the responsibility for making the programs work on the newly installed IBM 360/30 in Basinghall Street in the City. A team had been assembled with a Computer Room Head overseeing the installing a head of data input who had to employ and train keypunch operators and me in charge of programming and development.

Before I could start any implementation I had to get the whole system into London from Paris where we had completed the development. The Company agreed that I should take my car to Paris for the last two weeks of my stint there and load it with the boxes of punched cards. We had definite reservations as to whether as this was now a complete bookkeeping system we should apply for an import licence but we decided that the Computer Industry was so new that this would not be covered and that we would leave it to customs to decide if we were acting properly or not when we got to the border. I say we glibly as when it came to it I loaded in excess of 35000 cards into my boot and set off for the late night ferry from Dunkirk. Not wishing to create questions I decided to leave the boot unlocked so that when customs ask for it to be opened I could just say 'it is open'. A long day and along night and so at six in the morning when the customs ask me to open the boot I jumped out to open an already open boot. The Customs Official asked me what was in all of the boxes and could I open one. This I did and prayed that he would not take random samples and I would have find where they had come from to make the system work in London. I need not have worried as he looked at one and ask me if I REALLY understood what the holes meant and I explained that I probably knew what was on each card. He was obviously totally bemused and said well good luck to you I hope it all works. I took the cards to the office on the Monday and when I got back home I realised that the rear springs had not, at that point, returned to the raised position. I pointed this out to my manager and he agreed that if it was still the same in a one weeks' time he would pay to have it put right.

This was the start of a long journey through data processing from the early days. I had become reasonably competent at programming in COBOL but my first task was to load the system we had written in Paris onto the IBM/360.and get it working and tested for implementation. We had excellent support from our IBM rep and with dedicated staff we got up and running in quite a short time. It was our boss's job to work with the senior management and auditors to arrange test and parallel runs with the existing manual systems. We had staff from the main office and our data centre to cross check all the results for several weeks and particularly over the month ends. Most people were very sceptical of the new technology and the day we stopped the manual systems was definitely a red letter day. It was not long however before the system was accepted and it looked like the promise of a paperless office was on the way. Not quite what happened! Once the front office realised that although the system only mathematically replaced the manual ledgers it held out great potential for quick and useful analytic output. One of the first enhancements was to provide analysis of the regular overdrafts split and distributed to the individual managers responsible for the accounts. After that the requests seemed endless. At this time I converted all of the Bank of England weekly and monthly returns into computer generated reports. As for the paperless society I was the first person in England to order a million sheets of music score from our particular supplier. Definitely unheard of. As with all systems you are dependent on manual input and although we wrote extensive edit programs to cut out bad data some wrinkles in the system occasionally came to light. Also all the controls were dependent on control cards. These sometimes got chewed by the reading machines and could be transcribed wrongly by the computer operator. When problems occurred overnight then my phone would ring and I would attempt to solve the problem there and then. If this was not possible then I would get in the car and do a 'hands on job'. This usually caused delays in the distribution of the reports the next morning and it was wise for me to either stay at work or go home and be back early so as to support my boss in handling the wroth of the traders and front office.

Year-end always meant that I was in the Data Centre for at least 36 hours non-stop but this also happened when we decimalised our currency. On this occasion I had written and tested all of the conversion programs and asked my boss to find out from the Management and Auditors what amount of monies I could write-off or accrue at maximum. Their first reaction was why did I need any but I pointed out that we were dealing in at least 35 different currencies and thousands of individual accounts each with its own sterling equivalent and each would have to be either rounded up or down. They then came back and asked if £10 would be enough but indicated that I could not argue. As I was to be the Officer in charge of the conversion I agreed on the knowledge that I could if necessary make my own decision on the day. As it turned out the whole process went like clockwork and to my amazement the final rounding figure at the bottom of the balance sheet was less than a pound.

Having come up through the ranks I was often in a position to change the input to reject the bad entry and redirect it to an exception report. Over time some people realised that bad entries went to exceptions for next day correction and took to trying to vary their month end figures in their reports through this route. They were not happy when I had a program written to identify particularly large errors and have them corrected to ensure inclusion in budgets. This did not make me popular and some years later I found out that the first item on the Operations Joint monthly meeting was 'how can we get Terry out of the Data Centre', this was to give them more ability to fudge returns. I actually stayed in my job and worked up eventually to head of Data Processing and Systems. Outside systems development staff in Europe and New York would write programs for implementation as additions to our packages. This was not always totally successful and on one year end our local European Systems team asked to run a newly developed program. I refused as it had not been seen and tested by my staff but was overruled by more senior management. The outcome was that we retained the programmer on site in case of problems and when it went down we thought we had done the right thing. Not true when we returned the dump of the process to the programmer he insisted that there was nothing wrong with his program and that it was our system. I had to insist that his manager send him home and said I would solve the program error myself with the help of my systems manager. We both decided that the instructions to the printer were the problem and all turned out for the best. Another event was when New York came to London and put what they thought were the finishing touches to a budget reallocation program. I was told that I could not refuse to implement this package as it was going to go worldwide and that they had spent 3 million dollars developing it. I persuaded my boss that we must have a chance over a weekend to test the system as first I did not know that it would work with live data and more important to me I felt it would take up so much space and time in processing overnight that all my important output would be delayed. I spoke to my systems programmer who was close to a genius with several maths degrees and ask if he could provide some really good test data as a combination of our own live file and some specially created test data (e g Blank records all Alpha or all Numeric etc.). He agreed to come in at 10 o'clock on the Sunday morning and told me he would be going back home in time for lunch. I emphasised that I was looking for his continued support and he said that he had had an opportunity to see the program and that the formula that it was based on came from a Cambridge University Book of Formulae and that this was not efficient to handle our situation. He said that within five minutes of running the whole machine would go into lockdown. He was true to his word and in this case by the time he was due to leave for lunch the N Y team had been convinced by his argument and by Monday the whole world wide development had been cancelled never to resurrect.

Alongside running the Data Centre I was fortunate enough to get to a number of in house training programs and was taught Effective Speaking, Credit Control, Change Management and various other goodies. One day I heard I had been given a travel award. This was generally a four week trip to New York with three weeks working with various departments in the Operations Division and a fourth week on visits to customers' warehouses and offices in other parts of the States. Just my luck that budgets were tight and they cancelled the prestigious fourth week and then told me that I would have to attend a new notorious course called Operations Management. I was given several books to study before the course which was to start on the Sunday I arrived in N Y and cover the next ten working days. This turned into a memorable experience as we were divided into four teams of six. My six became a five as one person was sick with Operations Management Sickness which seemed to hit lots of the locals who had heard of the horrors of the course. Our team included a man from a New York State branch, two from elsewhere in the States and a Woman Brooklyn Jew. We actually made a very good team and on the first night agreed that regardless of what we had heard about the need to work late into the night we would shut up shop at 7 O'clock each evening and go for a good meal before retiring and meet for an early breakfast to discuss the day ahead. We based our thinking on the fact that we had to have the computer input available for 6 o'clock and we could not effectively alter anything. The course was computer based and each day the work representing a month in the real world of an operations department. Our job was to convert a poor mismanaged and badly budgeted area into well-oiled one. The general way success was identified was in the reduction achieved in the overall budget. We felt that this was not desperately important and spent our time making a good presentation and presenting as a team. We also had a fridge in our work room which was always full of Buds and Cokes and on the last day of the course we were presented with a Brick for the team that had drunk the most Buds and were told that we had far exceeded any previous teams although there were only two mainly and occasionally four of us drinking alcohol. On the Wednesday evening we reviewed our work and completely reproduced all our charts for the final presentation which made all the others done with overtired eyes and voices fade in our wake. The next day after the team efforts each player had to make an individual presentation for the further month to a New York, Vice President. My own presentation done from a ring bound folder obtained the comment, (What can anybody say to a presentation like that done fully prepared and articulate in English by a very English man, thank you). During the following weeks the task that remains in my mind is that I was asked to predict staff requirements for totally unpredictable events. I pointed this out and was advised when the New York management asked for something to be done you had to do it. I explained my case but the response told me why many staff in N Y were in total fear for their jobs and were in fact the worst example of how staff could be demoralised but also needed to have a job.

I was fortunate that for one weekend I was invited to stay with the family in New Jersey and share their hospitality. For other Sundays I took the opportunity to visit the only really green area in N Y, Central Park. I found that the park appeared to be divided by the lake. The lake itself was constantly being circumvented by joggers and the paths full of cyclists but if you stayed on the city side although not obvious the grass area made up the concert bowl where the recent Paul Simon and Art Garfunkal Concert had been performed. On a Sunday afternoon this area was occupied by groups of people playing softball and baseball. Move further and you came across the Tennis Club and also a two rink Bowling Club. Go to the right you find the tunnel that features in lots of films and nearby a fully sculptured representation of the Mad Hatter's Tea Party from Alice in Wonderland. Also nearby was the Zoo. Move up past the side of the lake towards the Penitentiary and after a while the sport changes to basketball and American football and atmosphere changes to where I got a feeling of the hairs on the back of my head rising. At this point I returned to the city. I visited Bloomingdales the American Harrods, Macey's the dime store, the Staten Island Ferry and walked from Battery Park to my Hotel via the site where they were to build the

119

original World Trade Centre (the Twin Towers) and China Town and the Diamond Centre

Later a junior manager was asked to go to New York to participate in a new development of the local bookkeeping. He had only just returned from an overseas assignment and his wife was unhappy that he should be away for a further ten weeks. In the event I was asked to take on the assignment and found myself heading once again for the Big Apple.

When I started in the training centre on Long Island I discovered that it was not the start of the system but that all of the major decisions had already been made. Many of the key benefits of the European system had been ignored and interest and value dating were not included. More important the accounting and General Ledger were run separately with one system feeding the other and the packages being kept independent of each other. It was obvious that I could not affect this situation which was a very big disappointment but I was given specific tasks to achieve which I completed with time to spare and by giving up a trip home it was agreed that I could return to London after only eight weeks.

Again I only had weekends to discover New York and on one of these a colleague invited me to his home and I watched his son play roller hockey league and exchanged a little league baseball glove and a baseball for a cricket ball and bat. The young lad was amazed at how hard the cricket ball was and that we caught it with bare hands. Another weekend there were some other Londoners in town and we hired a car and drove to Washington. Early on Saturday morning we went to where the tourist touts were plying their trade. A man standing next to a coach told us he could give us a combined tour to include the Museum, the White House, The Senate, Lincoln Memorial and Kennedy's Grave in Arlington Cemetery. We debated the price and as we were visiting on education visas he agreed we pay only student rates. We followed him to the coach and he redirected us to a minibus nearby. He then took us to The Smithsonian Museum and arranged to meet us on the other side of the road at an agreed time. When we came out we found the driver and he was now driving a limo. We proceeded to the Capital Hill and the White House and the guided tour was very good but when it was over and we reappeared on the street the driver was nowhere to be seen. We had just decided that we had been conned when I spotted his car and he was about to pick up some new tourists. I ran over and collared him and he said he thought we had given up. We got into his car and from then on he was excellent and when we got to the Cemetery he told me I was to go with him to the gate house and advise them that one of our group was an invalid. This meant that he could save us a long walk and take us right to the side of the Grave. The changing of the guard was spectacular and completed our tour.

During the final days of my visit I did get quite involved in how the proposed software would be implemented and on the ability of the proposed hardware to cope with the necessary partitions and volumes. In this case I identified major shortcomings both in the available hardware and software support for multiply simultaneous processing. As the expectation was to implement the system within six months into the Middle Eastern Branches I felt a compulsion to ensure senior management were aware. On the Thursday prior to the end of my assignment I penned a letter laying out my doubts and listed the shortcomings of the chosen hard and software. That evening I invited the Head of the Data processing area to have dinner with me. Before we started the main meal I showed him my missive and asked him to consider it. I pointed out that I realised that he was recently promoted and was the first coloured person to have achieved such success. His simple comment was to ask was it all factual and on a solid basis. I confirmed this and he said I should distribute the letter if I felt that strongly. I again asked about his involvement and he said that he had not got where he was without knowing how to look after himself.

On the following Monday I left for work and my last words to Margaret were that with what I had done I could be home by 11 O'clock without a job. Her comment was simply 'never mind we will cope'.

At work well before nine I met my boss and gave him a copy of the letter. He was distraught and told me I had had a very good future and asked why I had written it. He said that the phone would ring at exactly 9 O'clock and we would be summoned to the sixth floor where the Head of European Operations had his office. He was right and off we went.

We were asked to sit down facing him at his desk and he said very solemnly that he had had a telex that morning from New York with regard to my recent assignment on the computer development project. My boss was waiting for the worst and kicked me gently under my seat.

'I hear they were very pleased with your participation in this project and could not understand why you were not as yet a senior officer of the Bank and recommended that at my next review this be properly addressed. In the meantime they had arranged for $1000 to be sent to London for payment to me and apologised that tax had to be deducted.

With a short well done I am sure London are pleased with you we were dismissed.

This gave a big boost to my career and many things turned for the better. I was lucky enough to be in the right place for a number of different salaries reviews in a very short period of time and one day as I came home from work and approached the front door Margaret opened it for me. She seemed better than I did at knowing when I would get home and regularly did this. This time I walked up the path and asked her to pinch me. Her response was 'You haven't got another pay rise have you'. She was of course right.

I was asked to accompany my boss to Athens to attend an area 3 budget meeting as his numbers man. I was once again the most junior member of the team and all the other countries had high level participants. I had learnt my numbers and was thanked for my efforts when I returned to London. It must have been positive as I was invited a year later to a similar get together in Brussels. This was hosted in style and at the end of each day we were taken out for a particularly special meal to end the proceedings. On the last night we were bussed to a Chateau on the outskirts of Brussels and as we left the coach we were welcomed by a local group facing the castle walls and playing hunting horns.

During the meal the kitchen staff paraded round the tables and introduced each course. The salmon was on a silver platter and decorated with the Citibank Logo. I was introduced to what must have been Premier Cru Chablis to which I have unsuccessfully compared future white wines. After the meal we all retired to the balcony over the Keep and chatted and shared drinks and at one point my boss caught up with me and at this point he again proved to me that he was the only American that really understood the English and particularly their sense of humour. He put his arm around my shoulder and asked me intensely if I could recall who I had been speaking to during the evening and then asked who I had been sitting next to at the table. I named those I could think of and he just nodded and then said 'anyone else'. I was quite nervous at this point as I had had a reasonable amount to drink and he took his arm from my shoulder and said 'don't try any harder, all I have heard is good reports'. A memory I will always treasure.

The time did come when they found it prudent to offer me a job out of Data Processing and I moved on to the Internal Audit Department. Whilst I was starting to get the hang of the ropes I heard that the chosen replacement for me had found the job more difficult than he thought and was off with a breakdown and to replace him they had split the area into two Departments to avoid a recurrence. My new job was interesting and challenging but the team were good and as I knew most of them quite well I felt I made a good start. This group were responsible for UK, Ireland, Channel Islands and Scandinavia. It was not long before I was lucky enough to head up Audits in Dublin and St Helier. I discovered that

Audits were always done abroad out of season so as to have fully staffed offices (to avoid the obvious excuse for shortcomings) and to suit the tight budget we always had to work within. The end product meant that on the first two occasions I visited Jersey it actually snowed. The amount of snow was so little as to be insignificant but on one visit I finished up ferrying the staff home in relays as none of them would drive on the snow. In Dublin I got into trouble with my boss when I entered the trading room and got involved in the banter. This was commonplace for me and I treated everyone the same and all seemed to go well but when I got back to our allotted office I was informed that only recently the Belfast trading room had been closed and the staff moved to merge with the Dublin Traders. I was advised to be very aware of the differences. As it happened when we neared the end of the Audit some staff including the Traders invited us out to a pub in the docks. This is before the regeneration exercise and the pub was full of locals and on stage there were people singing and playing the spoons and penny whistles. All very pleasant and sociable. A little before what I thought was to be closing time, one of the traders got up and decided to introduce his friends from England. This was immediately accepted as a gesture of good will and I think showed that the perceived animosity in the Branch did not really exist. I had by now been given a responsibility for Scandinavia and got involved in the auditing of the new office being opened in Helsinki. I found out that the Finnish did not consider themselves Scandinavian and were proud of their independence. Later I did a three week trip to Audit Helsinki, Stockholm, Oslo and Copenhagen. I fell in love with Copenhagen and visited it on a number of audits. When I returned with Margaret after I retired I was very disappointed as it had become a university town like Brighton and the walking road and the fountains were littered and over populated with students.

I had two assignments when I was co-opted as 'A DP Specialist' to assist the local Audit team. In Zurich again I found the place quite exciting and made up my mind to take Margaret there on a part of a holiday. I was respected for my involvement and only had one major difference of opinion on which I was eventually overruled.

In Athens it was a different story except that I was again introduced specifically for Data Processing to address Implementation, Back-up and Fire & Safety but also had responsibility for presenting the final Audit report. I had met the Athens Operations Head when he was in London and clashed with his opinions and on one occasion embarrassed him into accepting that I was right. One time he left a meeting to go to mass and confession and returned to the meeting and lied through his teeth which prompted me to suggest he return to the confessional. Not a good start and things got worse as I made major comments on one problem, the fact that the back-up power supply entered the Data Centre through the same duct as the mains power supply and two that a program under test was being run as a live function in the Operations Area. Additionally the second computer authorisation was being performed on an open and not a blank screen. These among other things encouraged me to downgrade all the sections of the audit from Excellent to satisfactory. I had arranged a meeting with the Operations Head and the Head of the Country for early on the day that I intended to return to London, to discuss and present my final report. The Ops Head immediately objected to the whole report but after about two hours he was pleading that he would accept all the downgrades except that of Management which he insisted should stay as outstanding. I argued that he was responsible and with his vast experience in London he was aware of these shortcomings. The Head of the European Audit, who I was representing, was attending the discussions and after my return trip had been put back several times he intervened and said that I had made my point and that he would handle the rest of the meeting and I should go for the last plane of the day.

I heard that on his next presentation to Head Office the Ops Head ignored my report and presented the earlier one as the current one. The head of Audit in New York apparently took him to task and said his presentation did not appear to reflect the updates that Terry had presented recently. His response was that he had not accepted the report, but he was made to amend his records.

I have mentioned earlier that I have met only a few nasty people in my career and this man was one of them and when he came through London at a later date he refused to speak to me except through an intermediary.

Not too long after this there was a potential fraud in the Purchasing Department and I was seconded down there to look into it and report to the Head of Premises Dept. The whole thing was strange as the particular reason I was sent to the area turned out to be relatively insignificant but actually opened up a different alley and caused the resignation of the Head of Purchasing. The Head of Premises was short of a manager at this time and I was transferred from Audit to run Payments and Expenses Area. In this capacity I ran a full audit of furniture and fittings and paintings. I upgraded the Inventory Control System and identified a massive difference in the list of paintings and furniture which led to a write-off of nearly one million dollars but the system was back under control. We also identified a management group that appeared to be duplicating their Expenses. It was agreed that this was the result of miscommunication within the area and a couple of individuals returned several hundreds of pounds to make amends for specifically identified double accounting. I was also at this time managing the writing of a new computer system for the whole of the Premises, Purchasing, remote ordering and inventory. I was head hunted to work with the control department in the Investment Bank and at first told them I would like to complete the implementation of the new system. However as a massive coincidence my cousin was working for the computer company in Birmingham who were writing our system and he was seconded to London to work at Citibank. I declared the possible conflict of interest and although I was advised it was relatively unimportant I arranged to follow my instincts and apply for the job in the Investment Bank.

I was transferred and moved to The Strand and took over the running of the Reconcilements which was run on Desktop computers using a small database system. I spent a lot of time and effort with the Department Head amending and streaming this into a simple and proficient process. An outcome of the better reconcilement identified an apparent non-payment of Can$ 1million. The manager of the area concerned assured us that there was no discrepancy and signed off the difference. John in the other side of the Control, whom I had worked with before agreed with me that this should not be treated in this manner and that we should continue to investigate. The end product was that John, his team and I received a one dollar Canadian bill each presented in a picture frame with the notation 'thanks a million' when the money was recovered. A great gesture by the Art Dept. and Head of Operations.

It was about this time that our daughter Christine was working in the Off Licence in Bromley and ask me to help her to set up a stall outside Bromley Station for Beaujolais Nouveau and her manager gave me three bottles as a thank you. I drove on to work and bought eighteen croissants and on entering the office I went to the kitchens and borrowed a tray, glasses and a tea towel. I then set myself up and as each member of staff came in I offered them a croissant and a glass of wine. All was going well when one of my staff told me that somebody was going to report me to the Head of Operations as alcohol was banned. My reaction was to go immediately to his office and speak to him and offer him a croissant and wine. He accepted and said it was a nice gesture.

One of the senior managers in international audit asked me if, as I had a vacancy, would I interview his son? This was not a practice of mine but in this case I agreed. When I interviewed the young man I found out that he had been employed straight out of school by a local motor engineering firm on the Government guaranteed two years training on a fixed nominal wage. At the end of this he was expecting to be offered a real job but was actually told his employment was to terminate. They were to con another young into cheap labour apparently supporting a sponsored Government Scheme. I did employ him and he proved very capable but was obviously more interested in working with his hands and not sitting all day using his wits. He got to know the engineers who serviced the computer and after a short spell of working in the City he was offered a job as one of their engineers which he accepted and as far as I know it worked out well. This lad had done a lot of his schooling in Greece and one of his school friends got a job with us in London. While he was working for me the two of them went back to Greece for a holiday which ended in tragedy as his friend was found dead as he was sunbathing on the beach (another death to somebody I worked alongside). It did not end there as his father later died while out jogging when he felt he was getting a bit overweight. I spent a number of evenings after work playing snooker with him and hope this helped him along. Later his mother re-married and the family seemed to get on really well and on moving down to work in Lewisham I then lost touch.

Not long after this the Control Dept. was audited by the company's outside Auditors. The overall area was rated unsatisfactory and although we had a good report in our section it was not long before the dept. was closed down and merged with Citibank. This indicated that I would probably be made redundant and to take early retirement. At this time someone must have felt it wrong for me to go and found someone else to offer me a post. I worked next door to the training centre for a while and with the Control Dept. and then moved into the section handling year-end company returns. There was again a local desktop database system managing this process and it was particularly cumbersome. There were five girls operating six terminals and an order was in for a further one. Each girl would input on one terminal and while waiting for it to process input another transaction into a second machine. My first reaction was to see if there was a purge program and had it been used. Nobody knew the answer to either and it was down to me to find the documentation. There was if fact a purge program but no evidence that it had been used since the system had been set up several years earlier. I decided to gamble and see if the program would work and ensured the staff stopped work early one day and set the program to start the purge. By nearly 8 o'clock it was still running and I did not know what was happening but decided to put warning notices to the cleaners and anyone else not to switch the plug off which was standard practice. When I arrived early the next morning the program was still running and so I told the girls not to start until I was ready. By just after ten I felt I had to make another decision and pull the plug on the program. That evening I returned to the terminal and looked at the records and to my surprise it looked as if the purge had been working well and I was able to restart and stayed to see it complete the purge and rewrite the master records. The girls were amazed the next day to find that the one terminal was ample to keep up with their input speeds. I looked closer at the keying process and saw that although in more than ninety per cent of the cases only the front page was needed but a further six pages had to be accessed, accepted and verified. I studied the Database System and decided to modify the programming so as to exit the system at the end of the first page if appropriate. The end result of these actions meant that we reduced the five terminal operators to three.

At this point early retirement again reared its head and this time it was really going to happen. I was quite happy with the process but disappointed that as of the previous April the terms had changed significantly and not in my favour. The main impact was that I had to repay my mortgage and loan on the day of my retirement. The previous system had allowed you to complete the repayments as long as you lived in the same house and only had to repay if you sold up and moved.

CHAPTER ELEVEN

Business Events

Life was not all work as we know it and from early in my business life I got involved in helping to organise staff social events. This chapter will detail both social and business that I was either involved in organisationally or simply attended either personally or with the family.

My first effort in Martins Bank arranging an evening jazz riverboat trip which started at the Tower of London and travelled to Teddington and back, which proved to be a great success and was repeated in later years. I started an athletics club and we managed to participate in a number of inter club events and also the Junior Banks Competition at Motspur Park annually.

At FNCB of NY there were established events both in the company and within the American Banks Organisation. As you have heard I played football in the Banks League and took part in Bank evenings out which included an annual stag night for the men. I only went twice but the second one was at The Hilton in Hyde Park which typifies how the Bank treated its staff to top level quality events. We also learnt that the stripper who danced at our table was only part time and had a full time job at Midland Bank.

Early memories to come to mind are the Children's Christmas Parties which were run by some of the ladies who bought and wrapped presents for each child. These excellent presents were supplemented by tea, of course, but also at least a couple of professional entertainers. One year however they were short of either money or an entertainer and two staff and I stepped in to do some slapstick comedy. I never really liked the idea of climbing a ladder and putting paper on a wall only for it to come down over your head but then I was absolutely amazed to hear the excited screams from the kids. I also remember the party was arranged for the day after the Brixton riots in Railton Road. I had to take the children to the West End Branch and this meant driving through Loughborough Junction just alongside the end of Railton Road. My neighbour advised me to go by a different route but I decided that this was not necessary and at the traffic lights approaching Camberwell Green the man in front having stopped for the red light was unable to start his car. He got out and was looking for someone to help give the car a push. At this point I wondered if I was in the right place as the driver and his passenger were dressed I army fatigues and the nearby bus stop was attended by three large coloured lads. Low and behold these three ran over the road and with a quick push and a wave set the car and its occupants on their way. You would not have known that there had been carnage there overnight. What spur of the moment hospitality!

We also had an annual Family Day and the first to come to mind was when Thorpe Park had just opened and we took over the whole complex for the day. All the rides were free and there was a water skiing display on the lake and of course free food. There was another time when I was fully involved in the organisation and then the activities on the day. This was an 'It's a Knockout' over water. We ran it at Harrow Leisure in the outdoor pool area. On this day I saw the best and worst of people. It was my job to announce each event and demonstrate it prior to the teams competing. The teams were representing the various sections of the Bank. We had Operations, Human Resources, Marketing etc. and many senior managers actually took part in the actual events. We had a well- known band and DJ, John Peel playing all afternoon in one corner and we had built a stand for spectator viewing and we provided an Ice Cream Van, a Mobile Fish and Chip Shop and further food outlets. The competitive side of the management came through and in the last event of the day, which was a straight forward dinghy relay race. Not so! The bung on the HR dinghy was removed by the Operations team and in the following melee the Head of HR had an oar hit him in the face which gave him a bloody nose. I abandoned this race and said it would be replaced by a simple swimming relay. The Head of HR said he was ahead and going to win when he got hit and he should be given a walkover even if the others raced for the other places. I risked my future loan approvals by insisting he took part or came last. We completed the tournament and my children rallied around to collect all the balls, bats and other paraphernalia while I took a welcome rest on one of the benches by the side of the pool. I had my eyes closed when someone put there arm round my shoulder and thanked me profusely for my efforts. I will always remember this gesture from Andy Ripley who I looked up to as an outstanding rugby player who was to represent his Country later. No one else said any words of thanks but this gesture gave me all the thanks I needed. After the whole thing finished and we were in the car park preparing to go home we saw the sad side of life. Many of the staff who had been to these occasions before had brought ice boxes and had filled them with the free food and were taking it home. These people were to my surprise not the low paid workers.

On another occasion we took over the whole of the Albert Hall and took out alternate rows of seats and fitted tables so that food could be eaten at your allocated seat. My job at this event was to sort out the seating and bar arrangements where the aim was to get the front office and the support staff to share a bar but not in those days share the same section of seating. At this event we had the stage cast of IPI TOMBI perform for us but as we were an American Bank and at that time going topless was infra dig we had to insist on the girls covering up. The three forces band played and marched for us and the evening finished with dancing to a popular big band. Until this particular day it had been the practice to offer a staff member who was unavailable or perhaps did not want to come, to be given a cash allowance to entertain his or her partner to dinner. The Head of Human Resources came up with this idea of using the Albert Hall and as it was prestigious and expensive he put out a notice that you either came or not. No alternatives. I happened to be at a management dinner at an offsite do in Winchester and sat next to Mr HR. I was next to my boss when I told him that it was not as clear cut as he thought as on that night I and others would have to have staff manning the office on planned shift work .My boss felt I should not create a fuss and told me so but I persisted. I was told that the HR man was like god and could not be challenged and did not bend to popular opinion. However the next day at my lunch break I received a call from the Office to be told that a circular had been sent out to say that any staff member who was on shift on the night of the Albert Hall function would be contacted and offered an alternative. Another chance of being refused a loan (it never happened and I finished up getting on quite well with our Mr HR). We ran a similar event the next year at the Alexander Palace and the meal was provided by one of the best restaurants in London and when our blue collar workers tasted the soup they complained that it was cold; not realising that it was in fact a cold soup which they had never heard of.

For a few years a chap called Terry Fitt ran a swimming gala and for some reason asked if I could help. This was held at the Indoor Baths in Holborn and I acted as M.C. while Terry and others kept track of the results and the prize giving.

Each area was allowed to run its own Christmas outing and I attended one in Shepherds Market where a conjurer/illusionist relieved a number of the staff of watches and wallets etc. and music was provided by Tudor Minstrels and a violinist. Another do was held under the arches at Tower Bridge where the food was served on pewter platters accompanied by mead and music.

Later the Christmas parties were to be organised at departmental level and as my area had to work particularly hard over that period in preparation for the Year-end I decided to have my do in February. This was arranged at my house as we had our own bar and a swimming pool (all be it very small) and we had outside caterers cook the food on the premises. This went well but one husband tried to insist to my daughter that he only ever drank double gins and she said that I had told only to issue measured singles so all knew where they stood with regard to driving. He was upset but I and his wife put him in his place. Another idiot tried diving into the pool, against advice, which was only 5ft deep. He was relatively unhurt but had a rather nasty graze down most of his chest. I did feel after this that it was better to give a less generous allowance of food and drink and go to themed restaurants in future.

The American Banks at some point decided to organise a London to Brighton walk. This was to be in teams of four with any number of teams being entered by each Bank. The event was to start at The Guildhall but the ladies started at Merstham near Redhill. In those days charity had not become a big thing and most walkers entered for the fun of it. We started at Guildhall at about 8 O'clock in the evening and walked overnight. Each four were supported by at least two helpers and one or two cars to provide drinks, moral support and even accompaniment at times. When I walked I had failed to do any real practice but we all four got as far as Crawley without mishap and with our best man striding ahead of the rest of us. I needed a change of footwear and got left behind to do 'running' repairs. At this point we were averaging over 4 miles per hour. The chaps in the car kept me up-to-date with our position as medals were to be given to the four with the shortest net time. As I approached the big pillars marking the five miles to the Brighton Pier I understood that we were possibly in the lead but that the two walkers behind were in contention. Not quite disaster but at the pillars I met one of our team members sitting on the grass verge declaring he could not go any further. I pleaded with him to not let the team down and eventually he looked up at me and asked if I was really going to finish and when I said definitely he replied that if I was going to finish in the state I looked he could surely reach the Pier. By this time we had been passed by one of our opposition and I had stiffened with standing around. We did however get going and after what must have been at least two more hours we kissed the railings of the Pier. We heard that one of the other team had got left behind and was not sure he would finish but on the next Monday we heard that we had come in the first three teams and at the prize giving evening we each received a proper silver medal. I believe we won but being as the medals were not engraved and each of the members of the first three team's home got a similar medal I think today we all think we won. The next year I joined with one of our team to become an escort car. We drove from Lingfield to Brighton and left his car there while we then drove to London for the start of the walk. One of the team we were supporting dropped out just outside of Purley but we still helped the other three. When we got to Horley we caught up with one of our lady's team and I was asked by her as I was her boss to give her moral support and walk with her. My car partner thought it was a good idea as at that point she appeared to be at the head of the ladies event. This was a more than brave decision as I finished up walking the whole of the rest of the walk with her where she was greeted as the first lady home. My legs were killing me after 25 miles and I still had to pick up two of our men's team and deliver them back to their homes in London before driving back to

Lingfield. By the time I got home I had been out for very nearly 24 hours and driven 150 miles as well as walking with both the lady and each of the men for several miles. I vowed never to do it again but was back again the next year with a different co-driver.

A special event was the celebrations for the 25th anniversary off my time at Citibank. This went in three stages. The Company sponsored a lunch and a cocktail party and I arranged a get together in a pub. The lunch was for me to invite eleven members of staff to join with me which was expected to reflect who had been an impact on my career and was still around. At this event, prior to the meal I was presented with a 25 years pin and a silver platter and the event took place in the Senior Officers dining room in the Strand. The cocktail party was an after work event also in the dining rooms in the Strand and the invite was sent out by the Human Resources Dept. This was less formal and attended by those who thought they had a working relationship with me and of course a few hangers on who came for the free snacks and drinks. A Senior Officer of the Bank attended at my request to give a potted-history address to all present. My own do was in the Cheshire Cheese in Fetter Lane off Fleet Street. This was known for its Real Ale and Pie and Mash. I ordered several barrels of ale and invited Work Colleagues, Friends and Family with no speeches but a very convivial atmosphere. A great time from what I remember of it.

In 1986 the two country Annual Board Meeting was set to be held in Scotland and England and I was co-opted to look after Security, Data Processing Facilities, Secretarial Support and Luggage transport from Scotland to London.

This whole process started nearly a year in advance and the first of my tasks was to get the security set up. I was told that I would have to provide guards on a 24 hour basis as well as medical support on the same basis. The head of the task force arranged for helicopter support for all the time in Scotland and to support the rail trip down to London. Early on I met some of the largest and well-known companies that provided these services but I eventually settled for a firm in Woking run by an ex forces man. The price was sensible and we became a good team. We worked with about sixteen staff and in Scotland where our base was The Gleneagles Hotel the guards hot-bedded at a B & B in Auchterarder which was within walking distance. Special events had been arranged for the first weekend and each evening and it fell to me to visit all these places with the New York Protocol team. One week they came over and I picked them up at Prestwick Airport and drove first to Gleneagles and then over subsequent days to a restaurant in Edinburgh, Royal Residences north of Edinburgh and Balmoral and St Andrews Golf Course. Each evening we shared dinner and of course they wanted the experience of Eagles Nest (the hotel restaurant) which was renowned worldwide. I felt that I had eaten better and the next evening I took them to a recently opened French Restaurant near the Hotel and this was voted better than the previous night. The next night I took them by minicab to Glendeveron and this proved to better again. While we were out the following day, thankfully for me their last night, they were betting that there was no way I could again improve on the evening meal. Always up for a challenge I settled on booking in at a small hotel with a small bar and run by a husband and wife in Crieff. Guess what! I won. This was then selected for the team dinner for the night prior to the start of events proper. On this occasion I booked the whole restaurant and agreed a limited menu. We were in the bar ordering our various meals when the head of Protocol advised me that she was vegetarian and could not eat any of the arranged meals. I sought out the wife and told her my problem and she said that I should not worry as she herself was vegetarian and she would do me proud. She was right and to this day I have not seen a better veggy meal, it had fruit, nuts, root veg and red and green salad. It looked absolutely grand and the New York lady apologised and then personally thanked the hotel.

As part of the hospitality I was tasked with purchasing cigars basically for breakfast, lunch and dinner. The recommendations were built up based on previous meetings and did not include the British popular King Edward. I spoke to Protocol in N Y and they agreed I could make amendments as appropriate. I then realised that as I understood that only green cigars were approved in the state of N Y it would be correct for us to include these in our selection even if they were not used. I got agreement and bought lots of cigars in a shop in St. James and they loaned me a humidor for the week and agreed a sale of return for all unopened boxes.

In the run up to the event I went with the Security Manager to visit the planned venues and when we got to St. Andrew's we pulled up next to the eighteenth green and the driver asked me very politely whether he could get out of the car and walk over to the green. I agreed and he left the car and walked right on to the green and got down on his knees and kissed the ground. This action provided the prelude to the actual golf morning as on that day I had to provide security and this man was selected to drive a minibus with golf gear while the twelve who we had managed to book tee times for went in three limousines arranged by the lad in charge of travel. Don't ask me, but somehow they had put thirteen men into the three cars and we had one too many players. It was good fortune that the assigned driver for the minibus was our golf enthusiast and he summed up the situation and managed to find a three who were willing to take our spare player along. Seeing his keenness our Bank's Board member decided to invite him to caddy for him and this not only made his day his man also finished up with the winning score. He became my backbone when help of any sort was needed even if it did not relate to security or he was officially not on shift. In fact when we were leaving for London all the Board were to travel by a chartered 125 Express to York where they would transfer to the Orient Express for the onward trip to Kings Cross. I had arranged for medical staff to be on standby at all the major hospitals en-route and the helicopter was to escort both trains in case of an emergency. As breakfast was to be served on the train all baggage was to be left outside the rooms in Gleneagles for security to collect and put into a removals van for the next step of the journey. The van had been organised by our self-proclaimed excellent travel man and having got an extra man to golf he appeared not to have managed to get the van to Gleneagles. He of course felt bound to enjoy the experience of the train travel and was not available to solve the problem (no mobile phones in those days). I found out that the van was actually booked for the next day. Using the security intercoms we arranged for the coach to return from the station to be loaded with the luggage to be taken to Edinburgh Airport. I had leased a transport plane to leave Edinburgh at 11 o'clock for Southend where we had to transfer the luggage to vans and get it all into the correct rooms by 4 o'clock. It seemed a good compromise with ample time but as usual paddy's law came into play. We could not according to the coach driver put the bags in by the unused seats but had to stow them properly in the luggage compartment and so by the time we were on our way we arrived at the airport to find that the pilot had removed himself to the main building for refreshment. Next problem was that my helpful security bod started to try and load the plane which nearly caused the union rep to call a strike which would have stopped us for at least several hours. This solved we had an excellent turnaround at Southend only to hear that The Orient Express was running 30 minutes early. I slept well that night as we had completed all tasks to please our team manager and the Board Members.

On the last morning before we returned them all to the Concorde Lounge at Heathrow one of our Board members made a point a finding me a thanking me for the work we had done and implied that it was the best Board experience he had had. I told him that there were others who had made up the team and he asked me to introduce him to them so that he could thank them personally, which he did. Again just one single person thanking me but also again a gesture to be treasured. When we arrived at the Concorde Lounge one of the board members from Texas had his six shooter returned by British security. We had relieved him of it at Prestwick when he came in and insisted he had not had it away from his sight since he was a small boy.

When retirement came it was customary for the company to provide a cocktail party for the retiree and his invited friends which normally was not expected to exceed forty of fifty. At the time of my going we had a system called Citimail which was similar to email in today's world. I decided to take advantage and sent my invite to everyone who owned a Citimail link (known as a mailbox). On the night well over 100 people turned up and John McFarlane gave a speech at my request. I understand this was probably the last party held as the cost significantly broke the budget but who was I to care! Onward to a happy retirement.

CHAPTER TWELVE

Holidays/Trips

My first memory of a holiday was as previously mentioned when I came out of hospital about 1948, in Brighton. We went to Brighton on several occasions as we had a fraternal uncle up near the race course and my father liked an early September break during what was known as the Sussex Fortnight. We would spend the mornings on the beach and at the Pitch and Putt courses at Brighton and Rottingdean. For the first few days we would visit Brighton Races and then go on to Lewes where the horses on the longer races ran right along the horizon. At Brighton the races could be seen for free from the open downs which stretched for miles to the pub in the distance at Woodingdean and had its name (Downs Hotel) painted in large letters on the roof. While we were still small we might go into the stands and we were lifted over the turnstiles for free. When we were bigger we found a point where the railings were badly made and we could work our way through, again for free. On the outside there was one bookie who took sixpences and did not worry if you were underage. One day one of the bookies must have had a bad day and decided to scarper across the Downs with what was left in his bag. A number of us gave chase and he was soon caught. If the betting went well we went to Folkestone races later. I seem to remember that Goodwood was to be an option in the second week but do not think I ever went but we did visit Brighton Dog Track at times. The B & B was quite cheap but near the front and on our first visit I seem to remember we were offered Cod and Chips for dinner and Mick took one look at it and said it was not Cod but was Coley and we only fed that to the cat. He was told to be quiet and eat up but we all knew it was Coley.

We progressed from the Guest House to renting Bungalows first in Peacehaven and then in Ferring. I bowled my first wood with an uncle in the Peacehaven Club which had several Billiards Tables a Dart Board and a bowling green. I remember my father was asked to play Billiards and he suggested that it would be better to play Snooker. I realised why when he had all three balls in one corner of the table and simply kept making cannons. There was one year a friend of Mick's came with us to Ferring and when he spotted me asleep with my eyes open he thought the worst but his shout woke me up and all was well. My last family holiday was the week before I started work at Martins Bank.

There were several holidays with friends usually with at least Adrian and Chris and mainly at Holiday Camps and they all consisted of sport and dancing with beach games and swimming. There were no lasting relations from these and we all returned to the Youth Club.

Adrian and I cycled to the Isle of Wight one Friday evening and found a friendly landlady who was willing to put us up in her conservatory if she was fully booked. On the Friday and Saturday we went to the local jazz club in Shanklin where the singer was in my opinion better than Ottilie Patterson. In order to afford to go on a reasonably frequent basis we managed to get part time work on the Saturday's in the Café on the Pier.

No special holidays until my honeymoon, which has already been mentioned. We did have the Holiday at the time we were moving in at Crowborough but the next step was my own family events. The first I remember is our first boating trip on the Thames which came about by accident as one of our staff members had booked a boat for himself, his girlfriend and two or three more couples. At quite a late date one girl discovered she was pregnant and they could not afford to go and a break up and sickness left him with facing paying the full bill and not being able to go because the boat was too big for just two to handle. He offered for me to pay half the cost and bring all my family. The boat was rented from Maidenhead and although it was not totally harmonious we all fell in love with the idea of boat hire.

Our next trip started from Market Harborough and went through the Oxford and Grand Union Canals. We learnt how important it was to make sure you closed all the locks properly as that year there was little rain and the Oxford Canal was very low and at times almost un-passable. Having gone south for the first few days we wondered if we would get back. We did but only with some quite severe groundings. This would not have happened if everybody had paid attention to the canal etiquette. We became braver and again rented a craft from Maidenhead and travelled on the longer journey as far as the boat would go to the bridge at Letchlade. We had developed a pattern by now similar to my cycle trip around Holland. We would do all the boat checks in the early morning and travel until around lunchtime when we

149

would seek out a pub for a pub lunch. At some time before or after lunch we would discover the town or village and hoped among other things to find a good eating place for dinner. In some cases this did not work out and we carried on from place to place and stopped when we were happy with the dinner arrangements. On this trip I do not recall any significant incidences but when we went with friends on another occasion I recall that Chris was having a strop and was last off the boat as we left for dinner. I was in front of her and all I heard was her entering the water behind the boat. I think she was hoping to get sympathy but all I did was hook her out, take her back on the boat and put on a dry set of clothes and then catch up with the others. We were also at Goring on the Thames when we bought new wellingtons for the girls and then went fishing. I do not know how but Christine lost one of her new boots into the bottom of the river never to be recovered. She was less than happy.

Later we rented a 78ft narrow boat from a yard in Tewksbury for a two week trip. The first part saw us travel along the Avon where many anglers were fishing from the bank. This was the first time I had seen cluster hooks in multiples on fishing lines and I felt it was a barbaric way to fish but I understand it was popular and was allowed in competition. We got to Stratford and looked round before next day entering the canal system. First we encountered a large bank of locks and as we had learnt on the Oxford canal the boaters have to work all the locks themselves. We did not have the luxuries of the Thames. Actually we found lots of fun in this exercise and were to get quite experienced. We got to the Birmingham canal system after going through what seemed a very long tunnel where we had to cut the engine and work our way by walking our hands along the ceiling of the tunnel. It was very dark and we kept the children inside the cabin area but it sounded as though they enjoyed it. Arriving in Birmingham two things struck us (we were there before the re-development). The first was the amount of debris that was dumped into the water from bicycles to shopping trollies. The second was that the water was as black as ink but we could anyway make out many thousands of small fry obviously surviving in the pollution. Leaving there we came to Wolverhampton Racecourse but the real challenge was the almost twenty locks with a large pool area half way down where we could take a rest and prepare for the next stint. We had thought our first set of locks had been strenuous but this lot were actually very exhausting. Our next incidents were at Stourport-on-Severn where we were to have our toilets cleared and refilled with chemicals. We had completed this satisfactorily but as we crossed back across the harbour and tried to moor Karen did not quite get it right and managed to fall into the water between the boat and the wall. There was so much oil in the water that when we got her out her face was black and her clothes absolutely coated. We cleaned her up and decided to have a really nice meal that evening to make up. The other incident which has been recounted more times than Peter would care to remember was in the five star hotel restaurant. He was put in a high chair so that he could reach the table and we all ordered our meals. We had got a bowl of soup for Peter and he obviously enjoyed it as when we looked over from our own starters he was seen to be raising the soup bowl like a cup and drinking the last remains. We all learnt a lot by visiting places like this

151

and on this occasion although we chastised him the staff were amused and quite proud of what he had done. We travelled on from here to Worcester and moored on the bank of the Severn on the far side from the town. All seemed well and I was at the helm and the kids were sunbathing on the foredeck. Suddenly there was a shout 'Peter's fallen in the water'. I run into the boat and banged my head on the roof of the Galley, banged my leg in the saloon and then tripped up the steps to the deck area. With my shin grazed and my head halfway through the door I heard the next shout 'But we have got him out'. They all had buoyancy aids and I think they thought all my efforts and cuts were a reason for a good laugh. We explored the town and visited the ceramic factory and saw the cricket ground almost under water. We were near the end of our journey but had to go through the commercial lock at Tewksbury which was a frightening experience. We pulled in as the first craft and the lockkeeper took our ropes and told us to stay where we were and all would be looked after by the men on the quay. The next thing that happened was a fully loaded container ship drew in alongside us. It appeared to me that the wall of the lock and the side of the ship towered at least twenty feet above me on either side and I was in an eight or nine foot gap. The lockkeeper must have realised my novice level and came round and assured me that, honestly, we were very safe. He was right! Before leaving we visited the cathedral and had to traipse through a couple of inches of water which went right up to the entrance doors. Something I always remember when the flooding is shown on television.

We returned to again rent the ten berth wooden boat 'Gay Roberta' from Maidenhead for a week's break in October. It had rained very heavily for a whole week just a week before we were due to leave and I phoned the boatyard to enquire whether the Thames would have a swell as a result of this and was assured that we could take the boat out. We were two families on board and not long before approaching Goring we were passed by a very large converted barge. The Barge had moored just short of Goring Lock and as we were passing it I thought that one of our 2000 cc Perkin Elmer motors had failed and shouted to Peter, our friend, to check for any blockages. There were no apparent problems but we not only stopped making headway but appeared to be about to go backwards. I checked the lock and the white flag was flying but at that moment the lockkeeper came running out from his house with a red flag to close the lock. Reality dawned and we were using governed motors and the swell that I had asked about had hit us and we were now travelling backwards at increasing speed. I tried to zigzag to keep the boat in midstream but looked back to see we were actually probably heading towards the small local craft or the very large converted barge. The very sizable gentleman with a big beard came on to the deck and started to send his many children to collect fenders from the far side of the boat and rest them over the side I was heading for. This made me feel sure he thought I would hit him. He had other ideas and called to me in a bold voice 'Keep going son. You're doing well'. He then kept up with instructions and encouragement and we moored gently alongside his craft. The children helped secure the ropes and with the usual, women and children first we disembarked across his boat to the bank. He

153

guided my crew and pointed out the nearest pub. As I was Captain and last off, he put a hand out and stopped me with a congratulatory comment and a large glass of Brandy and said 'you probably need this and the rest of your lot are in the pub over the road. I did need the tranquiliser and was happy to have met another of the unhailed gentlemen that add something special to life.

We never did get through the lock before it was time to return to Maidenhead but the experience gave me pleasure and encouraged me to later rent a Sunseeker type boat on the river Shannon in Ireland. This trip left me with three or four memories. First because of the weather we went up the river from Carrick-on-Shannon and when we moored to go into explore Boyle, Margaret rushed across the car park and tripped. By the time we had walked into the town it was obvious that she had done at least severe bruising so we went into the Chemist and while she spoke to the Pharmacist I visited the very convenient bar in the back of the shop. End product was at least a broken rib. The nearest hospital was over 50 miles away and our car was parked in Carrick. We made the decision to get the boat to Carrick that evening and to drive to Sligo hospital the next morning. Soon after we left the shelter of the mooring it was apparent that a strong wind had come up so Margaret went to the cabin to rest on a bunk. She must have been in a lot of pain, as we watched a tender boat appear to be crossing our path it completely disappeared from sight behind the waves created by the wind. The hospital said there was little they could do but if possible they would like to see her the following week. She made the appointment as asked for 9.00 am, as we were going to be staying with Shawn's family in Crossmalina at that time. I pointed out that this was a 50 mile journey and we would have to leave at 7.15 am at the latest and that normal practice was for me to be drinking and playing board games until at least 2.00 am. We did not return to change the appointment but returned to the boat and continued our holiday. We went down stream in the hope that the thick mist would clear so that we could go through the Loughs to Galway. We stopped at about 11.00 am and while Margaret and the kids walked round town I visited a local Inn to find out our hopes of navigating if the mist did not clear. The owner of the bar had bought the place on returning to Ireland to retire after working in England building roads for the previous 20 years. He told me there was no way we could expect to go downstream and I asked him how he was enjoying his retirement in his homeland. I was interested because I had an idea in the back of my mind that I might like to retire to Ireland. His actions and words clearly said it would not be for me. First he drew himself a large whiskey when pulling my pint and then he explained that the speed of life was so slow and back in the fifties that he was suffering with depression but could not afford to go back to England. I could see his point. After we returned the boat to Carrick we drove back round the lough that we could not navigate and had a drink in a local pub. The boys wanted to play pool but the table was occupied by a German father and son. I suggested they challenge them and we started to chat. The two of them had brought a boat across the lough and said it was easy and that they could have walked over the reeds if there was a problem. At this point I realised that they were drinking Guinness too quickly and that they had in fact scared themselves stiff. I was glad I had taken the barman's advice. We toured some of Ireland before going to North Mayo and this and another trip to Dingle get mixed but I do remember that I bought a blazer from a stall on the coast and that the man gave Tim a book of Irish Birds as he showed an interest at the time. We also took his visiting card and later bought from him again. In Mayo Shawn's father insisted we get up early each morning and he would show us round his surroundings. He took us to Ackle Island where he had been the Gangmaster when all the roads were laid and showed us the cemetery used especially for the potato famine and explained how the men went to Scotland and many got burnt to death in a fire on the farm they were lodging at. The boys Tim and Peter later returned and worked on the farm and we also returned later with Shawn and his wife. I did stay up half the night each night playing card games and drinking and I certainly did not have the energy left on the last day to climb Croix Patrick. On the morning of our return I was taken to meet the Matriarch of the family which entailed going to the local pub in her village where we changed a barrel of Harp and I was later invited into the main room of her house to share homemade Poitin (illegal distilled whiskey). I guess my car was doctored because when we got back to London I was told that I had imported at least nine bottles of the illegal whiskey and that for my trouble I could keep one. That was Shawn and the Irish for you.

Just one further boat trip and this was again on the Thames but with Robin's friend Paul joining us. This turned into a question of which of them could find a better evening meal than Mr. Fitzgerald. We lunched at the Copper Inn in

Pangbourne and Robin decided that the restaurant there was going to be his piece de resistance and we arranged to return in the evening. We had a starter drink and I asked Robin if we were eating in the bar area or the posh restaurant and, of course, he said 'posh'. He and I shared a Chateau Briand for the first time and became hooked on it. This is normally a full fillet cut up between two diners and was often the dearest item on the mains menu. The meal was excellent and we retired to the lounge area for coffee and platters of English Cheese with an after dinner drink. This was not only expensive but was more than I had ever paid per person and I am not sure that even to this day Robin has really got over the shock. He remembers to price to the penny. He still now always spots the best and usually the most expensive meal on a menu when I take him out, which nowadays is quite often thankfully.

Other holidays we enjoyed were when we used to just get in the car and stop each evening at a B & B which had to be within walking distance of a good eating house to avoid the need to limit the drinking because I would have to drive home. One trip took us all round Scotland where we visited a number of distilleries but also drove alongside the Lochs and visited John O'Groats. Leaving there we passed through the Highlands down to Loch Ness and we saw and I think at least one of the kids did a bungee jump. We stopped in a posh house on the side of Loch Lomond and found it was run by a member of the Duke of Argyle's family. I explained that I had worked with Lord Lorne in London and had been to his stag night and also was invited to his wedding in St. Giles in Edinburgh. As we were going to Inverarey the next day she offered to ring him and try to arrange a meeting. I foolishly did not accept and thought I could just surprise him. When we visited the Castle he was not available and I missed his return call that evening as we were out of signal range in a basement restaurant. Even worse he died suddenly later at quite a young age and I had not been able to get back to see him. This was not our only trip to Scotland but Chris was with us although she had missed our previous year's holiday in Cornwall (more later) and she was surprised that although she had felt too grown up to come she really enjoyed the stop at Aviemore and Ice Skating in Inverness and even the sightseeing. The other B & B trip that as interesting was round Wales. We started entering through Shropshire and went down the North and West Coastline. Somewhere near Harlech we noticed a big change. We could not easily find accommodation and went to the Tourist Centre. We paid a small fee and booked for a stay in a local B & B. We were given a ticket to present to the people who ran the place but as we pulled up outside the lady came running down the path and said there had been a mistake and she did not have rooms available. I think this was because she saw our number plate and did not welcome the English. We had already that morning been into a local grocery cum post office and as we entered the chatter changed from English to Welsh and we were only served after there were no more locals to be attended to. A further event on this trip was that in Abergavenny we knocked on a door which was answered by a young child who listened to our requirements and escorted us to some rooms on the third floor. Next morning we went down for breakfast and found there were just three young kids looking after us, they took our money which was a more than reasonable cost and we never did find out if any adults actually lived there. Anyway at the aftermath of this Peter returned to school and as was common was asked by the teacher where he had gone on holiday. He apparently said 'abroad Miss, to Wales'. She explained that Wales was not abroad and his reply was 'well they all spoke a foreign language'.

We decided that we should go back to Cornwall again and felt we would like to take the whole family and my mother to Heston on the tip of the toe. Christine had reached that age of supposed independence and wanted to make her own arrangements so she declined the offer to join us. We had booked into a good hotel and used each day to visit a place of interest after breakfast, have a pub lunch and do more visits in the afternoon before returning for dinner. I particularly remember visiting a closed tin mine where we all had to put on hard hats and we did take a photograph in which we looked a motley crowd. Mostly I remember my mother keep telling me I was spoiling the children and that I should not be spending all the money it was costing. Typical of a caring mother who knew what it had been like to be lucky enough to have come through many frugal years, which had included two wars and the loss of her husband. This holiday was however a great success and when Chris was told about it by her brothers and sister I am sure she regretted digging her heels in and staying at home and this probably contributed to her reluctantly agreeing to come to Scotland the next year. She was of course determined not to enjoy herself but in fact she turned out loving it.

Apart from formal holidays we did on occasions go out on day trips either to places of interest or the seaside. When Chris was very young you only had to show her the sea and even in February or October she wanted to go for a swim and being a responsible parent I had to get into a swimming costume and look after her. Not the part of the day I enjoyed most. In the early years we had second hand older (to say the least) cars which tended to break down. We lost a core plug on one of our outings and while we were waiting for the breakdown service Karen found a discarded cone with the reflective cladding gone. This made it look like a witch's hat and it helped to while away the time with the kids taking turns to pretend to wear it.

Going back to my visits to hospitals when we went to the playground behind the sea near Bexhill and Christine hit herself on one of the rocking horse elements and cut her face under her eye. When we got to the hospital she refused to have stitches and eventually the doctor gave up and mended it with what were known as butterfly plasters. On another occasion one of the children, I think it was Karen, ran on to the beach near where we now live, either East Preston or Climping and immediately stood on a piece of glass. When she had been stitched up the family felt that they had not really had a day at the seaside. The pleasures of fatherhood, such delights.

CHAPTER THIRTEEN

Family parties/Events

I think I should start with the close family get-togethers
which probably started with Chris's sixteenth birthday when I
thought it would be a good idea to take all the family out for
a proper meal, that is, to a real restaurant and not some
burger bar. I cannot recall where we went but when Karen
was sixteen I asked her where she would like to go and
stopped outside what I thought might be an acceptable
venue. She got out of the car and went to look at the menu in
the window and came back to say that it was no good as
there was no vegetarian dishes. This was the first I had heard
that she was that way inclined and she told me she had
decided only that day. These occasions were interspersed
with trips out to eat for any reasonable excuse and there are
a few special memories. The most lasting are that I went to
many local places from basic Italian to fairly high class like
the Napoleon in Croydon where they parked the car for you
and there was a proper sommelier, and I was never let down
by the children. Looking back I do not doubt that some of
these times were very wearing for the children but it appears
they learnt to appreciate this style in later life and I watch
them introducing their children and their friends' children to
a similar torture. Anyway nowadays they are always willing

to accept my dinner invites and even invite me out on days like Father's Day.

As mentioned Robin liked his food and on one of his birthdays we visited a local Italian restaurant with neighbours also with us and the owners knew us quite well. Early in the evening the subject of oysters came up and the owner said he had some in his kitchen and invited Robin to share some with him (he had never tasted oysters). Much later that same evening we were the only guests left and it was agreed we would test out Robin's appetite. We were each served our sweets except for Robin. The manager took a massive wooden spoon which he kept on display and cleaned it in the kitchen and returned with his wife pushing the sweets trolley and presented both to Robin and said that as he was the last person that day he should use the large spoon and clear the trolley. I do not think he quite made it but he gave it a shot.

On another challenge for Robin we went to a pub near Tonbridge which promised to put a framed photo of you on their wall if you ate a whole chicken. The catch was not that it was at least 3lb in weight but that you had to clear the plate including all the veg. I warned Robin not to drink heavily before the meal but he ignored me and when asked to slyly help his sisters happily refused and he lost. Not very often I can say that Robin lost.

When Karen was studying history and Peter was only three I settled on ensuring the children all had passports and I then obtained the documentation to travel to Europe. I decided to spend a few days in Paris and show the family around on an American style tour to include The Eiffel Tower, Champs

Elysees, Arc de Triomphe, Louvre, Notre Dame, Sacre-Coeur and a trip through the Bois-de-Boulogne and a visit to Port de Saint Cloud where I had shared an apartment during my stay in 1969. On our visit to Sacre-Coeur Peter was amazing and walked up all the steps to the top and back down without asking for a carry. We bought a painting of a French Boy and failed to buy anything in the Salvador Dali museum sadly. All went remarkably well until the lunchtime of the day we were coming home. We visited the shops behind the Elysees Palace and after going in and out of several shops we arrived at a side street and in true Terry style I spread my arms and stopped and counted the children, and, low and behold Peter was missing. We had actually only gone about 50 yards since we last saw him and I confidently went back up the road. At the last shop we had visited the lady said that she thought our boy was lost and had ask a Policeman to take him to the local police station. It sounded simple when she gave me the directions but I mistook 'tout droit' for 'a droite' and finished up asking a lorry driver with a map to direct me to the police station. We found the place just in time to see a young police lady offering Peter some chewing gum. Anyway, I had Chris with me and we returned via our previous route to collect Margaret and the rest of the children from where we had left them. At this point I told Karen that she would not be able to visit Les Invalides as we had run out of time. I guess it was both a result of losing Peter and not being able to brush up her History but she burst into tears. It was then agreed that we would run round the Museum and look at as much as we could. I was right that we would be running late and it had now started to pour with rain. We had to get to Dunkirk in short shrift and I put my foot down on the motorway. This

163

was fine until I saw our rear wiper disappear onto the side of the road. Never mind I carried on and we made the journey home safely.

A few years later Karen wanted to go to Paris on a student union organised race for charity. To cut a long story short at the last minute this was cancelled. I said as we had got the Green Card for the car and paid the extra insurance we could perhaps convert this into a family outing. We did just that but went to Belgium on the overnight ferry to Ostend. We visited Brussels where first thing in the morning we met a work colleague of mine but then went to the Autonium and saw a fair in Antwerp before staying overnight in Ghent. The girl at the Hotel was very helpful and sorted the best price for our rooms and advised us where to eat. Next day we visited the regular market and also a bird market before going back to Ostend where we were lucky enough to see a carnival passing through the streets with big floats and eight foot high men who we guessed were on stilts.

One Christmas Eve a friend of mine suggested that we join his family for an evening meal. It was a good idea but his wife's choice of restaurant did not come up to my children's standards and the boys still remember the greasy Turkish Café in Sydenham, however, the idea caught on and I started arranging Christmas Eve dinners from then on. We started as a small family group with a couple of friends but this regularly expanded and at times we had at least twenty which for some years included my twin brother. Being him, he liked to wear flashing light ties, and part way through the evening would disappear to his car and return dressed as Father Christmas with presents for everyone. One year we had our first introduction to Political Correctness and when Mick offered presents to the kids on the table next to us, the parents got quite uppity and told him not to talk to their children. Life has only got more difficult since then and everyone has to be careful what they say to whom. Still only this year Karen's Partner's daughter said she recalled these events and wanted her mother to organise an evening for the whole of the family who lived locally.

On a lot of the dinners that I hosted I would try and get a table gift for the ladies and men. It started with cuff links and gloves and after broaches, keyrings etc. I eventually settled for travel compendiums and then I just gave up.

I think I thought that I could cook and at times invited two couples round to dinner when I would prepare the meal. I got a lot of support from Margaret and Christine both in selection of food and table preparation. Chris became our cocktail maker and bar person (all part of her training for pub work and running an Off Licence). With a couple of my work colleagues we went to each other's houses in turn and this went on for a number of years even after I retired.

I particularly remember after Margaret's mother died we made special efforts to look out for her father and three happenings come to mind. We had a special dinner at the restaurant on the A24 outside of Worthing and it was a terribly stormy night. We sent Robin off to pick up his grandad and thought that he knew where he was going but after nearly an hour we were more than worried but he then turned up and said that he had turned too early and got lost in a private estate and could not get his bearings (pre satellite days). We all thought that Robin was clever until then and then decided that he only had a photographic memory and actually needed more savvy. Remaining with grandad Margaret and I took him on a short holiday for a short B & B break in my usual style and each evening we had wine with the meal. Grandad insisted that he only enjoyed sweet white wine and that Liebfraumilch was his choice and although I got him to try some French white he was adamant in his choice. We introduced him to a new version of alcohol when at the end of a meal at another dinner with Mary and Margaret we asked if he would like coffee and he agreed to have an Irish coffee and after tasting it said this seems to have alcohol in it and I thought he was going to order another. He had never had Irish coffee before. On what I think was his 80th birthday we went again as a family group to the Findon Manor Hotel and true to form we ordered his favourite white wine which he shared with Mary. I noticed that the bottle was empty and went to order another when he said he would try our red wine. Oh I like this he said and from then on it was never a problem buying him wine.

I had a couple of work related parties and Chris was in her element and had been instructed to only pour measured drinks and no doubles. One husband told her he only drank doubles and that she must serve him. This was the first time she threatened to have someone removed from 'her' bar. I was called and supported her and spoke to his wife and all was well.

The other kind of party was the extended family parties and I can never get these into order but will try to relate each and pass on some anecdotes. The parties included my mother's

166

75th birthday, Margaret's parent's diamond jubilee, another anniversary for Margaret's family and my 50th birthday. My mother's party was as described earlier and we had the usual knees-up and sing song. I think it was about then that her three boys started a trend of jointly singing the Guy Mitchell number 'She wears red feathers and a hoola-hoola skirt'. At one of Margaret's family parties her cousin sat in the corner and attempted to drink us out of beer and stuff his face all the time he was not supping, and going back to my surprises we managed to get Margaret's cousin Simon to collect her mother's brother from a hospital in Northampton and bring him in his wheelchair down to West Wickham. On this occasion I was standing outside the house when Margaret's mother said what a magnificent party but what a shame her brother was too ill to attend. At this point Simon drew up and took a wheelchair out of the boot of his car and settled her brother into it. I do think she shed a tear as she greeted him and was completely overwhelmed. The day before the diamond jubilee party we took Margaret's mother and father for a surprise outing. We drove to Waterloo Station and parked the car. We walked over the bridge and I pointed out that you could see down past St Paul's to The Tower of London one way and to Westminster the other. This is a great sight and we later did the return trip in the dark when the same view was there but totally different in the night lights. We continued over the bridge and entered The Savoy Hotel and had afternoon tea to the sound of the white piano in the corner of the lobby. Margret's mother was delighted and thought what a lovely thought but we then left the Hotel and walked to the Theatre and watched Evita. In the interval I found an usher and asked if she could get the cast to sign

167

our souvenir program. She said we should have asked earlier but suggested that I leave the program with her and she would, during the week get the autographs and send them to me. I did not expect what happened next. First as the second half started a gentleman came on stage and announced the presence of a couple celebrating their Diamond Jubilee and then within a couple of days the program turned up through the post with most of the cast having signed over their photographs. As I worked near the theatre I took a large bunch of flowers in for the cast to share and was thanked profusely.

My 50th birthday was, as I was a twin, sent out as an invite to a hundredth birthday party. When the invites had been sent I had a call from a cousin who said he would be coming but thought that his brother would have to decline as having been out of work for a while he had recently got a job that involved working Saturday nights. Denis would have only been in his new job a few weeks and would hardly be likely to be given time off. I had hardly put the phone down than I had Denis on the other end. Great idea I will be coming to your do. I said he must not take a sickie and he said 'no problem what a great invite, I showed my boss the invite to a 100th birthday party and he said I must not miss it and gave me the time off'. When the last family arrived with their young baby I calculated that we then had 100 guests at our 100th.

MIDI-LOGUE TWO

Life is about to change and will be more concerned with
Margaret and I reacquainting ourselves with each other and
sharing some of our aspirations. I will now proceed to ramble
more and take things as they come to mind and hopefully
interlace holidays, bowling and family together as I think of
them rather than in the specific order that they took place.

CHAPER FOURTEEN

Retirement

I had decided that I would definitely enjoy my new found freedom and planned to take Margaret on a tour of Europe before settling into a more regular pattern of life but first I had to put my finances in order and sell the house and in modern parlance, downsize. We also had Peter living with us and had to arrange how his future would pan out. Anyway, just as a start, I arranged to put the house on the market and to take Margaret to Athens. Whilst in Athens Margaret cut her foot and it became infected. Whether this was the start of her Diabetes we do not know but it was only a week or so later that she appeared to have a severe bout of flu. First one doctor then another evening locum gave this verdict and said we would have a difficult weekend. Later that evening Margaret wanted to go to the toilet and was unable to support herself. I again called the doctor and was told that there was a long queue and he would probably not come before the early hours of the morning and the operator asked if I reverted to calling 999 would I ring her back so as she could rearrange the doctor's round. Sadly I had to ring her back and not much later Margaret was on her way to hospital. When we arrived at the emergency ward there appeared to be some serious concern and I was not allowed to meet Margaret or the doctors. Eventually she was transferred to the intensive care ward where she remained for a further week or so and did not return home for a further week. At this point she was diagnosed with serious Diabetes and has been on Insulin every day since. We had enjoyed our first trip abroad as a couple and were determined to do more trips but getting to grips with handling the Diabetes meant that a long trip around Europe was out of the question.

Finding a property and moving was a priority as three years earlier when Peter was about to start his GCSE course we had searched the Worthing area for a bungalow and found only one that we liked and this was sold before we could put an offer in. I went down to Findon Valley to register with an Estate Agent and found that the property that we had missed out on was now back on the market. Without checking with Margaret I discussed with the Estate Agent how I could put a hold on the Bungalow as we had not marketed our house in West Wickham. His recommendation was that I put in a very low offer in order to delay the process and he would assure the seller that I was a genuine buyer. I talked to Robin and he said go the whole hog and drop by a round twenty thousand. We did this on a Friday and to our amazement the offer was accepted on the Monday. I had all my usual problems with selling houses but we did get the place and the next twenty years were underway.

We bought Peter a motorbike to commute to Croydon and although I thought it was a tough ride he tells me he enjoyed it. He had not seen the bungalow before he returned from work on the day we moved in and his first exclamation was 'I thought you had bought a bungalow, not a ranch'. He later moved to live with Robin as had Timothy before him. This reminds me that except for Robin, who was self-sufficient, we assisted each of the children onto the housing ladder. In Tim's case after he was married and was selling his flat we had trouble completing on the Freehold purchase and one day he rang me from a solicitor's office to ask could I get money into a specified Lloyds Bank account before noon that day, it was about 10.45 am at the time. No sooner the word than the deed and the transaction was complete to the surprise of the solicitor who wanted to know how we had managed it. He must have thought he was stalling again on behalf of his client but lost the gamble.

Margaret's diabetes was on a very fast learning curve and she had been registered with the senior Consultant in Sussex for special care. We called the ambulance on two occasions but by the time they arrived I had managed to get some serious amount of sugar into her and she was recovering rapidly. In truth it was somewhat like having a baby in the house again as I would lay half asleep and half awake and listen for changes in breathing patterns and or rising temperature. She could get up in the morning and knowing she had a low level count attempt to have some breakfast. I several times found her buttering and marmaladeing her bread over and over again and not eating anything. When challenged she insisted she was eating and it was quite difficult to get her to eat properly. I thought we would never win until one morning after we had visited the Lido in Paris she woke up and I asked if she needed sugar. She seemed not to hear me but suddenly of her own accord said 'I think I need some sugar'. This was a massive turning point in her personal control which was later enhanced when the consultant suggested she take control of her own insulin doses by taking injections before each meal as appropriate to her planned intake which by now she always measured.

Before we bought the place I had insisted that we pull down the existing conservatory and build a big one in place of it. We built the largest you could without going for planning permission and we also had the place double glazed. I also remember that the insurance company that I had used for probably thirty years asked me because I had had a claim for broken drains in my previous property to put locks on all the windows and special locks on all the outside doors before they would cover me. I phoned to explain that I was in a new property and that it had Crittall windows and doors. The outcome was that I insisted on getting a proper quote as I would not want to tell a new company that I had been refused cover. Immediately I got the quote I moved to another insurer.

One of the first things that happened was that a member of the bowls club called to say that he had changed his mind and could he buy one of my train sets for his kid's birthday present. This would have been easier if he had made his mind up before we moved but as it was I loaded the whole 8ft x 4ft layout on the roof rack and drove up the M23 where my heart was in my mouth when a police car passed but he did not pull us over. The other train set was given to a local lad who Peter had got to know and had later married someone with a couple of children. The doll's house went to the family on the other side of the road who had a daughter who later became a good dancer and was auditioned, and got the lead in Barnham on the Worthing Pier.

 On the side of building alongside Cissbury Gardens I got cheesed off with cutting the hedge and decided to put a fence above the wall on both sides of the double door entrance. This did the trick and I think enhance d the look of the property. Inside the fence and only about ten feet from the building stood a very large Canadian Blue Cedar. This did not look too sizable when we moved in but after a few years it was overhanging most of the roof. I remembered that this tree had a preservation order on it and applied for planning permission to take it down. This began a long running battle with the planning department. First they allowed me to only crown lift it which was a particularly short sighted action. It was several years before one day the planning manager called at the door and when I was about to start another argument he said I should be quiet and listen. For no apparent reason he had decided that we could remove the tree as long as we replaced it with a specimen tree. Low and behold he agreed we could plant a crab apple tree about 15 feet away in the front garden. I immediately arranged with a local tree surgeon to have the tree cut down and the root removed. He did this at a good price but was to regret his quote. First when he was about to walk along the bough over the roof he realised that the tree was rotting and he would have to use block and tackle. Maybe the planners had found this out on a tour of the district but I doubt it. Later when he was using a power saw to destroy the root he came across a lump of concrete and broke a tooth on the chain saw. He stuck to his word and honoured his quoted price. The

Planners gave me less hassle when a local one man builder arranged everything from plans to the final finished extension to our kitchen. This did not include the extra cabinets and white goods or the tiling. We had the area fitted out by a local kitchen shop and I completed all the tiling. The work was excellent and my tiling did not I am told let it down.

Although my boss told the world that he would re-employ me as a consultant it was obvious that he never really intended this to happen although he did later offer me a job on local staff in Oslo, which he knew, did not suit me. I was lucky however as another employee asked if I could help him out and I worked variously in Florence, Bahrain and exotic Newcastle and this helped pay for the alterations to the bungalow.

In 1993 soon after moving Christine and I arranged to go on a Beaujolais Nouveau run organised by the British Racing Club. We went out on the Sunday and stopped in the morning in Paris in the Champs Elysees for coffee and a croissant which cost us most of our spending money for the day. We did anyway find time to stop for a special lunch in a small family restaurant in a village outside Fontainebleau. We decided to start with oysters and picked a dish of 18 medium size to share. We had an excellent lamb dish and a sweet. When we got our oysters there were in fact 21 and this made me feel there had been a mistake. When I came to pay the bill to the little old lady who appeared to be the head of the household I queried 'why 21 oysters?' and she said that we had ordered medium but as that day they were fairly small she had given us three extra. Where else would this happen? We arrived at St. Etienne and next day found a tour shop that was preparing to open later in the year. The owner was not there and our joint language skills were limited but we agreed to return the next day. We met someone who had some English and we agreed to be escorted around several vineyards the next day. We were picked up late, just as we thought we had got the arrangements wrong, and the driver of the minibus had brought his girlfriend along as a translator. We heard that the local rugby team had just won a cup and that the team consisted of many of the vintner's sons. We visited a Castile and then were offered either a series of small or large commercial vineyards We opted for the small and felt by the end of the day we had met the whole rugby team but could not be sure as our girlfriend 'translator' was very drunk after the first three stops and we had to get by with my efforts at the French language. We got back to our hotel well after dinner had been served but had had a grand introduction to the Beaujolais Region and it now sat alongside St. Emillion as my choice of wine. After a Gala Dinner on the Thursday with a midnight firework display we obtained our wine and left to make the shortest journey back to Calais and the bungalow.

During this early spell in the bungalow I built an en suite shower in our main bedroom and then went on to completely strip the bathroom and with Robin's help move the bath and sink and find space to put in a proper shower. These tasks done and health manageable we did set off on a shortened motor tour of Europe which took us down to Florence up to Lake Garda, over to Innsbruck, Salzburg and Venice and back through Zurich and Brussels. Not what I had first intended but an excellent trip. With further regard to travel throughout retirement we walked, boated flew and trained around Norway and this was such a success that later we drove round with Mary. The whole trip was arranged through Norway Only and at one of the hotels we stopped at there were two helicopters doing pleasure rides over the fjords. It was nearly closing time but I convinced the salesman to get me on the last flight and went over and told Margaret and Mary to come with me as I had a surprise in store. Many of our family gatherings involved an element of surprise especially for Margaret. There were several times that we managed to get her right inside a restaurant and she was almost sat down before she realised that most of the restaurant was full with her relatives or friends. On one of her birthdays we visited the London Eye and the New Tate and I had arranged for call in at Peter's house on the journey home before meeting the family in a restaurant in Croydon. Margaret was expecting a short stay before the rest of the trip home. All did not go well as I had a problem with the car and only limped to Peter's so our delay and the repair that Peter and I effected locally meant that we could not follow our original plan and Peter would have to come with us to get to the restaurant on time. I then suggested to Margaret that we take Peter for a meal and drive home later. When we stopped in the car park all the children had parked their cars just by the entrance where we had to pass them in order to park. Margaret did not spot the cars and I asked Peter to choose a restaurant nearby. He of course selected the one where the rest of the family were gathered. As we entered we had to stop the waiter giving the game away and he ushered us to the table in the middle where it was not until she had had her coat taken that she realised she was attending her own birthday party. A similar event took place after we had celebrated our 40th wedding anniversary and arranged dinner, bed and breakfast in an hotel near Dorking. I had got to the bar and ordered pre-dinner drinks before Margaret was aware that her three Bridesmaids and partners were sitting in the corner waiting to share dinner with us. I think that it was not long after this that Margaret said she would prefer no more of these surprises. The actual wedding celebrations involved me arranging a coach to the Epsom Derby. I invited all of the guests who were still around and their and our children to join us. The coach started in Kent near where my brother Mick and our Tim's family lived and picked up in Croydon and Leatherhead before going to the parking space on the rails. We wanted to make a quick getaway so I prepared the driver and told anyone who had winnings to collect to get to the front of the queue and get to the coach with all haste. All went really well and as we were the very first vehicle out we attracted a mounted police escort to the temporary exit up by Tattenham Corner and my guests thought it was a good touch that I had organised for the close of the day.

Somewhere along the way I thought it would be a good idea to invite our near neighbours and some bowlers who lived in the valley to join me in welcoming the New Year in in traditional style with wine and snacks from noon until 3 o'clock on New Year's Day. This was a great event and went on for many years until we had about 30 odd people coming and I thought the original aim of bringing locals together had been abused by infiltrators and most of the near neighbours had died. One neighbour tried to replace this effort but it did not last long, sadly.

My 65th birthday came and for this I took over a complete Italian Restaurant in Shoreham and in this case invited who I wanted to and had ex colleagues, bowlers and family and long standing friends. I remember only that it was a great evening and I was given a cake. The next week Margaret and I flew to Rome for a short vacation. We walked all round and visited The Trevi Fountain, The Colosseum, The Vatican, and found a fantastic art studio in the middle of a park on our way back. It had life sized carved wooden horses and coaches really lifelike.

One of the couples who had attended the New Year Party from the start told me that he had never really seen Scotland and this resulted in me taking them on a Terry tour which we all found worthwhile and it certainly added to my whisky collection. I also proved that my B & B formula still worked and we covered lots of sights from Edinburgh to Balmoral, Inverness, Oban, Loch Lomond, Inverarey, Troon, Burns House and Gretna Green.

A couple of further holidays are when we visited Lucerne and we met up with my cousin's daughter for dinner and then ate at a restaurant near her apartment in Wagga and saw how she lived and had done for many years. It did not seem long after this that her mother Pam had a special birthday and we were fortunate enough to host the surprise occasion when some their family and ours got together and shared stories of the past parties and gatherings and a number of memories which if I remember rightly I got somewhat confused and was put right. I trust this narrative does not have those lapses.

We also travelled, as usual, with overnight stays but by now we were looking for more comfort and stayed in gourmet hotels each night. We managed for the second time to visit Robin's friend Paul who lived in Huddersfield but first travelled through the west of England and the Lake District which I thought was one of our better holidays.

I have not mentioned that when Christine was about a year old we were given a small rocking horse by a friend of Margaret's mother, and for some reason I wrote a letter to say we could not accept as a gift and enclosed some money to buy it. I had always wanted a rocking horse and did not want someone to ask for it back when they had grandchildren. I must have been clairvoyant as some years later we were asked to return it. I refused and we have still got it. It has had an interesting life as early on Christine thought that the mane and tail would grow and cut them both off.

Staying with Christine somewhere in the 90's we decided to take her to France for a birthday meal and of course, on the way, call in to Belgium to get her up to a year's supply of tobacco. These trips became annual and are still on the agenda. We have discovered some of the best restaurants within striking distance of Calais or Dunkirk. One particular place is in Le Wast near Boulogne and having found it Margaret and I thought it would be a good idea to spend our Christmases abroad. We first went to Bruges but later returned to Le Wast and have now organised a gathering of blood relations just prior to my 80th birthday which I and Christine are putting the final touches to. I guess that going away for Christmas was really my idea as for many years we had met up in the holiday period and as I did not like getting up in one of the children's houses on Christmas Day and I did not want to start visiting each child on successive years I took the easy way out. I must say I do not regret this and the places we have stayed have been excellent value and now sometimes on our return we then meet up with the kids and theirs for exchange of presents and to catch up with each other.

Later we started going on River Cruises which were also something new and good because I did not have to organise anything and we had organised outings and three meals every day, some with wine or beer. We did the Danube and visited places along the way including Budapest and Vienna. We actually returned to Vienna on a boat over the New Year and the fireworks were continuous from about 11.00pm until well after midnight and as we moored in the middle of the city we had 360 degree fireworks. We visited Holland which included Amsterdam, the tulips and the ceramics before visiting Ghent Brussels and Bruges. We got really ambitious and booked a trip off the coast of Scotland on a fairly small exploration boat. The idea was that we went from island to island and discovered the ancient history of the Vikings and the stones. It meant that most days we left the boat and via a small disembarkation area entered a ten person Zodiac. This was quite a difficult activity for people of our age but to our surprise we were among the younger half of the group and age told one day when a fellow passenger was actually blown over by the wind. We did manage to see much marine life and three golden eagles which gave a special memory to the trip which took us to the Isle of Man and back to Mull and through the Munches where the whirlpools were dramatic but not seen by all as the weather meant that only a few of us braved the deck. The Isle of Skye and the distillery had to be there to conclude the trip. Another time we went up river from Avignon to Lyons and on a later trip visited Bordeaux for trips around the vineyards and a harbour where we went into the village and enjoyed oysters, well I did as all the guests who did not like them allowed me to have their allocation.

Of course I also carried on bowling and joined both an Indoor and Outdoor club and got involved in competitions. Indoors I played in both the National and London and Southern Counties matches with the same skip and went two years without our rink losing a match. I think this helped when the club put my name forward for a County Badge which was by good fortune presented to me when we played against Kent and I was well acquainted with their President who said some nice words about me. I started to play more games with The Banks Bowling Association and did some committee work before being honoured to be President. As President you were expected to select an area for the tour during your year, so I started to tour in order to get to know the ropes. On my first tour Christine took the same week as holiday and stayed with her mother which turned out to be a great success as they got to know one another again and shared shopping and eating together. This continued for several years. Sometime later I was able to join the London Irish bowlers when they relaxed their rules of entitlement. These two commitments were shared with at least one other bowler and we took turns to drive or drink. I also joined the

Dennyside which was a charitable group that played on Mondays in the summer and usually raised lots of monies for their host's selected charity. This was a success until the others appeared to be a lot older than me and I started to do all of the driving which eventually became too much when compared to the returned pleasure of the bowling and socialising as I could not include a drink. I gave up bowling but not until I had served a number of years as President of The British Wheelchair Bowls Association. I met the Chairman of this organisation about the turn of the century and when I became captain of my outdoor club I ran a captain's day and raised enough money to buy a specially adapted wheelchair to be used at Stoke Mandeville during training weekends. As President I introduced the use of charity boxes and managed to get these placed in a number of petrol stations and shops. I ran an annual President's Day and with the help of other's and particularly Christine managed to always collect at least £1000 on the day. I like to think I did my bit while I was fully associated and involved with bowlers in the South East of England. I played my last game for the BBA at Newhaven and although I was particularly unwell I did manage to win on my rink on that day. The next morning I called the doctor and she seemed worried and prescribed antibiotics. The next day she rang to enquire how I was. I then discovered that she thought that I had pneumonia. It turned out that I had an Inhaled Infection and was still very ill. I was referred to the heart surgeon as she felt that she had also identified an irregular heartbeat. Having recovered it was now about the middle of June and raining and I thought maybe I would not bowl this summer. I did not miss bowling and when the indoor season came along I was not keen and when I collected my charity box monies from the clubs I was only interested in the company and not missing the competition. That was when I actually decided to quit.

In 2000 I had a hip replaced and in 2002 I had the other one done. These were both very successful and are still trouble free, which I think is due to fact that I worked hard at the advised exercise regime which in turn was helped by Karen keep turning up and insisting on taking me out for a walk which was then supplemented with some cycling. Before I moved to our apartment I was walking across the road when my knee gave way. This was later diagnosed as a rucked cartilage and when the surgeon was about to operate (a keyhole process scheduled to keep me in for only 3 to 4 hours) he said that although I had limped in I would leave able to walk and without pain. I said that this would be a result of the anaesthetist and he told me it would be repaired and that I would be able to drive next day if I had an automatic but must wait two days if I had a manual. The miracle he forecast was absolutely true and I still have no pain several years later. Staying with my problems I had a fall in early 2017 and finished up with a bleed on my brain and was rushed into hospital for a brain op. As I am telling you this it appears that it was a job well done.

Going back to Findon I had both the back and front drives re-laid with the idea that we might need better access for heavy vehicles. We first used the back drive for a builder to remove our chimney which appeared about to be blown over and then to provide access to a new garage in the back garden. We bought an Irish DIY garage that came as a flat pack and seemed to have at least 2000 nuts and bolts and multiple lengths of moulded alloy that had to be fitted together to form the frame. We did manage this reasonably. It was built particularly to house Robin's Midget. Some years earlier the police seemed to forever stop Robin when he was out and about in his Midget and he thought it would be a good idea to take it off the road and give it a full and proper restoration. I was still fairly fit in those days and contributed both with some of the work and what seemed, at the time, quite a lot of money. I made new leather seats from a kit and did some of the trim. I also remember that Robin was proud of the job he had done in restoring the original rear number plate and asked me to do an equally good job on the front one before he was next due down. It was not long before I realised that this plate got all the stone chippings and needed a lot of sanding and smoothing before being painted with Hammerite. I feel quite happy that some twenty years later he failed the MOT because the rear number plate was not clear enough. The front one was still fine. We did the work in my main garage but when I bought a convertible I needed the garage and moved the Midget to the new purpose built effort in the back garden. The end result was really good and is still in good condition and used by Robin as his only car. Having helped to restore the Midget I then got involved with Peter who, having restored an Imp really wanted to have an Imp Van. He found what was described as a partly restored one and we travelled to the Midlands and collected it. The van turned out to be in a terrible state but we put our heads down and with lots of help and again what appeared to be lots of my money we completed the project. This is also now shown every year at the annual Imp show weekend. In this case I did less work and more supervising by arranging for specialist work to be done and ensure the signage was done properly.

Staying with restoration we go back to the rocking horse which was looking very sorry for itself so I decided that it needed a spruce up. I did not get on well with the rocking horse company in Covent Garden and sought out a small husband and wife business in Whitchurch a town north of Andover. We took a couple of days away and took the horse with us. The lady there made us a saddle and stirrups and sold us matching horsehair for the mane and tail and extra leathers for the harness and reins. They could not put a provenance on the horse but thought it was probably made privately for a shop like Harrods. I was given plenty of advice as to how much or not to restore what and later came home to put it all into practice. As I have said we still have it and it grace's our hall until forever.

Our life was often varied and we always tried to get myself and my two brothers together about twice a year. This started as an after Christmas activity but some time did not happen until at least February and in fact it was normally the three boys and their partners but being particularly late one year Pat invited Mick and me to join him at the races. It started with Lingfield but was later changed to Epsom Downs just prior to the Derby. I also met Pat at Goodwood and Salisbury, where on one of his big number birthdays I organised a family meeting in the Bibury Suite with a free bar and snacks and we retired to a local Hotel in the evening for a celebration dinner.

I mentioned that it was after a visit to the Lido in Paris that Margaret started to manage her diabetes, well, the Lido still holds out as one of my favourite evenings and we took Mary there on one of her birthdays and later for no particular reason that I recall we went again with Robin and Christine. Basically any excuse will do.

This is really a snapshot of our 17 years in Findon and we had no real intention of leaving but guess what! I was on one of my regular trips around some of the local pubs when I saw an apartment development. I enquired and found it was coming on the market in a few weeks. I took Margaret to look at it with the full expectation that she would be totally unimpressed as she loved the bungalow. To both of our surprises we really liked one of the two bedroom two bathroom places and that was it. I had just bought a new carpet for the conservatory and fitted a patio doors to the lounge, which were a great success. Anyway we were on the move and are now settled within walking distance, even for old people, of good local facilities in Rustington, which were a somewhat thing of the past in Findon.

Moving to an apartment somewhat changed our way of life as we felt we could no longer entertain and would now eat out a bit more. I must have got ambitious and one day pointed out an offer in the paper for a stay at a gourmet Hotel and mentioned it to Robin. I think he felt that this was the only time he had heard me want something and not done it before he could make an offer. We shared this occasion with him and Chris and it led to other breaks where Robin took Christine and I to The Fat Duck and I hosted a stay at Le Manoir aux Quat' Saisons. I also felt bold and on Karen's 50th birthday I suggested that she pick any Hotel/Restaurant that we could both get to, to celebrate. She to my surprise selected one of the best in Sussex as she liked the chef. We stayed at South Lodge Hotel and dined in The Pass. Things can only get better and I am now preparing for my own 80th celebration with all of my blood relatives and partners and children in a Chateau in Boulogne.

CHAPTER FIFTEEN

A Small World

There have been many times in life when Margaret and I have had occasion to comment on the smallness of this very large globe and I will list some of those that I remember from our early days onward.

When we were courting we decided to go to the dance hall in Charing Cross Road and we met my cousin and from this day on Margaret seemed to think that wherever we went we would bump into somebody I knew. It is true that this did happen on many occasions.

Another odd event was when we were given two seats in a box at The Albert Hall and we arrived before the other two occupants. After they had come in Margaret needed something from her coat and was confused when it did not appear to be in her pocket. She had a distinctive coat with a beaver fur collar but it turned out that she was looking in the wrong coat as the other lady had hung an identical coat on a hook nearby.

People find it surprising that I actually met Margaret for the first time at primary school and it is reported that she put her tongue out at me. More surprising was that her Aunt and Uncle were bombed out in the same house as me as they were living in the flat above us and that after the war when we were rehoused to No. 6 another of her Aunts and Uncles were to move into their rebuilt house at No. 8 Nettlewood and that the ones that were bombed out with us then moved back to No.12. At this time I attended the same church as she did and when I served at the early morning mass I always met her mother. At the time I moved away I was only 12 and only knew Margaret as the very blonde girl who was among those who walked home together after Sunday services.

Later when I joined Citibank A chap called Peter came over and said that he knew me. I did not immediately recognise him but then realised that before I left Nettlewood Road we had met at various scouting events and competed against each other. He had also been in the cast of the Gang Show when I had visited with my own scoutmaster and Ralph Reader who produced the whole thing. Peter later shared a car as support for the London to Brighton Walk and after retirement shared a number of home and away dinner parties.

When driving to work in Lewisham we all seemed to use regular parking spaces and a chap called Alan used to arrive at about the same time as I did and we parked facing each other most days. We went on holiday to Devon one year and as we pulled up in the car park of a very remote textile factory low and behold who pulled up facing me as he did each day, Alan!

On one of my visits to Ireland I was chatting to some people in a pub in Crossmalina when a lady asked me if I came from London. When I said yes she said that her brother had not turned up at a recent family funeral and she was worried.

She explained that he was a doctor and maybe I knew him. I explained that London was a very big City and that it was highly improbable. After further dialogue it turned out that he was in fact my mother's doctor and had taken over from the doctor who had many years earlier taken my tonsils out. As I now lived miles from where he practiced I said I did not have current knowledge but would enquire.

The first time I went to New York I was crossing the road to buy my Sunday English paper and was greeted by a colleague form our London Office who was at that time relocated to the States. Better still that same person appeared on the other side of the road when I had the family with me at about 8 O'clock in the morning in Brussels. It was on this same short break that I stayed in a Hotel in Ghent and the women in reception was extremely helpful and when a few months later one of the group's hotels was opened in Croydon, I thought it would be a good idea to find out if this could be a reasonably priced place to recommend for our overseas visitors and took time out one evening to enquire about costs and view the facilities. I walked up to the reception and was greeted by the woman from Ghent and she actually recognised me.

I met lots of people when out and about bowling and at one game the subject of the war came up and a player in the opposition said that he had been bombed out by one of the first V 1 bombers. I asked where he had been living and he said Streatham and that the bomb had landed on an empty house five doors from where he lived. I thought for a little while and then said that he must have live at 39 Lewin Road. How did I km=now that he wanted to know and I explained that he could not have lived five doors away in the other direction as that was where I had lived. I also went to a Surrey President's Dinner and met two men at the bar before the meal. We discussed among other things, our early upbringing. It turned out that one of these two had been brought up in Tooting and said he went out with a girl who had lived in 144 Topsham Road. This seemed to be impossible but it would appear that she was the previous occupant to us. Next surprise the other man had lived in the same road as Margaret in Norbury. Later after I had moved to Rustington I was walking along the promenade at Littlehampton when someone stopped me and said 'I know you, Terry'. He was visiting friends in Worthing and he was out for a walk with his friend while their wives shopped, He was the lad that I had sold the Train Set to in West Wickham.

CHAPTER SIXTEEN

Major Social Events

These are a list of some of the major impacts on life in my time and my take on them

First almost immediately after the war our problem with doctor's fees was solved with the introduction of the National Health Service. A great innovation to heal the sick and wounded for free which has been overtaken dramatically by what I call do-gooders who want to help everyone but cannot think through the consequences of their good intentions. Certain wishes are not needs and should still be paid for or, if unaffordable, be foregone.

Grammar Schools were around when I took the eleven plus and this was a boon for me and I think even many of our modern day politicians. In my era, although not currently acknowledged, it was possible to move from Secondary Modern to Grammar at 13 or 14 and to leave Grammar for Apprenticeships or other education. I did not understand why further education colleges became Universities and why so many people had to go to University and pay for the privilege. I believe in meritocracy.

This brings me onto Equality which was, I believe, built on the idea of Inclusion. Inclusion as it appeared to be intended was to provide opportunities for all walks of life to accept all who wanted to enter and could compete equally and provide equal returns. Equality be it by sex or ethnicity by law will only slow the natural progression of Inclusion. I understand that by banning smoking by law has in reality slowed down the rate of people giving up and there is a good argument for things to be allowed to evolve by normal social pressures.

National Service (Conscription) was abolished in the late fifties and this can be argued as good or bad but before this our do-gooders were at work and argued that as a man could go to war for his country at 18 then the age of majority should be eighteen. This sounded good but when the Unions got going and insisted that a full wage was paid to eighteen year olds it priced most industry apprenticeships out as you did not get a man's output from a partly trained employee. Eventually no company could afford apprenticeships and they were discontinued. The vote was also accorded to one at 18 and this in my humble opinion is far too early. Many current MP's were natural student anti-establishment but have matured to form a personal opinion. I have always believed that it takes at least two years from completing an education to learn the realities of life, i.e. Completing National Service, Apprenticeship or University etc. and would not allow people to vote under the age of 25. I certainly do not understand why kids are forced to stay at school until they are eighteen when this is in law and practice considered the start of adulthood.

I strongly opposed the idea of selling Council Houses as this was selling freehold land which in the middle of a big town was irreplaceable and anyway monies gained should have been earmarked for further development not kept aside from it. That said I would not have objected to the opportunity if I was in a position to afford it.

When a small tax relief was changed on Mortgage Interest it seemed that the Building Societies jumped on a bandwagon and started to provide loans on joint incomes. This sounded good and helpful but in no time the realities caught up and where one income had supported buying a house the inflation created in house prices meant that this would never be true again and both partners in the majority of cases would now have to work full time. In my earlier years the traditional housewife was not looked down upon by most people.

The European Project which I have voted against on all opportunities was not and is not a way forward. I think that people are generally tribal in nature and trying to bring different cultures and economies together is unsustainable. At least we have kept our currency. That said I also think there are significant advantages to the old imperial system over the decimal one. I am probably biased as having two brothers I would not today be able to share a gift from a relative of a note or large coins into three equal parts. Being the youngest I would always lose out.

CHAPTER SEVENTEEN

Omissions

I am sure that I have forgotten a number of anecdotes but there are also a number of things that I think of as appropriate for other people to tell or which or I find that sharing them with myself is all I want.

I know that I have not found a space to refer to the red rose that was planted outside the front door in Topsham Road. I pulled a piece of this out of the ground after my Mother's funeral and this took root and flourished. It was transferred to Findon where it was variously hacked back and cut down by the lawnmower but survived to be established next to the patio doors in Findon. On our move to Rustington we gave this to Christine and this year it has after being attacked by an enthusiastic gardener just given off multiple blooms. This and the family must go on for many years to come.

Included omissions are Weddings, Funerals, Significant Friendships (like Shawn and Snowy, and later Eugene and Peter) and bizarre events like me falling off a ladder or going head over heels backwards downstairs.

In general I usually only remember the good things in life and have often told people that I live by the adage that 'happiness is the best medicine'.

CHAPTER EIGHTEEN

Epilogue

What have I gained from Life?

What have I given to Life?

I do not really know but maybe now that you have read this you may at least have an idea of your own.

What I do know is that Life can be:

Good or Bad.

Happy or Sad.

Rewarding or Destroying.

Sometimes all of these seem to come in one week and in conclusion I believe that Life is never fair, but, it is a worthwhile trip and you get more out of giving than receiving.

25117675R00114

Printed in Poland
by Amazon Fulfillment
Poland Sp. z o.o., Wrocław

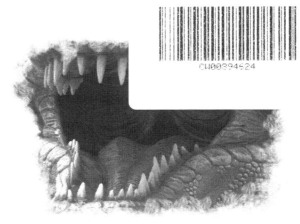

PLANET OF THE DINOSAURS
BOOK TWO:
THE JOURNEY NORTH

KEN PRESTON

Planet of the Dinosaurs

Book Two: The Journey North

Cover Design: Ken Preston

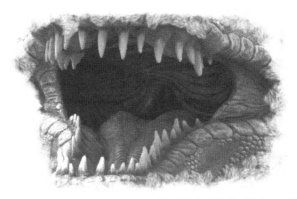

PLANET OF THE DINOSAURS BOOK TWO: THE JOURNEY NORTH

KEN PRESTON

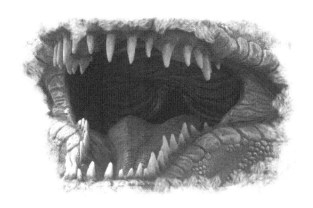

Chapter One

Daniel snapped awake from one nightmare to another. Before he could begin to recall any of the dream it drew away, out of reach. As if his mind was already deciding that Daniel had enough to deal with in the real world. He didn't need his imagination adding to his stress.

The teenage boy sat up, leaning against the cold wall. The perimeter of the sports hall was highly coveted, no one liked being in the middle, surrounded by a mass of stinking, filthy bodies. Here at least, at the edges, you could sit up, rest your back against the wall. And there was no one behind you. No feeling of vulnerability, you didn't have to fight the desire to turn around all the time, check what was happening.

Renton, of course, had got them the space by the wall. They had been here a day and a night and already the others knew to leave him alone. Knew to give him what he wanted.

His appearance terrified them. Daniel had never thought there might be an advantage to Renton's company, but here it was.

Then again, if it hadn't been for the thuggish American,

1

they probably wouldn't be in this situation at all.

The sports hall was part of the Blessed Robert Taylor Catholic Sports College. According to the welcome sign at the entrance, the school had achieved outstanding in their last Ofsted inspection. Daniel didn't know what they might use the rest of the school buildings for now, but the sports hall was a prison.

He had no idea how long any of the other 'inmates' had been here as no one was talking. The men and women huddled together in tight little groups. Sometimes whispering to each other, casting furtive glances around the hall. Some sat alone and apart, looking shell-shocked and scared. Daniel could relate to that look. Apart from the brief few days spent at the commune with Matt Hooper, that was how he permanently felt.

There were few children in the sports hall. Apart from Emily, and a pretty Chinese girl sitting across the other side of the hall, Daniel was the youngest by far. There were no old people, either.

Whenever he got the chance, Daniel would steal a glance around the hall. If you got caught looking at someone else, there could be trouble, the atmosphere was hostile and fearful. One man had become aggressive frighteningly quickly when he thought Daniel was staring at him. It was only because Renton had been there, had used his bulk and his power to intimidate the other man, that Daniel had not been beaten to a pulp.

Again, another reason to be grateful for Renton's company, for that charred, maimed face.

But now and then, Daniel still risked a quick peek at his companions. Some of them had obviously been in this dinosaur world a while, their weather-beaten, thin faces etched with exhaustion.

And then there were the newcomers.

2

There had been a storm. One of the huge, nasty, thunder and lightning end of the world displays that heralded another batch of dismayed newbies. The storm had been Renton's and Daniel's undoing, really. It had been night-time, raindrops the size of bullets driven against the van by a gale so powerful they had rocked from side to side like a boat at sea.

Renton and Emily had been arguing about going back to Keele service station. Daniel had hoped that Emily would know better than to argue with Renton by now, but, much like the American, the ten-year-old had no control over her temper.

The argument had been interrupted when the two men arrived with their guns and their attitude. Standing there in the storm, the rainwater running off their slickers, they had looked like monsters themselves, as though they had crawled out of a black, putrid lake only moments before.

They might have been human, but it turned out they were monsters after all.

That storm though, it had brought in some fresh time travellers. The men with the guns, it turned out they were hunting, gathering up the newcomers, herding them back here to the school sports hall. Some of them had been snatched up so quickly by their captors that they probably didn't even realise the true horror of their situation.

They didn't yet know about the dinosaurs.

Although the sports hall was filled with people, there was little sound. The mood was sullen and heavy. Very little sunlight penetrated the tall windows spaced out around the hall. Some of them had a fine tracery of cracks running across them, and some of those had traces of blood where a desperate escape attempt had been made. Daniel couldn't understand why anyone had bothered. The windows were covered with protective metal grills on the outside.

There was no chance of escape that way.

Someone started crying softly, and then another person joined in. Daniel couldn't tell if it was a man or a woman or both. In the gloom, in the stink and the misery of it all, his faculties and senses seemed to have dimmed. His limbs were heavy, his movements sluggish.

Why were they all being kept here? What was the point?

Renton had tried reasoning with the men when they ordered them out of the van, he'd even tried threatening them, but none of it had done any good. The three of them were herded silently through the night, the storm over by that point.

They had stumbled through mud and deep puddles, showered with drops of cold water as they shoved their way through gaps in the green, leafy undergrowth. Whenever Daniel paused to catch his breath, one of his captors prodded him in the back, the gun jammed forcefully against his ribs.

Daniel and Renton and Emily weren't the first to be captured that night. They soon joined a group of wet, miserable looking men and women, huddled together, eyes cast down.

Some of them tried asking what was going on. They were met with silence. All apart from one persistent man, dressed in a sodden suit and tie, expensive looking shoes caked in mud. He received a crack across the head from the butt of the shotgun for his persistence. He collapsed into the mud and their captors left him where he lay.

At the entrance to the school they were joined by more men in waterproof gear, shoving and jostling more captives before them. The iron school gates were pulled open, and the prisoners herded through. As a sanctuary from the dinosaur population, the Blessed Robert Taylor Catholic Sports College paled compared to the Botanical Gardens in Birmingham. There was a brick wall surrounding the school, but it was hardly tall enough, or strong enough, to withstand an assault from one of the larger dinosaurs. In the pale dawn light, Daniel could see that the wall finished by the sports fields, replaced by a chain-link fence, making them even more vulnerable.

But there was no damage anywhere. It was as though the residents of this commune had struck a deal with the returned monsters.

They shuffled between buildings and Daniel glimpsed sullen faces peering at them from behind windows. The place looked shabby and dirty, not at all like the sanctuary Hooper had taken them to. Daniel doubted these people had organised themselves enough to keep mussaurus as farm animals for food and milk.

They were taken to the sports hall where another figure wrapped in camouflage gear unbolted the door and swung it open. There was movement inside. With the others, Daniel and Renton and Emily were pushed through the door.

Those already held captive inside the hall sat down again as they saw they were being joined by new prisoners. Perhaps they had held out hope that they were about to be released, but as soon as they realised what was happening they lost interest.

Now it was morning, early by the looks of the pale light struggling through the grimy windows. No one had returned during the night to check on them. A few of the newcomers had tried to rouse the others, organise an escape plan, but that had come to nothing.

Daniel had tried talking to Emily, tried to reassure her that everything would be all right. He felt a sense of responsibility for her knowing her age. Knowing that they had taken her away from her mother. But Emily, usually so noisy, so ready with a snappy comeback, kept her mouth shut and her eyes fixed on the middle distance. Daniel couldn't tell if this was because she was angry with him, or if she was retreating somewhere inside herself, shutting out the nightmarish reality they had been dragged into.

The sports hall doors scraped open, and all heads turned in their direction. Three men walked inside, each of them holding a sawed-off shotgun. One of them, a huge, muscular man wearing a vest top, loose camouflage trousers and heavy boots, looked at the crowd.

"Back up everyone!" he shouted, waving the shotgun. "Get down the other end of the hall, now!"

Everyone backed up, shuffling as far from the armed men as they could.

The muscular man, he looked like the leader. His long, greasy hair, braided into tight lengths, and his mouth disfigured with scar tissue, the top lip curled up into a permanent sneer.

Renton hadn't spoken once since the men had shoved them into their makeshift prison camp, except to snarl at anyone who got in his way. He had sat brooding throughout the day and the night, cradling the stump of his arm in his lap. Daniel had wondered if he might say something now, maybe try to bargain or threaten his way out. But he kept silent.

Perhaps that was because the American knew there was no point in trying to reason with these men. If he'd had some kind of bargaining power on his side then maybe, but Renton had nothing to offer them.

"We need about twenty of them this morning," the leader said to the other two men. "Go get them."

Daniel's stomach tightened up at the thought of being picked by these men. This was like some hideous reminder of his schooldays, waiting to be picked to be on the team. Hoping he got picked to be on the winning team.

Only there would be no winners here, that was obvious.

The two men, one of them small, fat and sweaty, the other one wiry and limping heavily, approached their prisoners. They started separating people out, but Daniel could see no logic to their choices. The small fat man approached Daniel, looking him up and down.

"This one's hardly got any meat on him at all," he said.

"Then take him," the leader said. "We ain't got time to fatten him up."

The man grabbed Daniel by the arm and pulled him roughly to one side where he joined the others who had already been picked.

"Leave him be," Renton growled.

"You what?" the fat man said.

"I told you to leave him be," Renton said again, louder this time.

The wiry man limped towards them. "You having trouble, Dave?"

"This one here thinks he's a tough guy," Dave said, brandishing his gun at Renton.

"Looks like a piece of meat been left on the barbecue too long if you ask me," the other man said. "You're never going to win a beauty contest, mate."

A tear trickled down Renton's charred face, leaving a wet rail in the scar tissue. The two men looked at each other and laughed.

"Aww, the big soft sausage is crying," Dave said.

Daniel knew this wasn't true. The eyelids on Renton's right eye had been burnt away, and that eye watered all the time in an attempt to lubricate the exposed, bloodshot eyeball. And Renton's breathing was always laborious and forced, the air bubbling through the two holes in his face where his nose had once been. The teenage boy was still amazed to find that

7

Renton woke up every morning. He couldn't explain how the American was managing to live with his injuries.

"You're so worried about the lad, you can join him," Dave said, and prodded Renton with the shotgun.

Daniel thought Renton would lose it and attack the man called Dave. His left eyelid flickered, and his lips twitched, but he didn't retaliate. Just walked over and stood by Daniel and the others.

"That's enough!" the leader shouted. "Let's get them outside, we're running late."

Running late for what? Daniel thought.

The limping man stood by the entrance to the sports hall whilst their leader and the fat man pushed their prisoners through the doorway. Daniel risked one last glance at Emily left behind in the sports hall as he was shoved through the doorway. She looked small and frightened, alone amongst all the other adults. The limping man closed the door and bolted it shut once they were all through.

The morning air was cool and refreshing on Daniel's face. He was relieved to be free of the stink inside the hall. But his stomach was tied up in knots at the thought of where they were being taken, and what was waiting for them there.

The group of prisoners huddled together, waiting to be told what to do. The leader waved his gun at them.

"Go on, get moving," he snarled. "Over there."

They all began shuffling together, headed back for the gates where they had been brought in the morning before. There was a low mist hanging over the Victorian buildings. Something buzzed past Daniel's face and he flinched.

One of the men laughed. "Look at the boy, he's scared of a little flying thing."

Renton muttered something under his breath.

"Nige, go and unlock the gates," the leader said.

The man called Nige limped ahead of them and started the process of unlocking the padlock holding the gate shut. Daniel could only just see him through the white mist, but as they drew closer the limping man became more solid, more defined. The gate, wide enough to admit a car or a lorry, swung open with a rusty squeal. Daniel's stomach tightened up even more as they shuffled through the school's entrance.

They were being taken outside.

Where the dinosaurs lived.

"Come on, keep moving," the leader said, as everyone paused at the school's perimeter.

They walked them along the edge of the school grounds. The wall gave way to the chain-link fence. Through the slow swirls and eddies of the fog, Daniel could make out some of the sports field, part of the running track. Outside the school grounds he could see the shapes of houses and abandoned cars, some of them crushed whilst others looked untouched apart from the growth of creepers covering them. The jungle was everywhere, breaking through the tarmac beneath their feet, strangling the buildings beneath long, thick vines, their leaves dripping with moisture.

The school hadn't escaped the ravages of nature, but the buildings were mostly undamaged. Again, Daniel wondered how this could be. What was preventing the dinosaurs from crashing through the fragile defence of a fence to stomp around the school, eating everyone they found?

"All right, you can stop here," the leader said.

They were at a junction. There had been a smash up involving several cars, probably back when the dinosaurs first arrived, and the wrecks sat tangled together at the intersection of the two roads. The wreckage was rusted, the car tyres flat and the rubber rotting away.

But the blood splattered over the metal and plastic and glass was fresh. There were puddles of dark blood on the road, and a trail of it smeared on the tarmac and disappearing into the fog.

Nige limped over to the cars and started fiddling with something, the clatter of metal against metal only slightly muffled by the mist. Daniel didn't have long to wonder what the man was doing, or what the noise was. When the man called Nige moved along the wreckage to repeat the operation, Daniel saw the handcuffs hanging from the car's twisted door frame.

There were more handcuffs dangling from the wrecks, and Nige was unlocking them all. As he continued working, the other man, the one called Dave, selected one of the prisoners and pulled her over to the first set of handcuffs. She struggled and pulled, starting to cry as she realised what was happening.

Dave was too strong. He clipped the cuff around her wrist with a click and backed up, grinning.

"No, no, please!" the woman cried. "What are you doing? Please, please!"

She pulled against the cuffs, reaching out to the others, straining to reach them. Her face was smeared with dirt and her clothes hung from her thin frame. Looked like she had been here for a little while, but not born into this world.

Meanwhile, Dave had grabbed somebody else, an older man. To Daniel he looked completely shell-shocked, and he allowed himself to be led to another of the mangled cars and handcuffed to it. The woman was screaming and crying, sobbing helplessly. Daniel couldn't look at her, wanted to clap his hands over his ears to block out the sound of her cries. But he was scared that if he made any kind of movement, Dave or Nige would notice him and decide that he was next.

10

Daniel glanced at Renton. The big American looked on impassively at everything that was happening.

Dave selected his next victim, the young, pretty Chinese girl, Daniel had seen earlier. She struggled and spat at Dave and tried to claw at his face. Dave swore and slapped her so hard she fell over, into the tangle of undergrowth. Pulling her roughly to her feet, Dave dragged her over to the wreckage and snapped another set of cuffs around her wrist. The girl didn't cry out once, or beg for freedom. She just stared at the man called Dave, her eyes afire with hatred and anger.

"That's enough," the leader said. "Let's move on."

They continued walking beside the school's perimeter. Something rustled in the fog, a quick, darting movement. Dave and Nigel glanced nervously at each other.

"We're later than usual, that's all," their leader said. "Let's get this done quickly."

They urged the captives on, guns prodded into backs, commands barked at the prisoners. Soon they reached their next destination, more cars with empty handcuffs dangling from their frames.

And scarlet blood sprayed across the metalwork and over the ground.

"You," Nige said, and grabbed Daniel roughly by the arm, his grip tight.

He dragged the teenager to the nearest car, where Dave was already unlocking the handcuffs. Nige slipped them over Daniel's wrist and snapped them shut tight. The metal bit into his flesh, and Daniel had to clamp his mouth shut to keep from crying out in pain. He looked at the others, just visible in the fog.

Renton stared back at him, his one, bulging eye weeping.

Looked almost like he was crying after all.

11

When the two men had finished handcuffing victims to the various cars they rejoined the group, much smaller now than when they had left the school grounds. Renton was still with them.

"Okay, one more stop and then we're headed back in," the leader said.

The three men urged their remaining captives on, and Daniel watched as they disappeared into the swirling mist.

The mist quickly muffled the sounds of the group as well as hiding them from view. Daniel tugged at the handcuffs but, as he expected, they were firmly attached to the car. The other end of the cuffs had been locked around the passenger door frame. The window had been smashed in, and the seat was covered in shattered glass. Daniel pulled at the door and opened it wider, the hinges complaining noisily.

"Stop making all that noise! What are you doing?"

Daniel twisted around to see who had spoken.

"We've got to keep quiet," a man said. "There are things out there, I can hear them in the fog."

He was wearing a raincoat over a suit. Daniel remembered all the rain in Birmingham, the thunderstorm which brought the dinosaurs back from extinction in the blink of an eye. This man looked like he had been on his lunch break, or maybe he had been heading for the train station, running through the driving rain. Just another bad day at the office.

And then he had been deposited here. And his day got so very unimaginably worse.

The thing was, he might be new here, but he had already realised perhaps the most important of the key elements to survival. Stay quiet.

Daniel shuffled around the open car door. Quietly he sat down. Thought about climbing completely in and shutting the car door, but he didn't want to make any more noise.

Something clicked rapidly for several seconds, whatever it was hidden by the mist. Someone started sobbing.

"Be quiet!" the man hissed. "They can hear us!"

But the sobbing continued.

Whatever the thing was, hiding in the mist, started making its clicking noise again, like a cog or a plastic wheel with teeth being ratcheted around very fast.

Something shifted in the undergrowth, not far from them.

Daniel had finally realised why the school had been left undamaged by the dinosaur population. Because its inhabitants had been catching people and staking them out to be devoured every morning.

Daniel, Renton and the rest of them, they were sacrifices. Gifts to these ancient monsters from a faraway age, to ensure the safety of the commune in the school grounds.

Slowly, Daniel swung his legs inside the car. His feet crunched on the glass on the floor. Sitting like this his arm was stretched uncomfortably out to where it was cuffed to the door frame. He had to fight the urge to slam the door shut.

There was more movement in the fog.

And then, slowly, a creature appeared. At first Daniel thought it might be a raptor, but then he realised its neck was too long, and it was smaller than its deadly cousin. Its head flicked from side to side, its large eyes blinking as it examined its victims. Its eyes were like a cat's eyes, its pupils a long, dark vertical slit in its green irises.

The woman's sobbing grew louder as she saw the monster examining each of them in turn. The man in the business suit had backed up against the car, and he was yanking at the cuffs attached to his wrist.

The monster, attracted by the man's movement, darted for

him. The man screamed, lifting his free arm up to protect himself. The thing's thin jaws clamped over the man's forearm and the man screamed again. Daniel watched, frozen in the car seat as the dinosaur, about the size of the businessman, shook and chewed at its victim's arm.

The dinosaur let go of the bloody arm and backed up. It lifted its head, its snout pointing skyward, and let out a high chirping noise. Then it darted at the man again, this time sinking its teeth into his throat. The businessman screamed, and the scream swiftly turned into a wet gurgle.

The man's dying cries snapped Daniel back into action. With his free hand he grabbed the car door and slammed it shut. But, with the handcuff attached to the frame, the door wouldn't shut properly. And even if it had, the car offered him little protection with its smashed windows.

The dinosaur looked up at the sound of the slamming door and regarded Daniel quizzically with its cat's eyes, its teeth dripping with blood.

Daniel shuffled deeper inside the car, as far as the handcuffs would let him. Twisting and turning he started climbing over the seats to try to force his body into the back. He stopped when he saw the half-eaten corpse draped over the back seat.

Heart hammering in his chest, Daniel knew the car offered him no protection. That thing could get inside with him and tear him apart in just a few seconds. Maybe if he had something to defend himself with, something sharp and pointed. He looked around the inside of the car, but there was nothing.

The dinosaur made its high chirping noise again.

It turned and ran, disappearing into the mist.

Daniel let go of the breath he hadn't realised he was holding.

14

He was safe for the moment.

But how long before another beast with claws and teeth turned up, looking for something to eat?

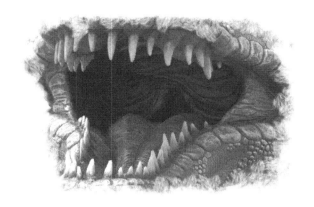

Chapter Two

Yesterday

"Do you know how to get to this District of Lakes then?" Lee said.

"It's called the Lake District," Will said. "We have to go north, and that's about all I know."

They were on foot, walking down Hagley Road. The opposite dual carriageway, the one headed out of the city, was jammed solid with rusted cars and buses. The road heading into the city was mostly free.

Lee cradled a rifle in her arms, and they both had rucksacks on their backs. It had been less than an hour since they left the safety of the commune at the Botanical Gardens, but already the bravado that Lee had felt was rapidly diminishing. There was so much foliage surrounding them, so many places to hide a hungry creature with sharp claws and even sharper teeth. Not for the first time, Lee found herself wondering what the hell they were doing.

We're going to rescue Dan, she thought.

They had been in this dangerous new world full of carnivorous creatures from the past for less than a week, and they had almost died within the first twenty-four hours and had to be rescued by Matt Hooper, and yet here she was thinking she could go all Rambo and set out on a rescue mission.

Lee glanced at Will, walking beside her. He was going to be more of a hindrance than a help, she knew that, but Lee also knew that with Dan the three of them were a team now. They had been thrown together by that freak storm into the future and together they had to work out how to get back to their own time again.

But the very first thing they had to do was rescue Dan from Renton's clutches. Hopefully they could catch up with them on the road. If not it was a case of heading for RAF Spadeadam, where Daniel's father had created the worm hole that got them into this trouble in the first place. Hopefully Professor Atherton was alive and well and had been working for the last twenty years on reversing the catastrophic events he had set in motion.

If he were here, Lee's daddy would have said that as plans go this one sucked big time. But it was the only plan they had. Best just to get on with it and not think further ahead than the next couple of hours.

So, the first thing to do was to find out where, exactly, they were headed and how they were going to get there.

"You know what we need?" Lee said.

"A time machine," Will said.

Lee glanced at him. She still hadn't figured Will out yet, and couldn't work out if he was trying to be funny or if he was just being sarcastic.

"We need a map," she said. "Then we can work out how we're actually going to to get to this place."

Will trudged along beside Lee and said nothing. Lee glanced

at him again. Everyone had taken Hooper's death hard. He had been a lovely guy, and he had been the one to rescue them from certain death from that thing that crawled out of the canal. But Will was suffering the most because he blamed himself, thought it was his fault that Hooper got killed. If Hooper hadn't taken him into the city centre to find a new pair of glasses, Renton would never have found them and blasted Hooper in the chest with his shotgun.

But Lee knew that was a stupid way of thinking. None of them could have known that Renton was still alive. From the look of him, with his missing hand and his charred flesh, he shouldn't have been. Lee couldn't understand how he was still breathing, let alone walking and talking. Maybe he was a robot underneath that burnt skin, an exoskeleton constructed of titanium.

Maybe he was a Terminator, sent from the future.

Made about as much sense as anything else that had happened in the last few days.

"Yeah, we need to find a map, that's what we need," Lee said. "You know where we could get one of those?"

Will shrugged, trudging along with his eyes cast to the ground. That was bad. Will needed to be alert, looking out for trouble at all times.

Looking out for dinosaurs.

"Hey man," Lee said, and stopped walking. She grabbed Will by the arm and pulled him roughly to face her. "I know you feel bad about Hooper, and I know you think it was your fault, but you gotta snap out of this funk, otherwise you're gonna get eaten."

Will shrugged again. "Maybe that would be for the best."

Lee punched him on the shoulder. "Don't be an idiot!"

Will rubbed at his shoulder and scowled at Lee. "That

hurt."

Good. She'd got a reaction from him at least.

"We need to stick together man, you and me, so we can find Dan."

Will shrugged again. "Renton's probably already killed Dan."

Lee punched him on the shoulder again, harder this time.

"Ouch! Will you stop doing that?"

"No, not until you stop talking like this," Lee said. "And next time I'm going to punch you in the head, maybe knock some sense into you."

Will glared at Lee, rubbing his shoulder.

"Renton's not going to kill Dan," Lee said. "Somehow he's got it into his twisted head that he still has to get Dan back to his father, like it doesn't matter that it was twenty years ago he got given that job, and that the world's been overtaken by giant lizards since then. Maybe it's because his brain got barbecued, but the guy's on a mission and nothing's gonna stop him. And that means Dan is still alive. Get it?"

Will shrugged.

Lee raised her fist again.

Will lifted his hands to fend her off, and said, "All right, all right, I get it!"

Lee lowered her fist. "So, even if we can't catch up with them, the thing is this, we know exactly where they are going. So all we need to do is find ourselves a map, work out the quickest way of getting there, and get moving. Capisce?"

"What?" Will said.

"Do. You. Under. Stand?"

"Yes, yes, I understand," Will said, glowering.

Lee placed her hands on her hips. "So, where can we find a map?"

19

Will sighed. "We need to head back into the city centre, look in the bookshops."

"Okay, great. Where's the city centre?"

Will pointed down the road. "We just keep heading that way."

They started walking again. Up ahead the dual carriageway widened along the middle and rose towards a large traffic island. The middle lane of the road they were walking along forked off to the right and down beneath the island. The entrance to the tunnel beneath the junction was obscured by trees with large leaves dipping to the ground, and a tangle of vines creeping around their trunks.

Lee and Will stopped walking.

"I'm not going down there," Will said.

"No, me neither," Lee replied, and then lifted her eyes to the traffic island. "That way's out of the question too, right?"

A dark mass of pterosaurs hovered over the traffic island, their wings a blur of motion in the bright morning sunshine. There were more on the ground, pecking at something they had found. As the two teenagers watched a couple of the prehistoric birds started fighting each other, squabbling over a scrap of food.

"What do you think they're eating?" Will said.

"I don't want to know, if I'm honest," Lee said. "Is there another way we can get into the city centre?"

Will looked to his left and right. "I suppose we could take one of the other roads and then double back once we'd got past the Five Ways island."

"You think you can do that without getting us lost?"

Will was silent for a few moments. "I'm not sure, everything looks so different now. It's like the city I once knew has been lifted up and planted in the middle of a jungle. Here, on the Hagley Road, I'm fine. But once we start diverting off the main route, I don't know, I'm not sure."

Lee could understand what he was saying. The last twenty years had ravaged this place. Another twenty and she was sure it would look different again. She thought back to what Hooper had told them, about how he thought maybe not just the dinosaurs had been transported from prehistory but how maybe spores, or something else too, something that had altered the climate. Because, although she had never been to England before, she was pretty damn sure it wasn't meant to look like a rain forest.

"Maybe we should just sit down and wait," Lee said. "Those big turkeys will finish eating eventually and get bored and fly away. Then we can carry on."

"Maybe," Will said.

They sat down where they were and eased their backpacks off. The tarmac was warm to the touch, pitted and broken up with eruptions of roots and weeds. Lee wondered what her hometown was like, back in America. She had a thought, that maybe it was just Britain that had been affected by the wormhole. That maybe the dinosaurs only returned here, and that the rest of the world was carrying on as normal. That Britain was quarantined off from the rest of the world.

Nah, she thought. That's a stupid idea.

The two teens both snapped their heads around at the same time when they heard the noise. A rustle in the undergrowth. Something moving, approaching them. Something hidden.

Lee picked up the rifle she had lain down beside her, gripping the unfamiliar stock so tight it made her knuckles hurt.

More rustling, more hidden movement.

"Shoot it," Will hissed. "Shoot it, Lee!"

Lee motioned him to keep quiet. She got on one knee and

levelled the rifle at the swaying mass of greenery at the side of the road. The rifle was a touch too long for her arms, and she struggled to hold it properly.

What were we thinking? We should have stayed back at the commune. We are going to die out here.

The rustling started up again, closer this time. Whatever it was, it was coming their way. Lee got the rifle positioned as best she could, hovered her finger over the trigger.

Don't be trigger happy, now, she thought. Don't want to go wasting bullets if that thing in there isn't any danger to us.

But how would she know? Lee couldn't see how she would have time to discuss with Will what type of dinosaur they were looking at, if it was a meat eater or not.

The long grass parted and Lee held her breath. A dark shape emerged from the undergrowth, its tongue hanging out, dark eyes staring right at them.

"Iggy!" Will said. "Don't shoot, it's Iggy!"

Lee was already lowering the rifle and letting out a deep breath she hadn't been aware she had been holding.

The black Labrador bounded over to them and knocked Will over onto his back. Incredibly, Will was laughing as the dog bounded around him, its tail wagging furiously. Lee started laughing too. Although he had given them a fright, it was good to see Hooper's dog. Good to see Will smiling and laughing again, too.

"Hey, boy, how did you get here?" Will said, sitting up now and rubbing the dog's head.

Iggy licked his hand in reply.

Lee suddenly scowled. She didn't like this, not one bit.

"What's wrong?" Will said, still fussing the dog.

"What's wrong?" she said. "We've gotta double back now, and take the dog back to its home, that's what's wrong."

22

"No we don't." Will scratched Iggy behind the ears, who arched his head back in pleasure. "He can come with us, we can look after him."

"Are you kidding me?" Lee said. "We can barely look after ourselves, let alone a dog too."

"But he'll look after us, he'll protect us," Will said.

"And what are we going to feed him with?" Lee snapped. "It's not like we can just drive into town and buy some dog food, right?"

Will was starting to look increasingly miserable again, and Lee hated herself for it. But they had to think about this. The dog could end up being more of a hindrance than a help.

At the sound of sudden movement behind them. Lee and Will both whirled around, Lee picking up her rifle again.

"Wait! It's me, don't shoot!"

Lee lowered her rifle again.

"I don't believe this," she said.

Matt Hooper's daughter, Helen, emerged from the high grass where Iggy had appeared from just moments before. She pushed back her long, blond hair and held up a hand in greeting.

"Hello," she said, giving them a sheepish smile.

"What are you doing here?" Will said, his arm around Iggy's neck, as though afraid that Helen had come to take him back.

"I was following Iggy," Helen said.

"You were following us," Lee said.

Helen screwed up her face. "Well, sort of."

"I can't believe you did this!" Lee said. "Look at you, you haven't even got a pack with you. You haven't brought a change of clothes, let alone a weapon, or food, or . . . or . . ."

"I know," Helen said. "It was kind of a spur-of-the-moment decision."

"We're going to have to take you back," Lee said.

"No!" Helen folded her arms. "I'm not going back. I'm coming with you, me and Iggy, we're both coming with you."

"It's a good idea," Will said. "We're better off if there's more of us, surely?"

Lee shook her head. "Uh-uh. No way. We've got enough to worry about without babysitting her."

"Babysitting!" Helen uncrossed her arms and jabbed a finger at Lee. "I'm the same age as you! I can look after myself, you know. I've been here longer than you, I know how this world works."

"Yeah, you know how to milk a dinosaur and sweep up, all in the safety of your compound, but out here it's different. Out here, you could get eaten."

Helen's eyes filled up, and she looked away. "You can't make me go back."

Lee looked at Will, who looked back helplessly and shrugged. Iggy licked her hand, and she looked down at the dog who gazed back up at her. She could imagine maybe taking the dog with them. He would be good company, and might be useful for defence.

But not Helen. Not only was she totally inexperienced in survival out here, but she was upset over her father's death. How on earth could they depend on her at a time like this? And why did she want to come with them? It had to be some kind of irrational response in the face of her loss. No way could Lee let Helen tag along.

"Come on, Will, we're going to have to head back the way we came," Lee said, and picked up her backpack.

Will's body visibly sagged at the thought of turning back. "Really?"

"Yeah, really."

Helen turned to look at them.

"I'm not coming with you," she said.

"That's up to you," Lee replied, shouldering her backpack on, whilst Will did the same. "But when we get back to the compound, we're telling them where you are and they'll send people out after you to bring you back. Your Mom will probably lock you in your room or something and then we'll head off again. There's absolutely no way you're coming with us."

Helen wiped roughly at her eyes. "My dad liked the three of you. He said you were tough, to have survived the way you did, and clever too. He said you made a good team together."

Lee glanced at Will. She could see the pain on his face, in his eyes. She knew exactly what he was thinking. Another good reason for Helen to not come with them, as she would be a constant reminder to Will of Hooper's death at the hands of Renton. A constant guilt trip.

Lee was about to open her mouth, even though she wasn't exactly sure what she was going to say, when she felt the tremor through the soles of her feet. Lee looked at Will, his eyes wide and staring right back at her.

Another tremor, this time accompanied by a low rumble.

Helen came and stood by Will and Lee.

"We have to go," Helen said. "It's the T-Rex."

Even before she had finished the speaking, the massive dinosaur appeared from behind a tall, wide building, the damaged words Tricorn House still visible at the top. The T-Rex paused, surveying its kingdom. It had a scar running down its head, across its jaws. Somehow, she wasn't sure how, Lee had the impression the tyrannosaur was old. But then what did she know? How many years did a creature like this live? How could she know how old it was?

25

The T-Rex hadn't spotted the teenagers. Lee was amazed at how calm Helen was. She had thought Hooper's daughter would have broken down into a screaming fit by now, but here she was standing stock still, hands out as though saying to the others, keep still. And Lee had an idea that the T-Rex had poor eyesight, that its vision was more attuned to detecting movement than anything else. But then how did she know that? Hollywood probably. And they just made stuff up.

For the moment though, keeping still seemed to be their best option. The tyrannosaur was swinging its head from side to side, completely oblivious to their presence.

It was the pterosaurs that caught its attention, flapping their broad wings and rising and descending over whatever it was they were feeding on and fighting over. The T-Rex immediately lumbered into motion, the ground shivering with each of its massive footsteps, heading straight for its prey.

The only problem with that was, the teenagers were directly in its path.

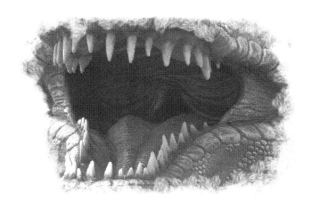

Chapter Three

Daniel had slept badly, contorted into the back seat of a small car, and had woken up with a stiff, sore neck. The temperature had suddenly dropped during the night, and he had spent the last few hours shivering, awkwardly curled up and trying to get warm.

Renton had spent the night in the front passenger seat, the shotgun laid across his lap. He hadn't seemed to mind the cold. Daniel wasn't sure if the American had slept at all. The teenager had toyed with the idea of making an escape when, or if, Renton had fallen asleep but eventually he had abandoned the idea. Renton had chosen the small car with Daniel in mind. There were no rear doors, and the teenager would have had to fold down a front seat and climb over it to open a door and get out of the car. All of which would have made too much noise and woken Renton up.

The previous evening, after the escape from the commune at the Botanical Gardens, Renton had finally stopped driving the jeep when they were out of the city and on one of the motorways. With the jeep roof squashed after the tyrannosaurus attack, Renton had been forced into leaning forward over the steering wheel. Daniel had been contorted into an awkward sitting position too, and each bump and furrow that the jeep bounced over was more painful than normal.

By the time they got out of the city, night had gathered around them. Only one of the jeep's headlights was working, and that was skewed, its beam shining off at an angle. Driving in these conditions was obviously too dangerous, although at least the storm had finished pounding them with rain.

Renton had climbed out of the jeep and Daniel mutely followed him. He was still in shock at the terrifying events of the last couple of hours. Renton, somehow, was alive still. A shambling, deformed monster, flakes of charred skin dropping from him, pus running from open sores, his one bulging eye weeping constantly. The sound of every breath the American took whistled and gurgled from the holes in his face where his nose used to be, making Daniel feel sick with revulsion. And a heat emanated constantly from Renton's body, as though the American was still burning up inside.

Without uttering a word, Renton began walking along the motorway, weaving between the wreckage of crashed cars. Now Daniel could see why Renton had stopped the jeep, their way was blocked by the road carnage ahead. Looked like there had been a major pile up all those years ago when the dinosaurs returned, and since then nature had taken over. Long fronds of sharp edged grass had grown between the cars, in some places almost hiding them from view, only the hint of moonlight on glass or metal giving away their presence.

Daniel looked up at the sky, at the stars shining brilliantly. He couldn't remember ever seeing stars so bright before. Then he returned his attention to his surroundings once more, suddenly acutely aware of the monsters that might be hiding in the long grass.

"Kid, over here."

Renton's guttural croak, alien and harsh in normal surroundings, seemed to fit their current situation perfectly.

The American pulled open a car door and lowered the passenger seat back.

"We'll spend the night in here, get moving again in the morning," he said.

Daniel climbed reluctantly into the car. Renton struggled in after him and slammed the door shut.

Inside the confined space of the small car, no broken windows to let fresh air in, Daniel quickly became aware of the smell of burnt flesh. He scooted around in the back seat, his face tucked into the crook of his arm, and tried to get to sleep.

Somehow, despite everything, he managed it, even though his sleep was interrupted with nightmarish visions of hungry mouths lined with sharp teeth, and Renton stumbling after him down a long, dark tunnel lit only by the flames dancing on the American's body.

When Daniel had woken up, shivering and badly needing to pee, he struggled at first to get his limbs working. Both his arms and his legs had stiffened up during the night, while he slept. Working slowly, carefully, Daniel had managed to turn over and sit up.

It was then he noticed that Renton was no longer sitting in the front seat. One thought after another tumbled through his mind. Renton had left him, he had gone somewhere else to die during the night, a dinosaur had taken him, or maybe Daniel was still asleep and dreaming.

The car windows were all misted up, but Daniel thought he saw movement outside. He rubbed slowly at the misted window, clearing a small, round patch, and peered through it at the outside world.

It was Renton, searching the other cars. He pulled open a passenger door, the hinges protesting with a loud screech. Daniel looked anxiously around, rubbing at the misted glass with his fist and peering through each of the car windows, expecting to see a reptilian head popping up out of the long grass. Baring its teeth in a wicked grin.

Nothing.

Daniel returned his attention to Renton, who was pulling a rucksack out of a car. He opened it up and emptied the contents on the ground.

What was he doing?

Looking for food and drink, maybe?

They needed something, and soon. Only his desperate thirst overpowered the gnawing hunger in Daniel's belly.

Renton left the contents of the rucksack lying where they were. He tried another car, but the door was locked.

Using a tyre iron, Renton smashed in the driver's window on the Audi. There were two skeletons sat inside, clothed in the tattered remains of trousers and shirts. Renton reached through the broken window and unlocked the door. He pulled the two skeletons out and dropped them on the ground, climbed into the car and rummaged through the contents of the rear seats.

When the American climbed back out, Daniel saw he had hold of a can of soft drink. Daniel's mouth suddenly filled with saliva. He pressed himself against the window, watching as Renton pulled the tab on the can and sank its contents in one.

Daniel pressed his face against the wet glass, hardly believing what he was seeing. How could he do that? How could he have drunk it all, leaving nothing for Daniel?

Renton squashed the empty can in his hand and dropped it onto the ground. Reaching inside the car he pulled out a second can.

Daniel scrambled over the front seat and fell out of the passenger doorway and onto the ruptured tarmac. Something called out through the fog, its cry strange and eerie in the silence. Daniel scrambled to his feet and then stopped.

What was he going to do? Fight Renton for the drink? Even in Renton's current state, Daniel knew the big man could overpower him. And did he really want to get any closer to that stinking mass of burnt flesh and suppurating wounds?

Renton looked at him, standing by the car. He held out the can of drink, a Fanta, and then tossed it to the teenager. Daniel caught it. Popped the tab and drank greedily. It was flat and tasteless.

Picking up the tyre iron, Renton shuffled around to the back of the car and smashed in the rear window. The sound of shattering glass was almost instantly swallowed up by the fog. The big man reached inside and pulled out a suitcase. Unzipping it, he pulled it open and once more emptied the contents onto the ground. With his foot he sorted through the clothes and toiletries, but there was nothing in there to eat or drink.

He moved on to the next car.

Daniel tipped the can back, letting the last few drops of precious liquid dribble into his mouth.

Dropped the empty can on the ground.

Thought about making a run for it, into the fog. Renton wouldn't be able to keep up with him, not in the state he was in. And the fog would quickly hide him from view, from Renton's shotgun. It was tempting. Although Daniel didn't know where he was right now, he was sure they hadn't driven too far. With the help of road signs and landmarks he was reasonably sure he could find his way back to the Botanical Gardens.

31

But there were things out there in the fog. Rustlings in the undergrowth, suggesting monsters with teeth and claws.

Daniel decided maybe he was better off sticking with the American for the moment. At least until he saw a better option.

Poking his head inside the car that Renton had broken into and retrieved the drinks from, Daniel had a quick look to see if he could find any more cans. As he suspected, there were no more. That was why Renton had moved on, searching for more food and drink. Anything that might have survived the last twenty years.

Daniel followed Renton at a little distance, not wanting to lose sight of him, but not wanting to get too close either. It was a strange predicament to be in. The American was Daniel's captor and a murderer, and yet he was also his protector and taking him to the very place he wanted to go.

But if Daniel found a decent opportunity to escape and get to safety, he was going to take it. Who knew for how long Renton would continue to see it as his mission to get Daniel safely to Spadeadam? The man had obviously lost his mind when the jet crashed and burst into flames, trapping him inside. For all Daniel knew, Renton might suddenly decide to kill him instead.

Daniel kept Renton in sight, but made sure not to get too close to him. The stink of his burnt flesh made Daniel feel ill if he got too close. Renton continued weaving his way between the cars. He was past the pile up now, and ahead of them lay an orderly queue of traffic, disappearing into the fog. Apart from the fact that some of the car doors had been left wide open, it could have been a normal day at rush hour on the motorway.

Except for the cracked tarmac, and the long fronds of grass and other vegetation climbing around the stationary cars.

Renton continued climbing into abandoned cars, rooting

32

around inside, or searching the boot. Daniel thought maybe he should help out, and search through a few cars too.

Some of the abandoned vehicles still held the remains of dessicated corpses, whilst others held a jumble of bones. Daniel wasn't sure why the rate of decomposition in some cars was slower than others. For the moment he decided to concentrate on searching the cars that had been abandoned by their owners. He didn't really fancy the idea of disturbing someone's long dead remains.

Renton had no such qualms. He simply opened up each vehicle's doors and dragged the occupants out, no matter their state of decomposition. The sound the bones made as they clattered against the tarmac sent a shiver through Daniel every single time.

After turning up empty handed from several searches, Daniel found a child's lunch box on the rear seat of an abandoned Zafira. Captain America stared back at Daniel from the lunch box, shield in hand, fist raised ready to take on the enemies of freedom and liberty. Daniel sighed heavily.

Hands trembling, he pulled open the zip and looked inside. There was an indescribable mess wrapped in cling film that had obviously once been a sandwich. A bottle filled with scummy, green water. A packet of crisps and a chocolate bar. Neither of which Daniel was prepared to investigate.

Daniel looked out of the front windscreen at Renton, just visible in the fog, climbing empty handed out of a car. This was pointless. Those two cans of drink that they found earlier had been a lucky fluke. But what were the chances they would find anything else they could eat or drink out here after twenty years? Barely any chance at all, Daniel decided. They were going to die out here. Either they would die of starvation and thirst, or they would be eaten.

Daniel thumped the passenger seat back in frustration and disturbed a cloud of dust. Only yesterday morning he had thought they were safe, that they had found a sanctuary in this dangerous new world, and that they could make a new life for themselves. But now here he was, separated from his friends and at the mercy of prehistoric creatures roaming the countryside.

Daniel climbed slowly out of the car. Although he couldn't see Renton anymore, he could still hear him, slamming car doors, obviously becoming frustrated and angry as he searched car after car and found nothing.

Run! Daniel thought, as he stood by the car. *Run now, get away. You're going to die if you stay with Renton, he can't protect you. Get out of here, find your way back to Birmingham, back to the Botanical Gardens. Do it now!*

Daniel turned, looked back the way they had come, at the bulk of the wreckage just visible in the fog.

Froze as he heard the clicking noise, like plastic cogs being turned on a child's toy, and steadily growing in intensity.

What could it be?

Whatever it was, the teenager didn't like the sound of it and started backing up. He bumped up against a car and sidled around it, his hand running over the wet glass and car body. The rapid clicking noise continued growing louder, drawing closer. Not just to his front anymore, but to his left as well, on the opposite carriageway. And now that he looked he could see small, dark shapes in the fog. Fast little movements, like low-flying birds.

Or . . .

Rats!

They appeared from the fog, scurrying beneath and around and over the cars, their claws making the clicking noise on the

34

metal and glass. They looked bigger than normal rats, about the size of a large cat, and their spiked fur was dark brown and glistening with drops of moisture. As they scurried over the cars they nipped at each other with their sharp teeth.

Daniel started running. If that horde of rats caught him they would pull him to the ground and swarm over him.

And eat him alive.

He stumbled between the stationary cars, resisting the urge to look back, doing his best to stay focused on keeping his eyes locked forward. The noise of the claws skittering over metal and glass had become intolerable, surrounding him and filling his head until he wanted to scream.

There was no way he could outrun them. Daniel knew the only way he could escape being devoured by these nasty looking creatures was to get off the motorway and out of their path. But in the time it would take to do that they would be on top of him, their claws ripping at his flesh, their teeth tearing at him.

Wait! The cars! If he could get inside one of the abandoned cars, he would be safe. He could sit inside and wait until the rats had passed him by. As he ran, Daniel tugged at a car door, but it was locked. Hardly pausing at all, he stumbled on grabbing the car door handles and pulling at them.

Something ran across his foot. And then another.

He was too late. Pausing, even if ever so briefly, to try at the car doors passed had slowed him down enough that the rats had caught up with him. They swarmed around him, over his feet and across the cars on either side. The skittering noise their claws made on the glass and metal was deafening, like a storm of hailstones on greenhouse windows.

Daniel clapped his hands over his mouth and nose. The stink of their wet bodies was suffocating.

Maybe if he stood still. Maybe they would swarm past him.

The nip of teeth on his ankle told him that was out of the question. Daniel kicked out at the rat on his trainer, but at the sudden movement it seemed that the pack as a whole noticed him. Another rat leapt on his trouser leg and he could feel its claws through the material. There was another nip of teeth on his other foot, more sharp pain from his ankle.

Daniel hit out at the rat on his leg and sent it flying into its companions. He started kicking out at the creatures, stomping at them. A sharp tide of panic flushed through his system as he realised he was surrounded by a mass of rats, carpeting the road and the cars as far as he could see in the fog.

"Get away from me!" he screamed, as more rats tried clawing their way up his legs.

There were too many of them to dislodge. In just a few more moments he would be covered in them, and they would drag him to the ground and eat him alive.

Staggering backwards, screaming at the rats, Daniel's back connected with a solid surface. A car, more rats flowing across its roof, stopping to chew at his hair and grab at his ears. The teenager swung his arms wildly, dislodging the ferocious creatures. He grabbed at the door handle and pulled. This time, thankfully, the door swung open and Daniel launched himself inside.

He landed face down on the rear seat. Squirming onto his back he kicked out at the rats scrambling into the car with him. If he was going to survive this, he had to get the car door shut, before too many of them got inside. Gripping the driver's seat head rest, he pulled himself upright and reached out for the open door. As his hand closed around the door handle, he had to keep kicking out at the rats trying to get inside.

Finally he got enough of a grip on the handle that he was able to slam the door shut. But not all the way. Two of the rats were squashed between the door and its frame, squealing in pain before they burst open and their guts decorated the car's floor. Working quickly, feverishly, Daniel opened the door enough to kick the two bodies out and then he slammed the door shut again.

This time it caught, the catch clicking into place.

Breathing heavily, his heart thumping hard, Daniel lay down on his back and listened to the rats climbing over the car, their skittering claws on the roof like the heaviest thunderstorm imaginable.

All he could now was to wait until they had passed. He wondered how many there were, how long it would take before they were gone.

And then he remembered Renton.

Had the American managed to find refuge in an abandoned vehicle?

Or was he dead?

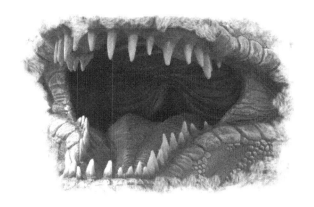

Chapter Four

The three teens ran. They didn't stop to look where they were going, or to even think about where they might go. They simply ran.

Will didn't need to turn around to know that the T-Rex was following them. He could feel its progress with every bone shivering tremor in the ground as it pounded after them. Whether it was still after the pterosaurs, or if it had spotted the tasty looking human snacks and was now after them instead, Will wasn't sure. He just knew they had to get out of the way. And fast.

Lee and Helen were both running on ahead of him, which was no surprise. Will had never been any good at running, or anything that involved physical exertion or coordination. As he ran he gasped for air, and his legs seemed to have turned into useless sticks of jelly. Never before had he wished that he had put more effort into PE lessons at school. This world of prehistoric man-eaters and other monstrosities, all of which they were sure to encounter the longer they stayed here, was no place for anyone lacking in strength and fitness.

And bravery.

Will thought he had proved himself to be brave and strong once, fighting off that monster in the boys' dorm before it slaughtered everyone. But then he had let himself and everyone else down by leading Hooper to his death. After all, if they hadn't gone into the city centre looking for a new pair of glasses for Will, Hooper would still be alive. And Will had done nothing to stop Renton killing Hooper.

Will knew he wasn't right for this world. He was a liability. He would be nothing but trouble for the others.

As Will ran, trying to keep up with the girls who were fitter and faster and stronger than him, and trying not to lose himself in a pit of black despair, he could see no reason to keep going. Why not give up and just sit down right where he was, and let whatever might happen, happen?

After all, there might be a few moments of searing pain, as the T-Rex snatched him up in its jaws, but then it would be over.

Forever.

And wouldn't the others be better off without him?

Will slowed down, a sensation of lightness and release coming over him as he realised his subconscious was making the decision for him. Yes, this was the best solution for everyone. Let the T-Rex devour him. That way he wouldn't have to continue the grim, unending work of surviving this nightmare, and his friends would be free of the need to look out for him all the time.

Will stopped running.

Closed his eyes.

The ground shook beneath his feet as the Tyrannosaur drew closer. It stopped, and Will couldn't tell if the monster was behind him or standing right over him. He knew it was close, he could hear its breath snorting from its nostrils, could feel its massive presence.

Now! Just do it now!

He heard movement, thick lizard skin folding and unfolding as it lowered its head, as he felt its hot breath on his back, rustling his hair.

Will tensed up, frozen, waiting for the monster's teeth to crush him, for the snap of his bones and the agonising pain.

The T-Rex spent a few moments examining him, seemingly not sure what to do with this thing that it had found. Twice, Will had to brace himself as the dinosaur nudged him with its snout.

Then, without any warning, Will sensed the T-Rex lifting its head. The ground began trembling again, the dull thud of its giant feet reverberating around the teenager, as the tyrannosaur began moving away.

Will opened his eyes. The T-Rex was pounding up the incline towards the pterosaurs. They were already flying away, their massive wings carrying them effortlessly skyward.

Will's knees gave way, and he sat down abruptly on the tarmac, shaking. Lee and Helen and Iggy had run down the incline towards the underpass. Lee was now running back to him.

"Wow, that was amazing!" she said, gasping for breath, as she approached him. "I can't believe how you managed to stay so still with that thing right in your face."

Maybe I should have jumped up and down and screamed, Will thought.

Lee reached out a hand and hauled him to his feet. "Come on, we need to get out of here before that thing decides you're a tasty snack after all."

"Lee . . ." Will said.

"No time," Lee said. "We've got to get moving."

They ran down the incline, although Will staggered more than ran. His legs still felt like sticks of jelly, seemed reluctant to do anything resembling walking or running. Lee pulled him on, towards the mass of greenery blocking the way into the tunnel beneath Five Ways. Iggy greeted Will with a wagging tail and a bark.

Above their heads the dinosaur stomped and roared, venting his frustration at being deprived of his prey.

"I guess we should wait here until Godzilla has finished having a tantrum," Lee said.

"Who is Godzilla?" Helen said, standing by the wall of vines and leaves.

"A Japanese monster from our time," Lee replied.

"I didn't think there were any monsters until the dinosaurs arrived?"

"Nah, we had plenty, but ours were all made up. Yours are real."

"What do we do now?" Will said. His legs were starting to feel stronger again, and the shakes were subsiding.

"Maybe we should wait here until Rex up there has moved on," Lee said.

Helen was stroking Iggy on his head. "He could be awhile. Sometimes he just likes to stay in one spot."

The ground shook again as the T-Rex stomped around and then roared.

"Well we can't stay here all day," Lee said.

"Why, you got somewhere important you need to be?" Will said, and then immediately regretted his sarcasm.

Lee gave him an odd look. "No, but we need to get somewhere safe, somewhere maybe we can spend the night. And we need to find a map book, work out how we're going to

41

get to this Lake place, zone, sector, whatever."

"District," Will said. "It's called the Lake District."

"We could go through there," Helen said, pointing at the underpass.

Will and Lee looked at each other and both shook their heads.

"I don't think so," Lee said, pointing at the wall of greenery. "How are we going to be able to hack our way through that?

"We could push our way in," Helen said. "Inside the tunnel we'll be free to move, nothing can grow in there without sunlight, can it?"

Lee looked at Will. "She's right, I hadn't thought of it like that."

"I still don't fancy it," Will said. "We don't know what might be living in there."

"Mushrooms?" Lee said.

"Giant cockroaches? Mutant spiders? Something we haven't even thought of yet?" Will said.

Lee looked at Helen. "Ignore my friend, he's a bottle half empty kind of guy."

"Does this mean you're letting me come with you?" Helen said.

Lee sighed. "Yeah, I suppose it does."

Will experienced a sense of relief at this. It was good for Lee to have another companion. At least then she wouldn't be on her own when Will got himself killed. Because there was no way that he could see how he was going to survive out here.

Lee looked at the tangled mass of vines and leaves blocking their way into the underpass. With every step the dinosaur took above them, the wall of greenery trembled.

Helen knelt down beneath a thick vine snaking at a right

angle across their path. Pulling and tearing at the leaves and hanging vines she started ripping a hole in the natural barrier blocking their way. Lee got down on her knees beside her and started helping. Even Iggy joined in.

Will stood and watched them. He seemed to have lost the ability to do anything, to feel anything, or think clearly. All he really wanted to do was lie down and go to sleep.

Forever.

* * *

Lee worked hard at creating a space for them to crawl through. Something like this, especially manual labour with a definite goal at the end, helped take her mind a little off their current situation. There was no way she could completely forget it, especially with Rex stomping around above them. But it helped.

The other thing it helped take her mind off was Will. He was still obviously upset about Hooper's death, still blamed himself. And Lee wasn't sure that it was a good idea to have Helen around as a constant reminder of that. But Helen had made up her mind she was staying, and Will didn't seem to care one way or the other, so there wasn't much to be done about it.

The work went quickly, and soon they had a hole large enough to crawl through and into the underpass. Lee went first, followed by Helen and Iggy, and then finally Will.

Lee switched on her torch, shone the beam around their surroundings. The air was cool and damp down here, and smelt of compost and stagnant water. She could hear water dripping, echoing around the underground space. There were pillars running down the middle of the tunnel, and on the other side was the opposite carriageway.

Helen had been right, there was very little to block their

way down here. Twisted roots hung from the ceiling, and the walls were coated with a green, wet slime. Underfoot felt soft and springy and damp. Apart from the steady drip of water, everything was silent.

The quiet was shattered by a tremendous thoom, as the T-Rex began moving once more. The three teens ducked as the tunnel vibrated around them, and the ceiling showered them in dirt.

"Oh man, I'd forgotten all about that thing up there," Lee said.

"Do you think the ceiling will hold with the T-Rex stomping around on top of it?" Will said.

"I don't know, but it's probably best not to hang around too long to find out, right?" Lee replied. "Come on, let's stick together."

The three teenagers and the dog started making their way through the underpass, their feet squelching on the soft, spongy surface. It wasn't long before Lee's trainers were soaked through.

The road continued sloping down gently.

A dark, bulky shadow slowly materialised out of the gloom ahead of them, almost blocking their route. Lee played the torch beam over it as the three teens slowed down and then stopped. She couldn't work out what it was, but she seriously did not want to draw any closer to investigate further.

"What's that?" Will whispered.

Lee shook her head. "Dunno."

Helen bent down and wrapped her arms around Iggy's neck and held him close.

Part of the wall above the thing had collapsed. Close up the smell of compost and earth was strong.

"Is it alive?" Will said.

"Don't think so," Lee said. "I haven't seen it move, have you?"

No one said anything.

"Damn it, we can't just stand around here forever," Lee said, and stepped closer, shining the torchlight over the strange monstrosity.

"It's a car," she said. "But look, it's covered in mushrooms."

Will stepped closer, but Helen stayed where she was, clinging onto Iggy. The outside of the car was covered in a layer of dirt and tiny mushrooms. Through the open windows, Lee could see bulbous mushrooms filling up the interior. Their flesh glistened beneath the light of the torch.

"That's gross," Lee said.

Will backed up. "I really would like to get out of here as soon as possible."

"Me too," Helen said.

There was another deafening boom from above, and more dirt showered them. Iggy barked and then lay down on his front, his tail between his legs.

Without saying another word the three teenagers began making their way through the tunnel once more. They had to edge their way past the mushroom filled car, and Lee made sure that no part of her body came in contact with any of the fungi sprouting from its sides.

There were more abandoned cars up ahead, some of them with their doors hanging open, some crashed into the sides of the underpass, others looking as though they had just been parked in the middle of the road. They skirted around them. Lee glanced in one of the cars, the torchlight illuminating the interior. There was a skeleton collapsed on the front seat, the skull turned upwards and facing the driver's side window. A bulbous mushroom was growing from one of the skull's empty eye sockets.

The T-Rex began moving again, the walls and the floor shivering with each impact of its feet. The three teens were showered with more dirt, and they stayed still, cowering beside the car, until the dinosaur stopped moving.

"We seriously need to get out of here now!" Will hissed.

Iggy whimpered his agreement.

"Come on then, let's go," Lee said.

They moved faster, running past the cars, Lee leading the way with her torch, the ground squelching beneath their feet. The decline of the road gradually turned into an incline, and it seemed to Lee that they were heading up to the exit. She just hoped the tyrannosaurus wasn't waiting for them at the other end.

They kept moving, slower now. There was no sign of light at the end of the underpass which meant that it was overgrown with vines too. The T-Rex began stomping around again, but this time the teenagers didn't stop. Lee just wanted to get out before the ceiling collapsed in on them, and she was sure the others felt exactly the same.

After a few moments of activity the huge creature above them stopped moving around, and only a second later Lee stopped too. Will and Helen bumped into her. Iggy started whining and pawing at the ground.

"What?" Will said. "Why have you stopped?"

"Didn't you hear the crunch?" Lee said.

Iggy was growling and whining, pawing even more frantically at the ground now.

Will took a step back. Lee saw his body stiffen up as they all heard the crunch beneath his feet. And she could hear something else, too. A shifting, a movement, within the darkness.

Lee swung her torch down and hissed as she sucked in a breath. The ground was covered in a mass of black beetles, scurrying in crazed circles and over one another as they tried to hide from the light. The carpet of shifting, shiny black bodies stretched as far as the torchlight would allow the teenagers to see.

Will started kicking his feet out, shaking them to try to get rid of the beetles climbing over his trainers. Iggy was barking and slapping his front paws down in jerky little movements.

"We've just got to walk through them," Lee said.

"Can't we go back the way we came?" Will said, still kicking his feet out. Every time he put a foot down they heard another crunch of bodies.

"No, we're almost there, let's go now," Lee said.

They started walking again, Helen dragging Iggy along by the scruff of his neck. Every step they took there were crunching and popping noises of beetle bodies exploding beneath their shoes. Lee felt sick. The insects began scurrying over her shoes and onto her ankles. She had to resist the urge to stop walking and bend down to brush them off.

Up above, the T-Rex began moving again, the gigantic thud of each footstep reverberating through the walls and the ground, through the teenagers' chests and stomachs. Lee had to resist the urge to crouch, get down low. She didn't fancy being face to face with the moving carpet of black beetles. Will grabbed her free hand and Helen grabbed her other arm with one hand, still holding onto Iggy.

The tyrannosaur seemed agitated, keeping up its pounding and roaring, showering the teens in dirt and wriggling, tiny insects. Did it know they were down here? Was it waiting for them to come out so that it could pluck them from the ground

47

and swallow them down in one go?

With a wrenching, grating noise, a section of the roof detached itself and smashed to the ground behind them. A ragged beam of sunshine penetrated the underpass, dust swirling crazily in its light.

"Run!" Lee screamed.

None of them needed telling twice. They charged for the exit, feet crunching over the carpet of beetles. Helen couldn't hold on to Iggy any longer and he bounded on ahead, barking. Small chunks of concrete began hitting the surrounding ground. Lee was amazed that none of them had been bashed on the head yet.

They got to the mass of vines and leaves, and all three of them immediately began tearing at it, creating a hole they could crawl through. Iggy went first, followed by Helen and then Will. Lee took one last look at the tunnel, softly illuminated by the ragged hole in the ceiling. She saw the cars, resembling alien monstrosities with their bulbous, twisted mushrooms covering them, and the mass of beetles scurrying around and around, like the surface of a black lake in a thunderstorm.

"What are you doing?" Will screamed. "Get out!"

Lee scrambled through the hole, back outside to sunshine. The light hurt her eyes, and she had to squint.

"Everyone okay?" she said.

Will and Helen nodded. They seemed dumbstruck by their narrow escape.

Behind and above them, on the Five Ways island, the T-Rex was pounding up and down, and roaring. It seemed frustrated, angry.

"I think we should get out of here, before it sees us," Helen said.

"I think you're right," Lee replied.

The dual carriageway continued on an incline back up to ground level, where it rejoined the main road. Lee could see an Odeon Cinema, its sign broken and missing the 'O', windows cracked and filthy. Lee wondered if they might have any old cans of pop left in there, or if it had been looted clean.

They started walking up the incline, casting anxious glances back at the T-Rex.

"Do you think he's looking for us?" Will said.

"Yes, I think he is," Helen replied. "He spotted us earlier, but decided the pterosaurs were more to his liking. But he didn't get to eat any of them, and now he's trying to work out where we went."

"I think he worked it out," Lee said.

Will and Helen turned and looked. The T-Rex was standing still, staring at them. The monster lifted its head and let out an ear-splitting roar. Then it began pounding towards them.

Before any of the teenagers had a chance to move, to turn and run, the tyrannosaur disappeared in a cloud of dust as the ground gave way beneath it with a thunderous rumble. A roar of pain and anguish echoed from the tunnel, as more concrete and steel collapsed on top of the T-Rex.

Without uttering a word the teens ran, not sparing even one backward glance to see if the dinosaur had survived its fall into the underpass.

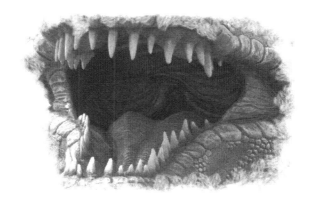

Chapter Five

Lying on his back in the rear of the car, Daniel waited.

And listened.

The last of the rats had finished scurrying across the car's roof but he could still hear them up ahead, scrambling over and around the other abandoned vehicles on the motorway. The noise they were making, that insistent scratching and scrabbling of claws on metal and glass, was slowly growing fainter. Daniel had already decided that he wasn't leaving his safe place until he could no longer hear the rats.

At least he was on his own in this car. He wasn't sure if he could have held out very long sharing his confined space with an old, dried out body, or a skeleton. He felt sure he would have gone mad, and started screaming and shouting, maybe even opening the door again to try to get out.

Of course, that would have been the end for him. There was no way he could have fought off all those rats once they started swarming inside the car.

Listening carefully, Daniel tried to pick out the sound of scraping claws in the distance. There was nothing, just the rustle of his clothes against the car seat as he moved. Almost reluctantly, Daniel sat up. The fog was starting to clear. He could see more cars now, a line of them stretching along the motorway, out of the city.

The opposite carriageway was mostly clear. There were a few cars here and there, but the road was free. Daniel wondered if they could get one of the cars started on the southbound side of the motorway and then continue their journey north unimpeded. But Daniel had no idea if they could find a car that would even start. Wouldn't their batteries be flat after all these years of just sitting here? Every car he had come across had flat tyres, so they would need pumping up at the very least before they could go anywhere.

Twisting around on the seat, Daniel tried looking for Renton. He couldn't see the American anywhere. He thought about opening his door, climbing out of the car and going looking for him. But the thought of being outside again didn't appeal one bit.

Leaning over the front seat, Daniel pulled open the glove box. There was a torch, which was dead, a bag of butterscotch which had turned into one horrible, gooey mess, car registration documents and a manual. Nothing of any use for him. Stuffed down the side of the passenger seat was a road atlas. Daniel pulled it out and tried to flip through it, see if he could locate where they might be. But the pages were all stuck together, and anytime he tried peeling them apart he just ripped it.

He pulled the rear seat backs down and looked in the boot. There was a suitcase, a foot pump, a bottle of car oil and another of screen wash. Daniel dragged the suitcase out and flipped the locks. Inside had been stuffed with hastily packed clothes, a hair dryer and a wash bag. Inside the wash bag were a combination of toiletries, both a man's and a woman's. Daniel thought about that hair dryer, wondering about the woman who had packed it. It looked like they had been heading out of the city, trying to find somewhere safe from the dinosaurs. And yet she had still stopped to think that, wherever they were going, she would still need her hair dryer.

Daniel wondered what had happened to them.

They were dead, obviously. But how had they died? They hadn't stayed inside the car which would have been the safest thing to do. Didn't look they had been seized by something with powerful jaws and sharp teeth and dragged out either. So what had impelled them to leave the safety of their vehicle?

There was nothing in the car of any use to him. Not unless he found a working electricity supply and had an urgent need to blow dry his hair.

Daniel shifted around, once more looking for Renton. The mist had almost completely dispersed. The view of all the abandoned cars, a long line of them extending up the motorway, was depressing.

Daniel thought about the decision he had made, just before the rats began swarming all around him. Now was his chance to get away from the American. For all Daniel knew he was dead, anyway. There was no point in trying to get north to the Lake District all by himself, he would never make it. Daniel knew his best option right now was to head back, try to find the Botanical Gardens again, the safety of the compound.

The thing was, this was the first time he had been alone in this world since he had stumbled out of the crashed jet, just before it exploded. And if not for meeting up with Lee and Will, he would be dead by now, he was sure.

Things are different now, he thought. *I've been here longer, I know more of what I'm up against.*

Daniel closed his fingers around the car's door handle, but

he didn't open it. He felt safe in here, protected from the outside world. But he knew he couldn't stay in here long. Already he was hungry, and soon he would be thirsty again. He had to get back out on the road and find his way back into Birmingham.

Daniel opened the car door. Poked his head outside.

Silence.

Up in the blue sky, Daniel saw a group of pterosaurs gliding on the currents. They were high and distant. Daniel wondered how good their eyesight was.

Slowly he clambered out of the car, little by little abandoning its protective environment for the dangers of the outside world. Once both of his feet were planted on the ruptured tarmac, and he considered himself to be properly out of the car, he took a deep, shaky breath.

You're okay, he told himself. *You can do this.*

Yes, but do what? He needed a plan. The drive down here in the wrecked jeep at night during a thunderstorm had completely confused and disoriented him. He had no idea how to get back to the commune, or how long it would take him. Daniel could see the jeep with its squashed roof at the back of the queue of traffic. From there they had searched the cars this morning for food and drink. Would it make sense to continue the search for a little while? It seemed to Daniel that he was more likely to find something out here than he would in the city centre which had surely been looted clean by now.

And that was even if he could find the city centre before he passed out from dehydration.

Daniel turned his back on the route into the city and looked once more at the line of cars stretching into the distance. All right, half an hour at the most searching the cars, and then turn back and head for Birmingham again whether he had found anything or not.

He began walking down between the line of cars, pushing through the undergrowth strangling the cars' wheels and bumpers. The tops of the cars, the bonnets and the windscreens were all covered in claw marks from where the rats had scrambled over them.

So many rats. Daniel shuddered at the thought of them.

He pulled open a door at random, although he checked to make sure there were no bodies inside first.

Nothing.

He walked around the back and pulled open the boot.

Nothing.

He moved onto the next car. No one in that one, either. He pulled at the door handle, but the car was locked. Thought about finding himself a tyre iron so that he could smash the window just like Renton had done, but decided against it. Didn't want to attract attention by making all that noise.

Who knew what was lurking, hidden in the long grass?

Daniel moved on to the next car. Pulled at the door handle. It opened easily and Daniel staggered back at the stink of rotting flesh. Renton was lying in the back seat, his arm ending in the bloody stump flung across his chest, the other dangling down by his side. His left eye was closed, but his right eye was open and staring.

Once he had calmed down from the initial shock of seeing the American, Daniel realised he was sleeping. Renton must have climbed in here for refuge from the giant rats and then he had fallen asleep. It hadn't occurred to the teenager that Renton might have stayed awake all of last night, guarding his prisoner. But he couldn't stay awake forever.

On the car floor lay the tyre iron and the shotgun.

Renton snorted softly, and a small mucus bubble formed at

the hole where his nose used to be and then popped.

Daniel wondered if he could gather the courage to reach inside the car and take the shotgun. Daniel had opened the front passenger side door, which meant he either had to kneel on the seat and reach into the back, or risk opening another door.

Neither option appealed to him. It was that single staring eye. How could he sleep without any eyelids to block the light out in that one eye? Was he even really asleep?

Renton snorted again and shifted position slightly.

He looked asleep.

But still, doubt nagged at the frayed edges of Daniel's nerves. He should just get out of here, leave now and run as far as he could away from the American before he woke up. Forget about the shotgun, just go now.

Daniel hesitated, paralysed by indecision.

Something roared in the distance, snapping him alert.

Get the shotgun, he thought. *And the tyre iron. You'll need them both.*

Daniel quickly glanced all around, as though he was about to commit a crime and he was checking for passers-by who might be watching him. He climbed inside the car, kneeling on the passenger seat. With one hand on the seat's headrest, he leaned into the rear of the car, reaching down for the shotgun. It was further away than he had thought and he had to stretch until his fingertips brushed the metal.

Renton's hand closed around his wrist in a tight, painful grip. Daniel jerked in surprise and tried to pull away, but Renton was too strong and held on to him.

Both his eyes were open, staring at Daniel.

"What do you think you're doing?" he said, his voice a harsh rasp.

Daniel said nothing. He couldn't think of a response. Renton's stink, and the heat that still rolled off his charred body in waves, seized Daniel's brain up, made him incapable of a single thought.

"Please," he said eventually, "let me go."

Renton seemed to be struggling to breathe. He lay on his back, the breath whistling and gurgling in and out of his mangled mouth, and continued staring at Daniel.

"You're staying with me," he said.

He let go of Daniel's wrist, and the teenager fell back and out of the car, landing on his back on the grass covered tarmac. He scrambled to his feet, scared that there might still be rats hidden in the undergrowth.

Renton slowly climbed out of the car, carefully holding his bandaged stump out away from anything it might bump into. In his right hand he held the shotgun. He leaned against the car, breathing heavily.

Daniel felt sick just looking at him.

"Don't think you can get away from me again," Renton said.

Using the arm that finished in the bloody stump, he wiped sweat off his bald head. He looked up and down the motorway.

"Those rats, they've gone?" he said.

Daniel nodded.

"You don't say much, do you? Not that you ever did." Renton straightened up. "Come on kid, we're going."

"Where?" Daniel said.

Renton looked at him. "You know where."

"Back to my father?"

"Yeah."

Daniel wanted to challenge him, tell him how impossible their situation was, that there was no point in heading back to the nuclear power plant where his father had set up base. Or rather, where the mysterious organisation known as *IntelliCorps* had set up base, with their top secret project, known only as Project Wormhole, that had most likely been the cause of all their problems.

But he couldn't find the words, couldn't see the sense in challenging Renton. The American had never been open to to being reasoned with even before the jet's crash landing in the city centre, but now he was positively crazy.

Renton straightened up and cradled the shotgun in his left arm. He turned and reached into the car and pulled out the tyre iron and hooked it into the belt of his ragged, filthy trousers. He took the shotgun back in his right hand and gestured with it along the motorway.

"Let's get going," he said. "We've got a long walk ahead of us."

Daniel turned his back on Renton and started walking, threading his way between the cars. He could hear the American shuffling along behind him, could hear his tortured breathing. And his back tingled at the thought of the shotgun in Renton's hand.

They walked past a slip road off the motorway, the lanes running down to a junction for Walsall and Wolverhampton. Daniel didn't have any idea of the motorways around Birmingham, or the distance they had travelled, but he felt they couldn't be too far out of the city. Whilst that was good in the sense that he still felt relatively near to his friends, it also meant that they still had a very long way to go to the Lake District.

Did Renton have a plan for how they were going to cover that distance? Daniel doubted it. He doubted the American was thinking clearly at all. The teenager wondered if it would be worthwhile asking him. Maybe try to get him to realise the situation they were in, the insurmountable odds they faced in travelling those hundreds of miles without food or water whilst being hunted down by hungry dinosaurs.

"Can I ask you something?" Daniel said.

"No," Renton replied.

They walked a little further. Despite the reply he had received, Daniel decided to risk another stab at talking. After all, surely he was safe with his former bodyguard? Renton, as much as he might hate Daniel, seemed to have made it his own personal mission to deliver the boy back to his father. Alive, presumably. Which meant he couldn't do anything drastic, like murdering Daniel because he talked too much.

"Are you planning on us walking all the way up to the Lake District?" Daniel said.

"I told you, no questions," Renton replied. "Now shut up, before I decide to shoot you."

Great, thought Daniel. He shut his mouth and kept walking.

The sun slowly rose in the clear blue sky, heating up the air and the ruptured tarmac of the motorway. Daniel's face and body soon became slick with sweat, and his thirst returned with a vengeance. Insects chirped and hummed, unseen in the undergrowth. Apart from a solitary pterosaur gliding high above them, the sky was empty of life. Had all the birds been killed and eaten? All the blackbirds, the robins, the magpies, even the pigeons, had they all gone forever?

They no longer stopped to check out the stationary cars. Daniel had started off looking in the windows as he passed them, but Renton told him not to bother. And Daniel, although puzzled as to why they weren't searching the cars for much needed supplies, was relieved. He'd had enough of coming across skeletons collapsed in their seats, or wizened corpse faces staring out of the windows with their blank eye sockets.

58

But still, they needed food, they needed drink.

And where else were they going to have a hope of finding anything like that on the motorway?

After another half an hour of mindless trudging along between the cars, Daniel got his answer. And of course it had been obvious all along, he just hadn't thought of it.

A motorway service station.

* * *

Keele Services looked like it had been torn apart by a bombing attack. The car parks and the access roads were strewn with mangled cars, squashed or blown apart, some upside down or on their sides, one car even jammed into the branches of a blackened, scorched tree. Parts of the building itself had collapsed, and the paved area at the front was covered in shattered glass.

Daniel and Renton walked carefully around the mangled cars, and past a squashed caravan lying on its side. Their feet crunched over broken glass, the sound frighteningly loud. Daniel kept turning his head from side to side, his eyes scanning his surroundings, looking out for predators alerted to their presence by all the noise.

They picked their way carefully through the main entrance, the sliding glass doors stuck permanently open, and into the main foyer.

Costa, McDonald's, WHSmith, all the familiar signs were there. But where once they had promised food and drink and entertainment, now their promises looked dull and dead, a faint echo from a previous life.

Daniel couldn't believe they would find anything of use here. The inside of the service station looked just as bad as the outside. Tables and chairs had been smashed up and scattered,

59

stands and shelves overturned and trampled on, the video game machines on their fronts, some of them blackened by fire.

But despite all the destruction, something stirred in Daniel's mind, something familiar about his surroundings.

"I think I recognise this place," he said.

Renton made a strange, strangled sort of noise. It took Daniel a moment to realise the American was laughing.

"You should," he said. "This is where you pulled your disappearing trick when me and Reece were taking you back to your father."

Daniel remembered now. Despite all the destruction and the thick layers of dirt, he could see it. Seemed strange to think that for him it had been less than a year since he was last here, hiding from Renton and Reece. But for the rest of the world, two decades had passed, and nature and time had done its best to obliterate it.

Renton walked deeper into the cool of the building. Daniel followed him.

Maybe here they would find something to drink at least.

Because if they didn't, he doubted they could survive long enough to walk up to the next services and look for food and drink there.

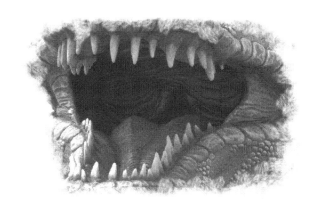

Chapter Six

The city centre was just as Lee remembered it. Quiet, deserted, but humming with hidden menace. By unspoken agreement they kept away from the crashed plane, from the Rotunda where someone had shot at them, and from the department store where they had been chased by raptors.

After living in the safety of the commune, if only for a few days even, it felt strange to be back in the city centre. Lee had thought they would never have to venture out here again, that they could live their days milking mussaurus cows and sweeping and tidying, all within the confines of what had once been the Botanical Gardens. She kind of wished she was back there now, somewhere nice and safe and boring.

But Hooper's death had changed all that. Even if they hadn't decided to leave anyway, to try to catch up with Daniel and rescue him, she doubted they would have stayed long. They would always have been blamed for Hooper's death, they would always have been excluded from friendship groups, would have remained outsiders no matter how long they stayed there.

Maybe, once they had got Daniel back, the four of them

61

could start up their own group. One that was run by their rules, and nobody else's.

First thing they had to do though was find Daniel, and rescue him. Lee wasn't sure which of those two was going to be the more difficult. Although they had a good idea as to where Renton was headed, Lee could immediately see two problems.

One, she had no way of knowing if Renton could still remember how to get to the Lake District and the nuclear power station where *IntelliCorps* had set up base. For all anyone knew, the fire in the jet had fried Renton's brain as well as cooking him on the outside. And even if he could remember how to get there, what was to stop him and Daniel being eaten on the way? Or dying of starvation and dehydration?

Of course all those things were problems for Lee and Will and Helen too. But that brought her to her second and more immediate problem. Renton might or might not know how to get to the Lake District, but Lee was certain of one thing, and that was that she didn't have a single idea where they were headed.

Her daddy came to mind then, and something he used to tell her.

Life's full of problems, he used to say. *One problem after another after another until some days you feel completely overwhelmed. The thing to do is, just take on one problem at a time and deal with it. Once you've got one of those problems out of the way, you can deal with the next one. Doesn't matter how many problems you've got, you can only deal with one at a time.*

So, focus. They were okay for food and drink for the moment with the supplies in their packs. They wouldn't last long, but finding more wasn't an absolute priority right now. What was a priority was sorting out a route to take them north. The most direct route possible. And for that they needed a map.

"Hey, Will," she said.

Will looked up. He was sitting cross legged next to the bull, outside the Bullring shopping centre. Helen was standing in front of it, hands on her hips, staring up at the bronze sculpture, as though challenging it to come to life. The bull had obviously seen better days. It was chipped and cracked and covered in filth.

Ahead of them, behind the bronze bull, was the entrance to the Bullring. On either side of them were shop windows, cracked and filthy but still, somehow, intact.

Will, in contrast to Helen, had been sitting with his arms resting on his knees, head hanging low. It looked to Lee as though he had given up.

"Yeah?" he said.

"We need to find a map, you know where we might get one?" Lee said.

Will shrugged.

"Aww, come on, man!" Lee said. "You know this city, better than me and Helen, anyway."

"What's the point?" Will said. "Even if we can find a map, you seriously think we can catch up with Renton and Daniel? And even if we do, you think we can *fight* Renton? He survived being trapped in that plane when it was on fire, and he cut his own hand off to get out of there. Do you seriously think we can go up against him?"

Lee stared at Will. He was on a bad downer, that was for sure. "What else are you gonna do? Sit here and wait until something out of your nightmares ambles by and decides to eat you? Is that your plan?"

Will shrugged again. "Can't think of anything better right now, to be honest."

Lee huffed in exasperation. Right at this moment she could

have strangled him. She knew he was hurting over Hooper's death, she knew that he felt guilty, and that maybe Helen's presence was exacerbating that guilt. But if they were going to have any chance of catching up with Daniel, and saving him from Renton, if they were to even have any chance of just staying alive, Will needed to snap out of his funk.

Lee looked to Helen for help, but she was still staring up at the bronze bull's face. Staring into its eyes, as though it was alive. The bull was huge, much larger-than-life size, and Helen appeared puny beside it.

Lee squatted down beside Will. "Come on, dude, help me out. We need a big book shop, or a supermarket, right? Somewhere they sell maps."

"Something like a road atlas?" Helen said.

"Yeah, yeah," Lee said, without even looking at Helen.

She punched Will on the shoulder.

"Ouch!" Will rubbed at his shoulder. "Don't start hitting me again."

"I'm gonna beat you black and blue until you stand up and help me find a map of this stupid country!"

"Are they big books, with maps inside them?" Helen said.

"So come on, big fella," Lee said, ignoring Helen. "I need you to help us out here. We're a team, remember?"

Will sighed. "I don't know, maybe."

"There's no maybe about it. You, me and Daniel, we can survive this place together, but we need to get Dan back, right?"

"And they cost nine pounds, ninety-nine pence, but sometimes they can be reduced down to two pounds, ninety-nine pence?" Helen said.

Lee didn't bother looking up. "Yeah, I guess so." She held out her hand to Will. "Come on, let's get you up on your feet and we can go find a map and then find Renton and we can kick his ass."

"I know where there is a road atlas," Helen said.

"Look, Helen, we don't have time to go back, okay?" Lee said.

"We don't have to go anywhere," Helen said. "Look."

Lee finally turned to look at Helen, saw her pointing at the shop window. And there, facing out in a display, were rows of road atlases.

"I don't believe it," Lee whispered.

She stood up, walked over to the window. Will and Helen followed her. They placed their hands against the glass and looked at the books.

This is like a sign, Lee thought. *A sign that we can do this, we can find Renton, we can rescue Dan.*

The first stirrings of hope blossomed inside Lee's chest. They could do this. They were going to be okay.

"Turn around, all of you."

Lee stiffened at the sound of the voice, all feelings of renewed hope draining away.

Slowly the three teens turned their backs to the shop window.

The man standing beside the bull was tall and thin. His long, grey hair was tied back in a ponytail. He was wearing camouflage trousers and shirt and a pair of heavy walking boots.

He was holding a rifle, but he wasn't pointing it at the teens. A young boy, maybe six or seven, was holding onto the man's other hand. He was grubby and thin, his dark hair sticking out in spikes. He had his thumb in his mouth and was regarding the teens silently.

"I thought you were dead," the man said.

Lee struggled to process what he was saying. The shock of

seeing another person had her thoughts whirling around in her head.

"What do you mean?" she said at last.

"The raptors, I thought they had killed you for sure."

"Were you the one shooting at us?" Will said.

"I was shooting at the raptors. I was trying to save you, not kill you."

Lee and Will looked at each other. Now Lee remembered. Daniel climbing into the plane wreck on New Street, looking for Renton. And then getting out, rejoining Lee and Will as the raptors began to surround them. Someone had fired a gun from the Rotunda tower, killing one of the raptors and giving the teens the chance they needed to run.

But Lee hadn't been entirely sure their mysterious rescuer had been aiming at the predator.

Had he been trying to rescue Lee and her friends, or kill them?

"You don't believe me?" the man said.

Lee looked back at him. "Yeah, sure, we believe you, of course we do."

"Nice dog you got there," the man said.

Helen clicked her fingers, summoned Iggy to her side. She put a protective hand on his head.

The man smiled, but it didn't do much to inspire trust. He was missing most of his teeth, and the ones he had left didn't look like they were going to last much longer.

"Don't worry, I don't want to hurt him," he said. "This is my boy, Kody."

Lee raised a hand in greeting. "Hi Kody."

The boy looked back at her, blank eyed. Sucking on his thumb.

"Say hello to the nice girls and boys, Kody," the man said.

66

Kody said nothing.

"He doesn't talk much," the man said. "But he can, when he needs to."

"My name's Lee, and this is Will and Helen."

Lee looked at the other two. They were all still standing with their back to the shop window, Helen with her hand on Iggy's head. Lee felt uncomfortable in this man's presence, and she wasn't sure why. The others felt the same way too, she was sure.

"You want to come back with me?" the man said. "We've got food, water, shelter. Even got a bed, and a fifty inch TV. TV doesn't work though, much like everything else these days."

"Um, I'm not sure," Lee said. She was starting to feel like the group's official spokesperson, although she hadn't asked to be and neither of the other two had told her that's what she was.

"What's not to be sure about?" the man said. "You stay here, you'll get eaten. Come with me, you won't. It's pretty simple really, when you think about it like that."

The sun was on Lee's face, and she could feel herself heating up. It wasn't even noon yet, but she knew they would have to find some shade soon. Whilst keeping an eye out for hungry predators.

"We're looking for our friend," Will said.

"Is he around here someplace?" the man said, swivelling his head, as though he might see Daniel from where he was standing.

"No, he's headed out of the city, we're trying to catch up with him," Lee said.

"Oh." The man looked down at Kody and then back at the teens. "Well, there's nothing I can do to help you there. I wish you would come back with us though. Even just for a night. I

67

can load you up with supplies, maybe even point you in the right direction if you know where your friend is headed." He paused, sucking on his rotten teeth. "It's been awfully lonely these past years, and Kody here, he's only ever known me and Megan. Megan's his sister, she's thirteen." He paused again. "At least I think she's thirteen. It's kind of difficult to keep track."

The man sighed and suddenly he looked very tired. Lee wondered if that little speech was the most he had spoken in one go for a long, long time.

Lee looked at Will again, trying to read his mind. It wasn't fair that she was having to make all the decisions.

"No, that's okay," she said, turning back to the man. "We need to keep moving, try and catch up with our friend."

The man said nothing, just kept on looking at them. His eyes flicked from Lee to Helen to Will and then to Iggy.

Finally he shrugged, and said, "All right. Come on Kody, let's get back home."

Lee heard a rustle in the undergrowth, behind the bronze bull. Everyone heard it. They all turned towards the sound. The fronds of tall grass parted, revealing a flash of orange and black.

A tiger appeared from the undergrowth.

No, not just a tiger.

A sabre-toothed tiger.

It peered at the children and the man, only its head and shoulders and front legs visible. The man raised his rifle, pointing it at the tiger and fired off a shot.

The crack of the gun cut through the air and everyone flinched. Iggy tried to bolt, pulling Helen over with him as she held onto his collar. Will grabbed him too whilst Helen calmed him down.

The tiger was nowhere to be seen.

"I missed him," the man said.

"You're not much of a marksman, are you?" Lee said.

"I got that raptor that was about to eat you," the man said.

Lee nodded.

"I reckon that tiger will be back soon," the man said. "He looked hungry. You sure you don't want to come back with me and Kody?"

"Maybe we should," Helen said. She looked scared. "Just for tonight?"

"I don't know," Lee said. "We need to keep moving."

"We could take the map book with us," Will said, looking at the rows of road atlases in the shop window. "We could plot our route and then head off in the morning."

Lee could see some sense in this. Carefully planning their route in the safety of the Rotunda. Heading out again in the morning, after a proper night's sleep. They were all exhausted still after the traumas of the night before.

"Okay," she said. "Just for tonight."

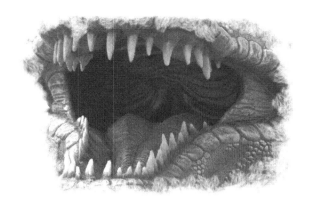

Chapter Seven

They wandered through the empty service station. The building seemed to echo with the ghosts of travellers. Daniel could hear them, talking, laughing, he could hear children crying. He could hear the roar of racing cars and the stutter of gunfire from the gaming area. The hiss of the coffeemakers from the Costa.

But he couldn't see it.

The vast service station might be deathly quiet now, but it was far from empty. The destruction here had obviously been swift and dramatic. The dinosaurs that had appeared here must have thought they were in dinosaur heaven when they saw the mass of screaming food, just waiting to be eaten.

The service station was now a graveyard. The floor was littered with broken bones and smashed skulls. The sound of crunching bone beneath Daniel's feet sickened him as he followed Renton. They passed familiar signs hanging from the ceiling, McDonalds, Subway, Burger King, M&S. All relics from a distant past.

Renton walked around the perimeter of the dining area, head arched up as he looked at all the signs. When they were almost back at the entrance, he stopped and looked through the filthy, cracked window at the car park. Somehow this sheet of glass had survived the devastation; most of the others had been completely shattered.

The service station had been busy when the dinosaurs made their sudden, shocking appearance. The car park was like a graveyard for cars and lorries and caravans.

Daniel looked up at Renton, still silently gazing through the window.

"Stop looking at me, kid," the American growled, his breath wheezing.

Daniel looked away, back out of the window. He could see something hovering, high up in the blue.

After a long, uncomfortable silence, Renton said, "You never should have run away."

Daniel kept his mouth shut. He didn't want to antagonise the big man.

"If you'd have done what you were supposed to do and stayed put at the base, we would both be there right now. Something to eat, something to drink, a bed to sleep in at night, protected from these monsters."

"Are you saying this is my fault?" Daniel said. He snapped his mouth shut, but it was too late, the words were out.

Renton turned his gaze on Daniel. He held up his arm, the bloody rag tied around the festering stump.

"This," he said, "this is your fault." He pointed at his scarred face, the charred holes where his nose used to be. "This is your fault."

Daniel looked away. Every time he saw the American's wounds his stomach turned over.

"I always knew you would be trouble, right from the very start," Renton said. "I told them, I said let him live with his granddad."

"Told who?" Daniel said.

Renton turned and started shuffling away, wheezing and gasping with each step.

"Told who?" Daniel shouted after him. "My father?"

Renton stopped walking and started making that strange, gurgling noise again. When he turned around, Daniel saw that he was laughing.

"Your father? What makes you think he had any choice in the matter? Sure, he wanted you with him, at the base where you would be safe. But he didn't get a say in that."

Daniel clenched his fists. "Then who did?"

"You ask too many questions, kid," Renton said, and turned away again.

Daniel punched his thighs in frustration. Did it even matter now? The whole world had gone to hell and there was nothing that could be done about it. So really, what did it matter?

It did matter, though. Somehow it did.

Daniel watched as Renton pushed his way past overturned tables, kicking his way through rubble and shards of bone and glass. He looked briefly at a long dead chiller cabinet, the glass smashed and the inside empty. Then he walked behind the serving counter of the Costa and into the back.

Daniel was torn between staying put, keeping as far away from Renton as he could, or following him and keeping close. As much as he hated the man, he knew he was better off sticking with him for the moment.

How long could they last, though, until they succumbed to thirst and hunger, or were attacked by a dinosaur? Their most urgent need was water, they had to find something to drink here.

Daniel decided to search one of the other eateries, instead

of following Renton around like a scared puppy.

He chose the McDonalds to start with. There was no chiller cabinet here, and he had to push his way through a door beside the serving counter to get into the back. The door gave way only a fraction when he first pushed it, and he had to shove hard before it scraped open enough for him to slip through into the kitchen area.

The ovens and the deep fryers were all black with grime and a thick layer of scum. A dark cloud of flies buzzed and hovered in a corner of the kitchen. One wall was mostly taken up with a huge set of shiny grey double doors. Long scratches had been gouged into their surfaces, as though something with claws had been trying to get inside. Daniel wondered if that might have been the chiller unit. The doors were shut, and the teenager wasn't sure he wanted to go in there. What would the inside of a closed fridge look and smell like after two decades without power? Especially an industrial sized one like this.

No, Daniel was pretty sure he didn't want to find out. But he knew he might have to. Something like that was worth investigating, definitely.

Maybe later. Maybe after he had searched the rest of the kitchens.

Daniel walked deeper into the disaster area that had once been a site of bustling, busy life. A skull lay on the floor, its lower jaw missing. More bones lay scattered across the cracked floor amongst the shredded, orange remains of polystyrene burger cartons.

A metallic clatter made Daniel jump, his heart suddenly thumping.

It's Renton, he told himself. *It's only Renton.*

But how could he be sure?

He turned and scanned the eating area, but could not see

Renton, could see no sign of life at all. Daniel's heart was thumping hard in his chest again. He had been living in a state of perpetual anxiety ever since the jet had crash landed him into this foreign, dangerous world that he had once thought of as home. There had been a brief interval of calm at Hooper's commune, but nothing more.

Daniel wasn't sure he could live like this. He wasn't sure he could survive what this world kept throwing at him.

He turned back to the kitchen, desperate to find something to drink. Anything.

The kitchen was cramped and small, much smaller than Daniel had expected. It didn't look like any kitchen he had seen before, and he could imagine the staff having to squeeze past each other back here, and how difficult it would be to keep from getting in each other's way during busy periods.

How trapped they must have been when the monsters from millions of years ago crashed into their lives, hungry for their flesh.

There was a door leading into a small office. A computer sat on its desk, the screen cracked. One wall was black with scorch marks and there was a fire extinguisher lying on its side on the floor.

Daniel pulled open a drawer in the desk and jumped when he saw a huge black beetle scurrying around inside, disturbed by the light and the sudden movement.

The drawer held a thin layer of grey, shredded paper and nothing else. Maybe the beetle had eaten all the contents. Maybe it had always been empty.

There was a filing cabinet standing against the opposite wall. Daniel tried the drawers, but they were locked shut. Hanging above it was a calender, a faded picture of Ed Sheeran, casually holding his guitar over one shoulder, the singer gazing back at Daniel.

Daniel turned his back on the pop star. There was nowhere else left to search in here except the chiller unit. The closed doors seemed to taunt him with empty promises of food and drink. Bottles of water, burgers, buns, fries.

A mountain of goodies waiting to be discovered.

Daniel knew it wasn't true. He knew that any food that might still be inside would have gone rotten many years ago. The best he could hope for were any unspoilt cans of soft drinks.

He approached the double doors. Slowly.

Seemed like his feet had suddenly turned into blocks of concrete and he had to force himself to drag them across the kitchen. He stopped before he had covered half of the short distance from the office to the chiller unit.

Maybe he should wait for Renton.

He could investigate the inside of the chiller while Daniel kept watch outside.

And where was Renton? What was taking him so long next door, in the Costa?

Daniel suddenly had a vision of the American surrounded by a stash of food and water he had discovered. He was eating and drinking and laughing to himself whilst Daniel stood here, hungry and thirsty and scared.

Another clatter, something falling over and this time much closer, shook Daniel from his thoughts.

Renton stepped into the kitchen. Daniel actually felt a moment of relief upon seeing him.

"Did you find anything?" he said.

Renton shook his head. "You?"

Daniel looked at the chiller unit's scarred doors. "I don't know."

Renton approached the doors, reached out and grasped a handle.

Daniel stepped back.

Renton pulled the door open. It moved slowly, haltingly, as Renton dragged it through the thick layer of scum and grit on the floor.

A putrid stink of decay hit Daniel and almost knocked him to the floor. He turned away, gagging. Renton stood immobile, seemingly unfazed by the foul smell, and stared into the unit's shadowed interior.

Daniel turned back, his hands over his mouth. He didn't know whether to breathe in through his mouth or his nose to try and minimise the stench. Neither seemed to work.

"Something must have got trapped in here recently and died," Renton muttered, bubbles of air popping from the hole in his face where his nose used to be as he spoke.

He took a step forward, towards the gloom.

Daniel stayed where he was.

There was no way he was going inside there. Besides the sickening stink of rotting flesh, there was also the possibility of something lurking in the darkness. Teeth bared, waiting for a victim.

Staying right where he was and watching Renton seemed like much the better option.

Renton walked deeper into the unit, slowly, seeming also to be very much aware of the possible dangers.

From behind Daniel there was a sudden eruption of clanging and banging. The teenager almost screamed as he imagined a horde of ferocious, hungry velociraptors charging towards him. Without looking back he bolted into the dark, stinking chiller unit.

Renton whirled around at the sound of the commotion.

"No!" he shouted.

Daniel looked behind him. The door was swinging shut, scraping over the filthy floor. The light from the narrowing gap in the doorway grew dimmer.

And Daniel thought, *Dinosaurs can't close doors, can they?*

Renton lunged for the door. They were almost in darkness now, and the gap between the doors was too narrow for the American to get through. He shoved his shoulder against the door and pushed, at the same time bellowing, a wordless expression of rage.

The door stopped swinging and immediately began opening up again.

No, thought Daniel. *Don't let it in here.*

Renton kept shoving, and the door swung wider. He lost his balance and almost fell over when the door suddenly swung free. Whatever had been pushing on the other side was no longer there.

Daniel caught a glimpse of a shadow darting out of the kitchen.

A small, human shadow.

Renton lumbered through the kitchen. He'd seen the movement too. Daniel followed him.

They ran into the large dining area. Saw a child dashing between overturned carts and bins. Daniel couldn't tell if it was a boy or a girl. Guessed the age at maybe ten or eleven.

They chased after the small figure, running for the exit. If they caught him, or her, what would Renton do, Daniel wondered. He couldn't imagine it would be anything pleasant. Like suggesting that he or she tagged along with them.

No, after having been almost trapped in that dark, stinking chiller unit Renton was most likely to take out his anger and frustration on the poor child.

Daniel had to stop him.

The child ran through the main entrance and outside to the car parking area. Through the shattered windows, Daniel saw the figure flash by. Renton ran outside.

Daniel followed close behind.

They ran along the outside of the large service station. The teenager overtook Renton, who was too slow to keep up. And he was gaining on the child too. Daniel put on an even faster burst of speed. They dodged between cars, some of them still looking undamaged whilst others were crushed and smashed.

The sun was high in the sky and Daniel was drenched in sweat. He suddenly realised this was doing him no good, that exerting himself like this was dangerous without any fresh water to drink. But he couldn't stop now, he had to catch that child.

Close behind the child now, Daniel reached out a hand and his fingers snagged clothing. But then the child swerved and Daniel crashed into a parked car, one that had somehow escaped damage. A skeleton in faded, tattered clothing lay crumpled in the driver's seat. When Daniel barrelled into the car and rocked it, the skull rolled over in a chilling imitation of life, as though it was looking at the teenager, annoyed at the intrusion.

He pushed himself off the car and ran again. He was pretty sure now that the child was a boy. And the boy was flagging too, the chase was too much for him. But Daniel was fit and strong from all the BMX biking he used to do. Even though his body was burning up with heat and his muscles were screaming at him to stop, he knew he had a little more in him to keep going.

He dashed between the cars, closing on the boy again. Reached out, snagging the back of his shirt once more. His fingers caught in the dirty material and when the boy tried switching direction again, Daniel was ready for him. He plowed into the boy, grabbing him with both hands and wrapping his arms around him as they crashed into another car.

The boy screamed and kicked and they both fell to the ground, kicking up clouds of dirt.

"Hey, stop! Stop!" Daniel hissed. "I'm not going to hurt you."

The boy twisted his head wildly, kicking and writhing.

"Get off me! Let me go!"

Daniel bore his weight down on the youngster, trying to get him to stop fighting.

"Please stop, we're not going to hurt you," he said.

Suddenly the boy stopped fighting and went limp. For a moment, Daniel thought the boy had listened to him, that he finally believed him. But then he heard the sound of Renton's whistling, gurgling breathing and he realised the child was simply terrified.

"Give the little bastard to me," Renton said.

"No," Daniel said, and shook his head.

"He tried to trap us, we would have died in that room. Give him to me."

"No."

Renton's charred lips drew back, and he growled quietly.

"If you try and hurt him I will run away," Daniel said. "You will never get me back to my father."

"Don't be an idiot, kid," Renton said.

The teenager stared back at the American. "I mean it."

Renton's one eye narrowed down into a slit, while the other remained bulging wide open.

"If that's how you want to play it," he said.

He took a step forward, his bulk casting a shadow over the two children as he loomed closer. Daniel got ready to let the boy go. He wouldn't be able to stop Renton for long, but he could give the child enough of a head start that the American would never catch up with him.

"No, wait!" the boy screamed in a high pitched voice. "I've got water! I've got water!"

Renton stepped back. Straightened up.

"Show us," he said.

The boy looked up at Renton, wide-eyed. "Promise you won't kill me first!"

"Show us where this water is before I rip your head off and drink your blood," Renton said.

Despite the heat of the day, a sudden chill ran through Daniel. Was Renton serious? Was he capable of something like that?

Keeping his eyes on Renton, Daniel let go of the boy.

"What's your name?" he said.

"Emily."

"You're a girl?"

"Well duh, yeah."

Daniel could see it now. Her dirty, blond hair had been chopped roughly short which made her look boyish. But more than that it was the jut of her chin and her narrowed eyes as she stared back at her two captors. Emily obviously wasn't the kind of girl who would play quietly with dolls and makeup.

"How old are you?" Daniel said.

"Shut up with the damn questions," Renton said. "Where's this water?"

Emily glanced at Renton. "I'm ten."

Emily pushed Daniel away and climbed to her feet. Stared up at Renton like she might run again.

Then turned her back on them and began walking towards the service station building.

Daniel stood up and followed her, Renton shuffling along behind.

I hope she's telling the truth about the water, Daniel thought.

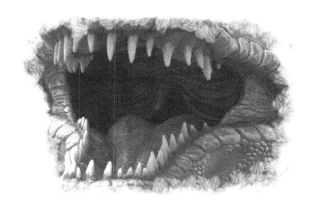

Chapter Eight

Will felt uneasy. He couldn't pin it down, couldn't explain it. He just had the feeling something was very wrong. Which was laughable in a way, because everything was very wrong. He had been catapulted from his own time and into a future ravaged by dinosaurs. They had been expelled from the one safe place they had found and were having to fend for themselves. They had little in the way of water, food and any real idea of where they were going or what they were going to do if they even got there.

And all the while they lived under the constant threat of being attacked and eaten by a hungry monster from their worst nightmares.

Still, despite all that, Will had the unhappy feeling that things had just taken a turn for the worse.

He just couldn't work out why.

The man, who still hadn't told them his name, took Will, Lee and Helen back to the Rotunda. When he was younger, Will had been fascinated by the cylindrical, high rise building. To him it had always looked like a fat Smarties tube of giant proportions stood on its end. He knew that originally the building had been used as offices and then later refurbished into apartments.

The man took them through a service entrance at the back of the building, and up a set of stairs. They climbed up and up, and around and around. The stairwell was gloomy, with only a little light entering from outside. Will wondered why the man had chosen to live so high up, when he could easily have taken an apartment nearer the ground. Surely having to carry food and water up here was energy sapping.

It was only when they got to his apartment and he opened the door into the large living space that Will understood. It wasn't just the view across the city, although that was spectacular enough through the floor to ceiling windows.

It was for defence.

Being up here, near the top floor, was how Will imagined it would have been like for knights defending a castle atop a hill.

The other two obviously felt the same. The three teens ignored the man and his son, they didn't see the grubby apartment with its ripped and dirty sofa, the stains on the walls or the holes in the carpet. They didn't even see the long scratches on the windows where things had tried to force their way in.

They just saw the view.

They dropped their rucksacks by the door and walked over to the windows and gazed out at the city. Will thought it was the strangest sight he had ever seen.

He recognised it still. It was Birmingham city centre all right. But much of it had been transformed into a jungle. The streets were filled with a dense layer of greenery, thick, tangled vines clogging up the thoroughfares and roads. Creepers strangled the shop frontages, climbing up the walls and through shattered windows. Will was amazed at how many of the windows had been broken, and the holes in the buildings. Had all the destruction been caused by the dinosaurs or had something else happened here?

In the distance was the tallest structure in Birmingham, the Post Office Tower. It towered over the cityscape like a giant, futuristic version of Cleopatra's Needle. As Will gazed at it, a pterosaur landed gracefully on the summit. It folded its large wings and sat hunched at the top.

"Bloody things are always perched on there," said the man. "I swear they're watching me, trying to figure out how to catch us."

Will didn't know what to say. The sight of the city strangled by a jungle that should never have been able to grow here, of the pterosaurs gliding overhead, had suddenly hammered home to him how complete and irrevocable the change had been.

"Wow," Lee whispered, as though echoing his thoughts. "I can't believe it."

"But this is how it's always been," Helen said.

"Not for us it hasn't," Lee said.

The man slid open a door and stepped out onto the balcony. The others followed him.

Will could imagine that this had once been the height of luxurious city living. A modern table, all curves without a single corner on it, still sat on the balcony, with two reclining chairs. Will could imagine sitting out here on a summer's night with a drink, looking out over the bright lights of the city below.

Now the balcony's floor and the outdoor furniture were covered in bird crap. Large, thick dollops of it lay everywhere. Most if it was dry and crusted over, but some patches looked fresh and sticky.

"Can't keep the sodding things away," the man said. "I used to clean it regular like, but I gave up in the end. It were a losing battle, and it's not like I were about to have visitors or anything."

Will took a deep breath. The air up here was clean and fresh. Down in the city, amongst all the vines and creepers and the thick leaves dripping with moisture, he found breathing uncomfortable.

A young woman stepped out onto the balcony with them. Her dark brown hair was long and straight, hanging down to her waist, almost. Her skin was white, as though she spent all her days inside. And she was rake thin.

"Who are they?" she said, staring at the teens warily.

"I found them wandering down by the Bullring," the man said.

"Why did you bring them back?" she said.

"Thought you and Kody might like the company, love."

"We don't."

"Now Megan, don't be like that," the man said.

"We're only staying the night," Lee said. "It'll be back to just the three of you again tomorrow morning."

"Are you the ones my father tried to shoot the other day?" Megan said.

"I already told you, I was shooting at the raptors."

Will caught the glance that Lee gave him. He didn't like this one bit. Maybe they should have stayed on their own, stuck with the plan of heading out of the city as soon as possible. They could still do that. Helen had the road atlas, was clutching it to her chest like it was a magical talisman whilst Iggy stood beside her. They had some food, some water.

They could leave now.

"Don't pay any attention to Megan, she's not used to visitors," the man said. "None of us are."

Kody started hooting, a strange bird like sound. He was

85

agitated, jumping up and down and pointing past them up at the sky.

Three pterosaurs were gliding towards them, blotting out the sky as they drew closer and closer.

"Everyone inside!" the man shouted.

No one needed telling. Megan was already through the door and back in the apartment. Kody was still jumping up and down and hooting. His father swept him up in his arms and carried him inside.

Will and Lee followed. The man was ready to slide the balcony doors shut, but Helen was still outside.

What was she doing? Why wasn't she running inside with everyone else?

Will saw why.

Iggy was standing at the glass balcony siding and barked furiously at the approaching monsters, his ears laid flat along his head and the hair on his back bristling.

"Iggy come on!" Helen wailed, pulling at his collar.

Iggy paid no attention to her, barking and snarling as the pterosaurs glided closer and closer.

The man started sliding the glass door shut.

"No!" Lee screamed.

Will watched with growing horror and despair as Lee shot outside, scrambling past the man and through the narrowed gap between the sliding window and the wall, and grabbed Iggy's collar. Megan screamed at her father to shut the door and Kody kept up his hooting and leaping up and down. Even over all of that noise, Will was sure he could hear the rustle of the pterosaurs' wings and the click of their teeth as they descended on their prey.

With their combined strength, Helen and Lee were able to start dragging Iggy towards the safety of the apartment. But they were taking too long. The first pterosaur would be on them in only a few moments.

And the man was closing the door again.

Will ran at him and shoved him away. He scrambled outside, slipping on a patch of fresh pterosaur excrement on the floor. Managing to keep upright, he grabbed Iggy's collar and the three teens were able to drag the dog inside.

Megan slid the door shut as the first pterosaur slammed into the window and started scrabbling at the glass.

Everyone screamed. They all retreated further into the apartment as the monstrosity outside beat its head against the window, wings flapping and claws scratching at the glass. The second pterosaur landed beside it and assaulted the window.

There was no room for the third one and it hovered above the other two, beating its wings and attempting to join them.

The man had fallen over when Will had pushed him away. It had been like pushing over a child, he was so light and weak. On his back, the man scrabbled like a crab away from the window and the frenzied monsters on the outside.

Megan rounded on Will and shoved him on the shoulder.

"That stupid dog of yours almost got us killed!" she screamed.

Iggy bared his teeth and growled.

"And your dad almost got my friends killed," Will yelled back.

"You would have trapped us out there, wouldn't you?" Lee said, looking down at the man on the stained, threadbare carpet.

"I had to," the man said, getting slowly to his feet. "Can't you see that?"

"We should go," Lee said to Will.

"No, no, don't go," the man said. "Stay here, please. Stay the night."

The pterosaurs hammered at the windows, their claws making screeching noises against the glass.

"Shouldn't we go somewhere else, another room maybe?" Helen said, looking anxiously at the window.

"It's all right, they'll get bored soon and leave," the man said. "They always do."

Lee was still looking at Will. He hated how she kept turning to him for confirmation of her decisions. Why would she do that? She knew he wasn't the decision making type, he wasn't a leader.

He shrugged. "I don't know."

"Stay, please stay," the man said.

The scrabbling noises at the window had stopped. Two of the pterosaurs had flown away. One still sat on the ledge, wings folded up, watching them.

"I suppose we should wait until that thing has gone and forgotten about us at least," Will said.

Iggy was still growling at the monster outside. Helen had hold of his collar, straining to keep him beside her.

"All right, we'll stay for a couple of hours maybe," Lee said. "But then we're heading off. We've got to find our friend."

Will sank into the sofa, suddenly exhausted. The excitement had drained him of energy. He pulled his rucksack off his back and dropped it on the floor by his feet.

"Maybe we could plan our route while we're here," he said.

"Good idea," Lee said. "Where's the road atlas?"

"I . . . I dropped it," Helen said, and pointed.

Everyone turned to look. The road atlas lay on the balcony floor, beneath the pterosaur still staring through the scratched glass at them.

"Oh great," Lee said.

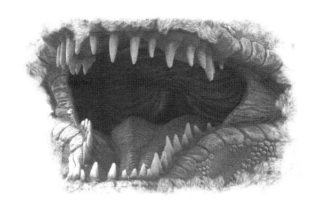

Chapter Nine

Emily took them back into the service station and up the stairs. As he followed the girl, Daniel remembered running up here. Escaping from Renton and Reece. They climbed the stairs and walked along a corridor, past toilets and another eating area until they arrived at the covered walkway across the motorway.

Daniel looked down, through broken windows at the carriageway of stalled traffic heading out of the city centre. The line of cars disappeared into the distance. The carriageway heading back into the city was clear of vehicles, but the tarmac surface was cracked and pitted and covered with a thick, twisting undergrowth. Daniel remembered the rats and shuddered.

"Get a move on, kid," Renton said as he appeared at the top of the steps. "If we let her out of our sight, we might never find her again."

Chasing Emily had obviously taken all of Renton's remaining strength. He was wheezing, the sound of his breath like a high-pitched whistle. His face had turned pale, and he looked even worse than Daniel had thought possible.

Still at the top of the stairs, Renton leaned against a wall, gasping for breath. He pointed down the covered walkway. Emily was standing at the other end, waiting for them.

"It's here," she said.

Daniel looked at her, unable to comprehend for a moment what she was telling him.

Emily held out her hands in a show of frustration. "The water, dummies. It's here."

Renton wheezed and grunted.

"I'm gonna kill that kid," he muttered.

Daniel walked towards Emily. He couldn't see any water. She was standing by an open door. A sign on the door said 'Staff only'.

"It's up there," she said.

"You're not going to lock me in there, are you?" Daniel said.

Emily rolled her eyes and sighed. For a ten-year-old she acted very much like an impatient adult dealing with an obstinate, naughty child.

She went through the doorway first.

Daniel glanced back at Renton, still shuffling along the walkway, and then followed her. More steps, plain concrete ones, heading up to another door. Daniel could barely see Emily, the space was so gloomy.

Already at the top, Emily pushed open the door, and the stairwell was flooded with sunlight. She stepped through the doorway, disappearing into the light like the heroine in a science fiction movie.

Now that he could see better, Daniel noticed a length of what looked like a garden hosepipe trailing down the side of the steps and out through the door at the bottom.

Daniel followed Emily up the stairs.

They were on the flat roof of the service station, the one on the opposite side of the motorway heading back into the city. Placed on the roof were barrels and crates and wheelie bins, all connected to each other with lengths of plastic tubing. The hosepipe that Daniel had noticed on the stairs was connected to the nearest, and largest, barrel.

"Take a look," Emily said.

The barrel was topped with a loose-fitting lid. Daniel lifted it off and peered inside.

It was full of water.

He looked across the rooftop at the other barrels.

"Are they all filled with water?"

Emily nodded, grinning.

Daniel placed a hand into the water. It was warm from the sunshine.

"Is it safe to drink?" he said.

"Duh, you have to boil it first," Emily said. "I've got bottles of water downstairs."

She ran back to the doorway, dodging around Renton as he appeared on the rooftop.

Daniel pulled his hand out of the barrel, the water dripping off it and splattering in dark shadows on the roof.

"The drinking water is downstairs," he said, as he passed Renton.

Emily was pulling plastic milk containers out of a cupboard. She unscrewed the top off one and handed it out for Daniel. He looked at it and his stomach tightened up at the thought of the water on his tongue, slipping down his throat.

But he couldn't take it. Despite the need to drink, his hands refused to reach out and take the container of water.

"It's safe, dummy," Emily said. "I've boiled it. I know what I'm doing, you know."

The mental block holding Daniel back from taking the water snapped. He grasped hold of the plastic bottle and lifted it to his dry lips, tipped it up. The water, although warm, tasted clean. Renton appeared beside Daniel. He pulled the bottle out of Daniel's hand and drank greedily from it.

Emily watched him chugging noisily at the water.

"Your friend doesn't look so good," she said.

"He's not my friend," Daniel said.

Emily handed him another bottle of water. "Here, take this."

"Thanks."

Daniel drank more of the water. He could feel his stomach swelling up with it, but he didn't care.

Renton stopped drinking and wiped his hand across his mouth. His breath whistled from the hole in his face where his nose used to be.

He held up the plastic container of water.

"This," he said. "You couldn't have organised this. Who set that water catching system up?"

Emily stared at Renton, her eyes ablaze with defiance, chin jutting out.

"What's the matter, kid? Cat got your tongue all of a sudden?"

"My mother did it," Emily said.

Renton turned and looked down the covered walkway, as though expecting to see Emily's mother walking towards them right at that moment.

"Where is she?" Daniel said.

Some of the defiance left Emily's face. "I don't know. I woke up one morning, and she was gone. But she's coming back, I know she is!"

Renton glugged at more of the water.

"How long have you been here?" Daniel said.

Emily shrugged. She seemed a little deflated, as though mention of her missing mother had taken some of the fight out of her.

"I don't know, it's hard to tell. Mum was here before me. We're just waiting for my Dad next and then we'll be together again."

Daniel glanced at Renton, but he wasn't paying attention, still drinking the water.

What Emily had said didn't sound right. Surely the chances of Emily and her mother being thrown forward into the future at different times and managing to find each other again were pretty small?

Renton wiped his mouth. His breathing had subsided a little, had become less tortuous.

"Your mother was clever," he said.

Emily stared at him, forehead scrunched up in a scowl.

Renton glanced up. "All that up there, the water catching system, that's something, it really is." He stared at Emily. "What did your mother used to do for a job? Before all this?"

Emily shrugged.

"You don't remember?" Daniel said.

"You two ask lots of questions," Emily said, and turned away from them.

"Yeah well, here's another one for you," Renton said. "You got any food?"

"Of course," Emily said, the contempt strong in her voice.

She turned and ran again. Daniel followed her. She didn't go far, into another eating area, on the Southbound side of the carriageway. She ran between the tables and around the food counter. Through a door into the back.

The kitchen was clean, shining almost. Everything laid out,

ready to start cooking the next meal. The cooker had been adapted, rigged up with plastic pipes snaking in coils onto large gas tanks. And there were more plastic containers full of clear water.

Someone had done a lot of work setting this up.

Emily pulled open a cupboard door.

The shelves were crammed with tins. Ham, potatoes, carrots, soups, stews. Daniel's eyes glanced over them, the coloured labels blurring into one.

Emily opened another cupboard. This one was filled with packets of dried food.

"We've got more like this," Emily said.

"This isn't regular service station food," Daniel said. "Where did you get all this from?"

Emily said nothing, just looked at Daniel with her big, round eyes.

"Your mum did this, didn't she?"

Emily nodded.

They heard a shout from outside. Renton, calling them.

Without a word, Emily ran. Daniel followed her.

Renton was standing on the bridge, looking through the scarred, filthy window. Daniel and Emily joined him, hands pressed against the glass.

A dark cloud swarmed over and around the cars on the motorway. The ground, the abandoned vehicles, even the motorway verge, and the fields seemed to be disappearing beneath the black, undulating shadow.

"Rats!" Renton hissed.

"So many of them," Daniel whispered.

"I've seen this before," Emily said. "Sometimes they just do this, it's like they're panicked or something."

The colony of rats swarmed beneath the bridge.

94

A mischief of rats, that's what a collection of rats is called. The thought had popped into Daniel's head out of nowhere. He couldn't remember ever being told this, but he was sure it was right.

"Don't worry, we'll be safe up here," Emily said.

Renton pointed. "Are you sure about that?"

Some of the rats, a part of the mischief, had separated from their companions. Although they seemed to have no destination in mind, they were headed to the service station car park. Daniel thought about the doors wide open, the shattered windows, thought about the rats swarming through the downstairs eating areas.

And he wondered if they could climb stairs. Maybe not climb, but he was sure they would be able to scurry and jump up them. He'd had a friend once, who had a pet mouse. Sometimes they would let it out of its cage and watch as it leaped up each step all the way to the first floor.

"I think we should leave," he said.

"Don't be an idiot," Emily said. "I told you, we're safe up here."

More and more of the rats were flowing like a river down the motorway. Daniel couldn't see an end to them.

A shadow swept across the ground, over the cars and the rats scurrying across them. Daniel craned his neck and looked up.

A pterosaur soared into view over the motorway, and then another and another.

This was why the rats were running.

They were being hunted.

The rats were fleeing away from the city, in the same direction that Daniel and Renton had been headed. Most of them just kept on scurrying down the motorway, but a significant number were breaking away from the main pack and heading for the service station.

Emily saw them too.

"We're safe," she said, but her voice lacked its usual tone of defiance.

"I'm going to see if they're coming inside," Daniel said.

He didn't wait for anyone to agree or disagree with him. He ran back along the covered bridge until he got to the top of the steps leading down to the area where he and Renton had found Emily. He paused at the top and listened.

The stairs only went so far before they turned a corner. The eating area was hidden from his view, but Daniel was reluctant to descend the stairs to the point where he could see if the rats were coming inside the service station.

After a few moments of standing rigidly still, he realised he was holding his breath. He sighed, softly. Took in a deep breath.

There was no noise from downstairs. Nothing at all.

Except . . .

Had he heard something? The sharp click of claws against concrete? The rustle of bodies scurrying inside?

There it was again. And Daniel could hear a low murmur of movement now, a scratching and scurrying and a dreadful, high pitched squeaking.

The rats were inside.

Daniel imagined their dark bodies flowing over the broken tables and chairs, the ripped fabric of the seating, and the counter tops. Imagined them crowding into the kitchens.

But would they come up the stairs?

Daniel looked back at Renton and Emily. They were standing side by side, little Emily dwarfed by Renton's bulk. Daniel put a finger to his lips. He didn't want either of them speaking, making any kind of noise that might alert the rats to their existence.

Turning his back on them, Daniel listened again at the rustling of bodies, the mass of crawling, scurrying, scratching, squeaking rats. Part of him, the sensible, rational part, wanted to run back across the covered bridge, back to Renton and Emily. Wanted to tell them that they needed to get out of here, to gather up as much water and food as they could carry and flee, before the rats found them.

But there was another side to him, and this one thought it would be a good idea to creep down the steps. Only to the point where the stairs turned a corner where he could stay hidden behind the wall. But he could peer around that corner from behind his hiding place. And he could take a quick look at the rats. See where they were inside. How far away from the steps they were.

Decide if they needed to run just yet, or if they could risk waiting it out.

Realising he was holding his breath again, Daniel gasped and took a deep lungful of air.

He should get back to the others, warn them. He knew that. It was the sensible thing to do.

But maybe if he risked one quick glance. Just to assess the situation.

After all, if he went back now to Renton and Emily and told them only what he had heard, they would argue about what to do next, he knew they would. But if Daniel could report back with something definite, something he had seen with his own eyes, then there would be less of a choice.

If the rats were coming up the stairs, Daniel, Renton and Emily had to run.

Without thinking about it anymore, Daniel took the first

step down. His legs were trembling, and he had to look down at his feet. Seemed like he was walking on a soft, spongy surface that could give way at any moment. He took another step, and another.

Drawing closer to the corner, he could hear the sound of scurrying and scratching growing louder, becoming more frenzied. Daniel didn't even have to take a look now to know that the service station was filled with scrambling, sharp clawed bodies crawling over everything in their search for safety.

Or food.

But still, he continued down the stairs. Couldn't stop himself.

He had to see.

Daniel reached the corner where the stairs turned. The sad remains of a fake plant stood in the corner, its plastic leaves dusty and nibbled at the edges.

The teenager braced his hands against the wall and slowly leaned forward so that he could see around the corner.

In that first moment his mind went blank at the sight that met him. It seemed as though the entire floor and everything in it had been replaced by a bubbling mass of dark brown bodies. There were even more rats here than he had seen earlier in the day when he had escaped them by diving into the car.

Overcome with a frenzy of some kind, the rats were biting and scratching at each other, their squealing an overpowering, maddening shriek. More of them were still flooding through the doorway and broken windows, even though it looked as though the service station could not fit any more rats inside.

Daniel watched, hypnotised by the gruesome spectacle before him. It almost seemed to have an appalling beauty to him, a fascination he could not explain.

Until the spell was broken by the sight of rats scurrying up the steps towards him.

Daniel turned and ran.

He sprinted up the steps, tripping as he neared the top, but regaining his feet before he fell over. At the opposite end of the covered bridge, Renton and Emily both stared at Daniel as he ran towards them.

"Run!" he screamed. "The rats are coming up here, run!"

Neither of them moved, simply watching him as he drew closer.

Daniel's trainers slapped against the walkway as he sprinted along the bridge. But over the sound of his running he could hear the rats, their claws clicking at the hard steps as they drew closer to the top.

"What's happening?" Renton said, shifting the shotgun in the crook of his arm.

"There're hundreds of rats, thousands of them, coming this way," Daniel gasped. "We've got to get away, down onto the other side."

Emily screamed.

Rats were pouring onto the walkway from the access to the bridge on the opposite side, nearest to them.

They were trapped.

Renton lifted his shotgun and fired with both barrels into the seething mass of rodents. The blast scattered them, bodies flying into the air in a shower of blood and fur.

Renton grunted as he lowered the shotgun.

Emily had clapped her hands over her ears, and she was staring wide eyed at Renton.

Daniel looked back the way he had just come. A thick carpet of bristling bodies was pouring towards them, a stream of death and disease.

Renton cracked open the shotgun and shoved two more

shells into it.

"I'll soon deal with these," he said, snapping the shotgun shut.

"It's no good," Daniel said, and pointed back to where Renton had fired into the mass of rats approaching them.

More rodents were clambering over and through the bloodied mess of dead rats, an unending deluge of them. Daniel glanced both ways. There was no way Renton could shoot them all, there were far too many of them. They only had moments left before the two hordes of rats overpowered Daniel, Renton and Emily. Claws and teeth ripping open their flesh, the rats feeding on them in a frenzy.

Emily bolted for the open door leading to the stairs up to the rooftop.

Daniel followed her, Renton behind him.

The rats were flowing all around them now, biting at their feet and ankles. Renton stamped at them, crushing their bodies beneath his boots. He started roaring wordlessly, adding more noise to the screech of the rats.

Daniel scrambled up the steps towards the rectangle of sunshine at the top. Emily was already through the door, urging him on.

"Hurry!" she screamed and started pushing the door closed.

Daniel threw himself through the narrowing gap, from the gloom of the stairwell and into bright sunshine. Renton was right behind him, barrelling past the door and shoving it open with his bulk.

The first of the rats quickly followed him. Daniel kicked out at one as it fastened itself onto his trousers. Its sharp claws stung at his leg through the material and he had to hit it with his fist to dislodge it.

Emily had given up on shoving the door closed and was

running across the rooftop, screaming.

Renton had broken open his shotgun and was fumbling with the shells as the rats began swarming around his feet.

The rooftop door was wide open, and the rats were pouring through it in a black mass. Bunched together, the rodents almost seemed like one living thing. An evil, monstrous river of fur and teeth and claws.

Renton snapped his shotgun closed and lifted it.

A massive, winged shape swooped down on him, knocking him to the floor and sending the shotgun flying.

Daniel looked up.

The bright blue sky was filling with pterosaurs.

Two of them broke from the pack and hurtled towards their prey.

Daniel screamed.

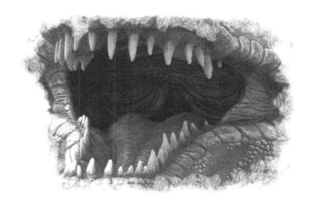

Chapter Ten

"Oh great," Lee said, looking at the pterosaur sitting on the balcony, hunched over the road atlas. "Now what do we do?"

The man collapsed into a chair and gazed blank eyed at the pterosaur. Kody was jumping up and down and hooting. Lee wasn't sure she had heard him say a proper word yet.

Will was standing with Helen and Iggy. Iggy was crouched low on the floor, his teeth bared at the pterosaur outside, his ears flat along his skull.

"We should go somewhere else in the building," Helen said. "Out of this thing's sight."

Megan went and stood by her dad, put a hand on his shoulder.

"Don't matter," she said. "It'll get bored soon and go. This happens lots."

Lee backed up against the door. The teenagers' rucksacks were lying in a row next to her, with her rifle propped up against the wall.

Lee couldn't take her eyes off the thing on the balcony. She'd always thought that pterosoars had beaks, but now that she could see one close up she realised it was almost a mouth. In fact, she could see its teeth. It still had a beak, or what looked like one, but those rows of sharp, serrated teeth made it look even more vicious than she could have imagined.

As fascinating as it was, like being in a dinosaur zoo maybe, Lee had had enough. She just wanted to get out, flee that monstrous looking thing and hope to never have such a close up view of one again.

She looked over at Will, but he was staring at the pterosaur too.

"Will!" she hissed.

He looked over at her, his eyes wide behind his lenses.

"We should go," she said. "We should get out of here."

The man stirred in the threadbare chair.

"No," he said. His voice was thick and slurred, like he was half asleep or drunk. "No, stay here."

Lee kept on looking at Will. Why the heck was the man so insistent all the time that they stay? Surely the last thing he wanted was more mouths to feed?

Will nodded, keeping his gaze fixed on Lee. He was with her. They were going.

"Helen," Lee said. "Come on, we're getting out of here."

Helen nodded too, took hold of Iggy's collar.

The man stood up, pushing Megan's hand off his shoulder.

"I told you, it's not safe out there. You should stay."

Lee shook her head. "Uh-uh, we've had enough of this. Thank you for your hospitality and all, but this is just too crazy for us. We need to get going, find our friend."

Megan suddenly grabbed her hair and started yanking at it. Her face all screwed up, she opened her mouth and screamed. Before Lee could even think about moving or getting out of the apartment, Megan rushed at her, still screaming, and slammed

103

into Lee's side.

Lee hit the floor and covered her head with her arms as Megan punched and kicked at her.

"Hey, hey! Somebody get this crazy freak off me!" Lee shouted.

Iggy was growling and straining at his collar. Helen let him go and he leapt on top of Megan, barking wildly.

The man picked up his gun and Will screamed at him, "No!"

"Iggy, here boy!" Helen shouted.

Iggy ran back to Helen's side, ears still lying flat. Megan climbed to her feet. She didn't look any the worse for wear for the encounter with the Labrador. Lee stood up too.

Megan stood in front of the door, blocking their exit.

The man was still holding his gun, pointing it at them.

"You should put the gun down," Will said. His voice trembled a little as he spoke, but Lee was impressed at how calm he sounded.

The man lowered the gun a little, but not much.

"You can go if you want," he said. "But you leave the dog here."

"What?" Lee said.

Helen put her arms around Iggy's neck. "No."

"What do you want the dog for?" Lee said.

"Company, for the children," the man said.

Kody was standing at the window, hooting and looking at the winged monster on the balcony. The pterosaur tapped the glass with its beak, but Kody didn't flinch.

Lee's stomach hurt. A sharp pang right deep down inside, where she couldn't do anything about it. And she thought she knew why, too.

It was obvious the man didn't want Iggy for company.

"You're lying," she said.

The man said nothing. He was holding the gun a little higher again, pointing it at Lee.

"Kill them, Daddy," Megan said. "Kill them now!"

"Now Megan, don't be like that," the man said. "They're going, and we'll keep the dog, and it'll be all right."

"What do you want Iggy for?" Lee said.

The man gave a little shrug of his shoulders. "Times are hard, you know that. Times've never been harder."

"What do you want Iggy for?" Lee said again.

"We want to eat him!" Megan hissed. "We want to kill him and cook him and eat him, that's why."

Kody hooted at the pterosaur.

The pterosaur tapped at the glass, growing more insistent and frantic. It lifted its wings, blocking out the daylight and throwing the apartment into a deep shade.

"No!" Helen shouted, holding Iggy closer. "I won't let you!"

Lee glanced at Megan, standing in front of their only way out. The girl was obviously crazy, and who could blame her having lived here her whole life? Just her father and mute brother for company all these years? Lee felt like she was falling off the deep end after only an hour or two in their presence.

But the father, he wasn't crazy. Desperate yes, but not crazy.

Maybe, maybe he could still be reasoned with.

The pterosaur was growing ever more frantic outside at the sight of Kody leaping up and down. It was bashing the glass with its beak. The sound, like a giant woodpecker, filled the room, making rational thought difficult.

"Can't we just get out of here and go somewhere where we can hear ourselves think?" Lee said. "We can talk about this, can't we?"

"Time for talking's over," the man said. "I'm taking your dog. Got mouths to feed, you can see that."

Lee's face went cold. He obviously couldn't be reasoned with after all.

"Now I don't want to hurt you children," he said. "I really don't. But you got to let me have the dog. You just got to."

Lee's eyes flicked towards her rifle, propped up beside her rucksack. It was too far away. By the time she had made a lunge for it the man could have shot and killed her.

The frantic tap-tap-tapping filled the room, filled Lee's head. She wanted to shut everything out, run away from these people and the pterosaur, get as far away as possible. Why had they even come up here? What had they been thinking?

The man shifted position slightly, lowering his gun.

Lee thought, *he's changed his mind, he's letting us go*.

The man pointed the gun at Iggy.

Helen wrapped herself around the dog, protecting him with her own body.

"Please don't make me shoot you, too," the man said.

Helen buried her face into Iggy's fur.

Will had turned a ghastly pale, looked like he was going to fall down in a faint at any moment.

Lee knew how he felt.

"Please, don't," she said.

The frantic tapping stopped and Megan screamed.

Kody had opened the balcony door.

Lee didn't properly see what happened next, everything was a blur of motion and panic. She saw Kody, already on the balcony. She was aware of sunlight filling the room once more as the pterosaur folded its wings in on itself. She saw the massive wings open up again as the pterosaur lifted from the

106

balcony.

And she saw Kody was no longer there.

Kody's father ran outside screaming his name. The pterosaur was already high above the city and being joined by others.

The man lifted his gun and fired into the sky. Megan was by his side, yanking at clumps of her hair, screaming wordlessly.

Lee looked at Will and Helen.

They didn't need telling.

Lee yanked open the door and the three of them grabbed their rucksacks and ran out of the apartment and down the stairs, Helen still holding Iggy by his collar. Lee stumbled and almost fell at the bottom, but regained her footing. They ran outside where they heard another gunshot. Surely the pterodactyl was far out of range now?

And if Kody wasn't dead already, he would be very soon.

* * *

"Where to now?" Will said when they got outside.

"Back to the Bullring, pick up another road atlas," Lee said. "Then we head north."

The three teens ran, Iggy padding along beside Helen.

"We should get out of the city as fast as we can," Will said. "I get the feeling Kody's dad will blame us for what happened, and might come looking for us."

"Yeah, I think you're right," Lee said.

They found their way back to the Bullring easily and quickly. Lee knew they were being careless, they weren't keeping alert for predators. Anything could be lurking in the undergrowth, waiting to pounce on them and rip them apart.

But Lee knew there was a human predator up there in the

107

Rotunda, and she had a feeling it wouldn't be long at all before he was hunting them down.

The huge bronze bull was standing where they had left it, where it always stood. And so were the map books in the shop display window.

Will ran inside and grabbed one.

"Let's take a look see where we need to go," he said.

Lee shook her head. "No, we should get moving as fast as we can. Get out of here before that crazy guy finds us."

Will nodded.

They ran through the Bullring and down a wide set of steps, past Harrods and Saint Martin's church. The old church building contrasted with the new and the modern even more starkly now that they were both covered in creeping ivy and surrounded by swaying fronds of green.

They kept running, sweat pouring off their faces. Iggy's tongue hung from his mouth as he panted.

Lee knew that although they needed to get away, they also need shelter and water. They had their packs with them still, and supplies of water and food, but they wouldn't last that long.

And Lee had her rifle. She thought of how she had left it, put it down without a thought, in the crazy family's apartment. What had she been thinking?

You weren't thinking at all, is what her dad would have said. She could imagine him talking to her now, guiding her through this dangerous new world.

You've got to stay on red alert, Lee. You're not playing games now, this is for real. Keep your eyes open and your ears listening. And don't give up your weapon to no one.

Her daddy was right.

From now on Lee was keeping her rifle by her side at all times.

No one would ever get the drop on her like that again.

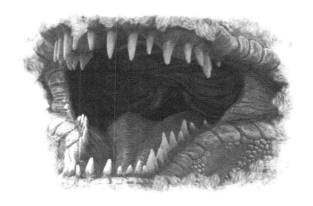

Chapter Eleven

The two pterosaurs hurtled towards Daniel, filling in the blue sky with their dark, winged mass. The teenager felt locked in place, every muscle and tendon in his body tight and rigid. The rats were swarming across the roof and around his feet. Daniel was vaguely aware of Renton screaming, but his hoarse, cracked voice seemed to be echoing up from a deep well.

The first pterosaur swooped past Daniel, almost knocking him over, and scattering the rats as it landed amongst them. The second was close behind and smashed into Daniel, knocking him down.

Day turned to night as Daniel was smothered in a stinking, hot mass of leathery flesh. He threw his arms up to defend himself, choking and coughing on the rank, overpowering smell of the pterosaur.

Its claws snagged at his clothes as it attempted to grab hold of its prey.

Daniel kicked out and flailed at the winged dinosaur with his fists, but it was no use, the pterosaur was too big and powerful. Its claws found purchase on his legs, like iron bands closing around his shins, growing ever tighter and tighter until the bones felt like they must snap.

The winged dinosaur began dragging Daniel across the roof, through the mass of swarming rats, as it attempted to lift him into the air. The teen kicked and struggled and screamed. Rats scurried over him, their claws pricking at his skin through his clothes, getting tangled up in his hair.

The pterosaur flapped its wings, washing fetid air over the boy fighting to free himself, the stink of it making him gag. He clawed at the roof as he felt his body being pulled upwards. Any moment now and he would be in the air, as the pterosaur carried him away.

But there was nothing to grab onto. He couldn't even see the rooftop, as it was covered in rats and he had to plunge his hands between their writhing bodies. Daniel's fingers scrabbled at the hard roof top beneath the mass of rats, ripping the skin off his fingertips.

His back lifted from the roof, and then his shoulders. A fresh wave of panic ran through the teenager. His head cracked against the hard roof surface, the pain like a lightning bolt through his skull. For a single moment the noise and the pain, the fight with the pterosaur, the squealing rats, all of it disappeared.

The world had turned dark and silent.

Before he could black out completely, Daniel was back, the noise and the pain and the sensation of being lifted into the sky overloading his senses.

Just at the moment he completely left the roof, arms stretched out and still trying to grab something to anchor him in place, his hands finally closed around a hard object beneath the mass of rats.

A moment later and he was in the air.

Waves of nausea washed over Daniel as his world turned upside down.

He was still holding the thing that he had latched on to in an attempt to keep from being lifted away.

It was Renton's shotgun.

He fumbled with the gun, suddenly scared of dropping it.

The pterosaur was having difficulty keeping airborne. Daniel's shoulder scraped along the roof of the service station as the winged dinosaur came back down.

Rats scurried out of the way. Daniel tried to keep his head away from the roof's hard surface as he was dragged along.

The pterosaur started gaining height again, lifting the teenager with it, its claws still clamped painfully around his shins. Daniel felt light headed, disoriented.

But he still had hold of the shotgun.

He pointed it up at the dark mass of movement above him, trying as hard as he could to keep his hands from shaking too much.

His finger found the trigger and he pulled it back.

The recoil from the shotgun wrenched it from his grip as the pterosaur seemed to explode and shower Daniel in blood and flesh and shards of bone.

He hit the roof hard on his back.

The dead pterosaur landed on top of him, and everything went black.

Daniel fought against the heavy mass of the stinking body of the dead pterosaur. Within seconds he had pulled himself free, emerging into the bright daylight, splattered with blood and bits of flesh.

The rats had scattered, scared by the shotgun blast.

But there were more pterosaurs swooping down from the bright blue sky, blotting out the sunlight with their broad wings.

112

Daniel dragged himself further out from under the dead pterosaur. If he could find the shotgun again, maybe he could use it to defend himself. Get back downstairs inside and find somewhere to hide, somewhere to protect himself.

He tried pulling himself shakily upright. Hot pain shot through his legs where the pterosaur's claws had gripped him tight and he sank to his knees again. He was by one of the wheelie bins of rainwater and he put his hand on it to steady himself.

A pterosaur swooped past, its beating wings washing warm air over Daniel. Another one followed it. They were both headed for the rats, which were scurrying around in a bunched up pack at the other end of the roof.

That meant Daniel had a breathing space for a few moments, whilst the pterosaurs were distracted. But what good would it do him? There were too many of the winged monstrosities circling overhead. As soon as he made any kind of movement, he would be spotted and they would be on him.

He needed somewhere to hide.

Next to him stood the black wheelie bin, full of rainwater. Of course, it would be ideal. All he had to do was get inside without being noticed by one of those giant turkeys, as Lee called them.

But that wasn't going to be easy with his ankles screaming in agony every time he tried to stand.

Still, it was either that, or be eaten.

On his knees, Daniel was able to reach up and flip the lid of the wheelie bin back. His luck was holding with the pterosaurs and the rats. The rats were too busy fleeing from the pterosaurs, and the pterosaurs too busy chasing the rats, for any of them to notice Daniel.

Gritting his teeth, preparing for the pain, Daniel hauled

himself upright. White hot pain surged through his ankles and up his lower legs. Were they broken? How would he be able to travel any further now, if he couldn't walk anymore?

Daniel shoved these thoughts away. First of all he had to survive the pterosaur attack, and the rats. Because right now, they were all swarming across the roof towards him.

Daniel looked inside the tall, plastic bin.

It was full of water.

If he wanted to hide in there, he would have to submerge himself in the water and hold his breath. What good was his hiding place if he had to keep revealing himself to take breaths of air? He would soon attract attention to himself with all that movement.

Daniel glanced back at the rats. He was too late anyway. The rats were fleeing, being chased by the pterosaurs. But as soon as the giant turkeys noticed Daniel they would forget all about the rats, and he would be their prey.

He would have to do it. He had no choice but to get inside the wheelie bin, submerge himself in the water and hold his breath for as long as he possibly could.

Just as he was about to haul his aching body up onto the wheelie bin, Daniel remembered its purpose. A rainwater collector, rigged up to drain down the stairs and into the upper level of the service station. Looking down at his feet he saw a hosepipe attached to the bottom of the black plastic bin, inserted into a crude hole in the side.

If he could pull the pipe out of its hole, the water would drain away.

A rat scurried past, squealing in terror, followed by more.

He had to act fast.

Bending down, Daniel gripped the hosepipe and yanked at it. It barely moved, but there had been some movement. He pulled again, this time with a twisting motion.

This time it moved even more, and tiny jets of water began spurting from the edges.

The rats were all around him now, some of them nipping at his feet and hands as they swarmed past. A large shadow fell over Daniel, blocking out the sun.

A pterosaur.

It soared past, intent still on its hunt.

Daniel gave the hosepipe another yank and this time it pulled free, water spurting out in a powerful stream.

Pulling himself up onto the wheelie bin, Daniel swung one leg over and then the other. The water inside was warm and gushed out of the top, splattering onto the roof, as he lowered himself inside. He risked a quick glance across the rooftop, looking for Renton and Emily.

Daniel could see no sign of either of them, and so he pulled the lid shut, submerging himself in the water.

For the first few moments the level of the water was above his head, and he had to hold his breath. But the level quickly dropped enough that he could breathe again.

The wheelie bin rocked and shuddered as the main bulk of the rats swarmed past. Daniel closed his eyes, squashed inside the hot, confined space of the dark wheelie bin, and waited.

* * *

Sometime later, Daniel awoke with a start. He hadn't even realised he had fallen asleep. For a moment or two he was disoriented and panicky. He couldn't remember where he was, why he was squashed into this hot, smelly space.

Just as the panic was threatening to overwhelm him, to swallow him whole and turn him into a gibbering, screaming wreck, he remembered.

Remembered everything.

The panic subsided a little, although not much. At least he knew where he was.

At least he was still alive, even if he was being stalked by carnivorous dinosaurs and giant rats.

There was something different now, though. Something had changed.

Daniel quickly realised what it was.

The silence.

No sounds of rats' claws clicking and scratching, no panicked squealing as a pterosaur landed on the roof and plucked at the rats with its sharp, teeth lined jaws.

Daniel placed his hands against the lid of the wheelie bin, but didn't push. The inside of the lid was coated with droplets of moisture, and more water ran down the sides of the bin. Daniel realised his hiding place was humid, like a sauna.

He thought about lifting the lid, letting some fresh air inside. And he needed to take a look, see what, if anything, was happening out there. But he couldn't.

Not right away.

What if the pterosaurs were still out there? If they noticed the movement of the lid swinging open, if they spotted Daniel, they would descend on him with their claws and their teeth and their broad wings blocking out the sun. And even if he got back inside the wheelie bin and closed the lid, the pterosaurs would know he was there, and they wouldn't give up. They would peck and claw at the wheelie bin until it was shredded apart enough that they could tear at him and eat him, like plucking a snail from its shell.

Daniel had survived this long because he was hidden, and the pterosaurs had forgotten all about him.

He couldn't risk losing that advantage.

But neither could he stay here forever. He had to leave the safety of the wheelie bin at some point.

He decided to risk it a look.

Slowly he pushed at the wheelie bin lid, opening it just a sliver. Bright sunlight stabbed at his eyes and Daniel let the lid drop shut, showering him in droplets of warm water. He waited, keeping very still, afraid that the sound of the lid dropping shut might have attracted a predator's attention.

And there it was, the sound of something approaching. The thump against the plastic as it hit the side of the bin. This was it then. Daniel was trapped inside this confined space, his limbs stiff and awkward. He had no chance to escape.

He screwed his eyes shut as he heard the lid being pulled back, felt his body bathed in sunshine.

Waited for teeth and claws to shred him apart, and hoped that it would be quick, at least.

"Hey," Emily said, "you're alive."

Daniel squinted at the blurred, dark shape above him, sunlight streaming into his eyes and hurting his head.

"Yeah," Daniel said, his voice little more than a croak. "I guess I am."

"What are you doing in there still? Those big birds left ages ago. They're stupid, you know. All you have to do is hide, and they get bored really easily and leave."

"Is that right?"

Daniel reached up, his hands shaking with the effort, and gripped the edges of the wheelie bin. He pulled himself upright, clamping his jaws together as his stiff limbs protested at the sudden movement.

The glare began to clear a little, helped as Daniel turned away from the direct sunlight shining into his eyes. The wheelie

117

bin cast a long shadow across the roof, littered with dead rats.

"Are you all right?" Daniel said.

Emily squinted at him. The sun was low in the sky, which meant it was late afternoon, evening maybe. How long had he been asleep?

"I'm fine," Emily said. "You don't look so good."

"Thanks, I don't feel so good either."

At least the pain in his ankles where the pterosaur had gripped him in its claws had lessened. They still hurt, but Daniel could support himself now.

"Where did you hide?" he said as he climbed out of the wheelie bin.

"Like you, in one of the water butts." Emily glanced around. "I haven't seen your friend."

"He's not my friend." Daniel reached out to Emily. "Here, give me a hand."

Emily helped Daniel clamber out of the wheelie bin and he collapsed on the floor.

"Are you sure you're all right?" she said.

"A pterosaur got me by the ankles, tried to take me away back to its nest or wherever they live."

Daniel pulled his trouser legs up. His ankles and his shins were swollen and covered in purple and yellow bruising.

"They look bad," Emily said.

Great, Daniel thought. *Tell me something I don't know.*

Gingerly he touched his ankles. They hurt, but not too much. Standing and walking was going to hurt more.

"We should go downstairs before those things come back," Emily said. "They're always hovering around here, looking for something to eat."

Daniel pulled himself up onto his feet.

"You're going to have to help me," he said, and put his arm

118

over Emily's shoulders.

Together they walked towards the door and the stairs leading back down into the service station. Daniel had to walk slowly. He was limping badly, each step sending spikes of pain through his lower legs. But he could walk.

Inside the stairwell was cool and dim. Small things scurried in the shadows, claws clicking against the floor. Daniel looked at Emily.

"We have to get inside," she said, but she looked worried.

They took the steps slowly down to the bridge over the motorway. Here they could see rats running from them, the floor littered with rat droppings. Daniel kicked out at a particularly large rat as it approached him. The rat scurried away, and Daniel cried out in pain caused by the sudden movement of his foot.

There were more rats in the kitchen and the dining area. Not the seething carpet of them that had swarmed up the motorway and into the service station, but enough that they were a problem still.

Daniel hobbled over to a chair and sat down.

If he could walk then didn't that mean he hadn't broken anything?

But then he seemed to remember hearing stories of people who had fractured a foot but not realised for a couple of days until the pain had got too intense, forcing them to go to hospital where the break was discovered.

There weren't any hospitals available anymore though, so Daniel would just have to hope his feet were just bruised, and not broken.

Emily was standing in the middle of the dining area gazing around at the rats scurrying between the chair legs and under the tables. For the first time since Daniel had met her she had

119

lost that look of toughness, and now she appeared vulnerable, like the little girl she really was.

"I'm sorry," he said.

"What for?" Emily said.

"For all this. Your safe place, you can't live here anymore, can you? Not with all these rats."

"I'll kill them all. When my mum gets back, we'll both kill them all, get rid of them."

Daniel flexed his feet, loosening them up. Now that the stiffness was leaving his joints his ankles were starting to feel a little better. It would still hurt to walk, but he was growing more confident that nothing was broken.

More rats came scurrying along the walkway and into the dining area. Daniel shuddered and lifted his feet off the floor, rested them on a table.

"There's too many of them, surely?" he said.

Emily screamed and kicked out at a rat by her feet. It tumbled over, squealing, and then ran away. Emily chased after it, kicking out at other rats as she ran, screaming.

Daniel took a deep breath and held it for a moment, before letting it go in a sigh of frustration.

With Renton missing, and surely dead, Daniel was alone now with only this precocious ten-year-old for company. At least they had food and water, but they couldn't stay here with all these rats. How long would it be before the rats got tired of being chased around by Emily and went on the attack instead?

But even if they did leave, where were they going to go? Daniel knew he couldn't walk far at all with his feet and ankles as painful as they were.

If only he had some way of contacting Lee and Will. If only they were here, right now.

Daniel imagined them, safe within the walls of what used to

be the Botanical Gardens.

He wished he was with them.

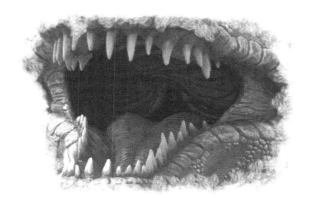

Chapter Twelve

They trudged on, walking along the motorway. They used the southbound carriageway where there were fewer obstructions. To their right, on the northbound road, the three lanes were clogged with cars jammed front to back against each other. The biggest traffic jam in the world.

Sometimes they came across huge pile-ups, like some modern art sculpted out of twisted metal and shattered glass.

Sometimes they saw the remains of mangled skeletons.

Will tried keeping his head down, did his best to concentrate on the pitted tarmac beneath his feet. But it seemed whenever he inadvertently glanced up he would find a grinning skull staring back at him, or a suitcase lying open, its contents scattered everywhere.

They were tired after their encounter with the man and his family at the Rotunda. Even Iggy seemed subdued, padding silently along beside Helen.

And it was growing late in the afternoon, turning into evening as the sun lowered towards the horizon.

Willy really did not want to be out here after dark.

"What did you say this road is called?" Lee said, breaking the silence.

"The M6," Will said. "It's the straightest route north."

"And how long's it going to take us to walk there?"

"I don't know." Will stopped and looked at the cars on the northbound carriageway. "If we were in a car, and there was no traffic, maybe a few hours, four or five. But walking?" He shrugged, helpless.

Helen looked anxiously up at the sky. "We should find shelter soon. The things, the monsters, they come out at night."

"Yeah, like we haven't seen any during the day," Will muttered.

"We could maybe use one of these cars to sleep in," Lee said.

Will started walking again. "Maybe."

"Hey, hold up," Lee said. "You can't just walk off like that. We've got to stick together, make a plan."

"Really?" Will said, still walking and not even looking back as he spoke. "What's the point of making plans? We're all going to die anyway, right?"

Iggy fell in step beside Will, gazing up at the boy as he trotted along beside him.

Will paused, patted Iggy on the head.

Poor Iggy, he had no idea what was going on. And yet maybe that was a good thing. Wasn't that what was dragging Will down, the knowledge of what they once had? Comfort, safety, food, water, shelter, entertainment even. Now they had lost all of that, and wasn't it that knowledge, those memories of the good things he had lost, that was filling him with a black void of depression?

Well, that and the fact that they might get eaten at any moment.

123

Iggy licked Will's hand.

Lee grabbed Will by the arm and pulled him roughly around, startling him from his thoughts.

"Is that what you think? That we're all going to die? You're just giving up that easily?"

Will pulled himself free of Lee's grasp. "Of course we are! I know you're the big, tough American, with the marine for a dad, but surely even you can see that we can't survive out here on our own. You can act like the Terminator as much as you want, but without help we are going to die!"

"Stop it!" Lee shouted and shoved Will in the chest. "We are not going to die! We're going to find Daniel and we'll be together again and we can—"

"Yeah? What?" Will shouted, up in Lee's face now. "What can we do? Get chased by more flesh eating monstrosities? Meet more scavengers who just want us so they can kill Iggy and roast him on a spit? Having Daniel with us doesn't make any difference, we're still in the same shit!"

"You're pathetic!" Lee hissed. "What do you suggest then, that we just curl up and wait for a raptor to find us and eat us? Is that it? Just curl up and die?"

Will looked away, said nothing.

On the horizon the sun was turning the sky a golden glow. Any other time it would have looked beautiful, but now that fiery horizon just seemed to Will a reminder of where they were. In the fires of Hell.

"At least it would be over quick," Will said. "All this running and hiding and scavenging for food, just seems like we're stretching out the inevitable, really."

"Hey, what's that?" Helen said.

Will and Lee looked at Helen. She was pointing, up into the deepening blue of the sky. Will's first thought was pterosaurs,

124

plunging to earth, claws outstretched and ready to pluck these morsels of food from the ground and away to wherever they nested.

But no, the sky was empty of threat.

Helen had seen something, though. And now Will could hear it, too. A distant drone, almost like the noise of an engine.

"It's a plane!" Lee cried.

Will saw it then. A tiny, dark shape silhouetted against the evening sky. It was only a small plane, a Cessna or something similar. Will had gone through a brief obsession with planes, even to the point where his father, in a rare show of paternal love and attention, had taken him to Halfpenny Green, where they had spent the afternoon watching the planes take off and land as customers had flying lessons.

Lee started jumping up and down and waving her arms in the air.

"Hey!" she shouted. "Hey! Down here!"

Iggy joined in, barking and wagging his tail.

"What are you doing?" Will said. "Shut up, will you? You're just going to attract every predator in the area with all that noise."

Helen had started shouting too, joining in with Lee.

"Please, be quiet," Will pleaded. "You're just going to attract the monsters with all that noise."

Lee fell quiet. "Yeah, you're right."

She shushed Helen, and they watched as the plane flew away, disappearing into a distant dot in the sky.

"He couldn't have heard you over the noise of his engine anyway," Will said.

"Could he have helped us?" Helen said.

"If we could get in a plane like that, we would be up in the Lake District in no time, right?" Lee said.

125

Will was still gazing up at the sky, his heart aching at the thought of being up there, far above all of this. Whoever was flying that plane must feel free. Free of all the misery and the danger down here. Free to roam the sky, fly wherever they wanted, amongst the clouds and under the sun.

Will envied them.

Except, they had to come back down to earth at some point, didn't they?

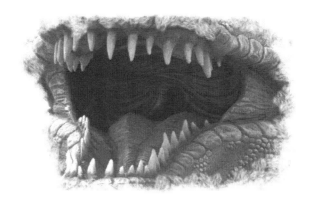

Chapter Thirteen

"No! I'm not leaving!"

Daniel sighed, gripped the sides of his head and closed his eyes. Arguing with Emily was like bashing your head against a brick wall.

They had been arguing over this for what felt like hours now. When they had first got down off the roof and back into the service station, Daniel had almost believed Emily when she told him that she could kill all the rats. Certainly the idea of staying inside and undercover, protected from the dinosaur population, and in particular the pterosaurs, roaming what was left of the English countryside, was attractive.

Except for the rats.

They swarmed everywhere and over everything. The maddening click of their claws and their incessant squeaking was driving Daniel mad. And then there was the stink, so rancid and powerful that he could taste it, thick on his tongue like a coating of putrid oil.

But Daniel had believed Emily when she told him that they could get rid of them, given enough time. That they were better off here, even with the rats, than they were outside.

Unfortunately, as the afternoon wore on and turned into evening, more and more rats appeared. It was as though they had gone into hiding when the pterosaurs first descended upon them, but now they were beginning to realise it was safe to come out.

Daniel, perched on a counter top in one of the service station eating areas, looked down at the moving carpet of rats. Emily was sitting cross legged on a table. Despite her determination to stay put, she didn't look at all keen to step down into the mass of vermin.

"What are we going to do then?" Daniel shouted. It was all he could do to think, let alone make himself heard above the squealing and click-clacking of the rats. "Are you just going to stay sitting on that table for the rest of your life?"

Emily looked down sulkily at the rats. "No."

"What did you say? I can't hear you!"

Emily lifted her head and stared with a fierce determination at Daniel. "I said no! When my mother gets back we can get rid of these rats together. She'll know what to do."

"Yeah? So when's she coming back? Because I don't know if you'd noticed but these things are starting to look hungry, and I don't rate our chances of sitting here much longer without them trying to take a bite out of us."

It was true. The more of the rats there were, the bolder they were becoming. Before Daniel had found his safe spot on the counter top a couple of the rats had tried taking a bite out of his swollen ankles. The nip of their claws and teeth on his tender legs had been excruciating.

Even if he could persuade Emily that they had to leave, he couldn't see how they would get through the mass of swarming vermin without being bitten and scratched.

Emily was sulking again. Daniel had the feeling that he was wearing her down. How many days had it been since her mother disappeared? Daniel was beginning to think that maybe Emily's mother didn't even exist, that she was a make believe parent conjured up from the girl's desperate imagination.

But then if that was the case, who had set up all the water catchers on the roof? And the system for piping it downstairs into the kitchen?

Maybe Emily had stumbled upon this setup left behind by somebody else, and her imagination had brought her mother to life. A way of making her feel safer.

There were so many of the rats now that they were tumbling over one another, some of them even taking bites out of each other. They were hungry, and they could sense food just out of their reach. How long before they found a way of scaling the sides of the counter to get to Daniel? Or, more likely, how long before Daniel was forced from his safe place because of thirst and hunger?

"We've got to get down and get out of here," Daniel shouted.

"I told you, I'm not leaving!" Emily shouted back.

"I don't care anymore whether you stay or leave, but we can't sit here for the rest of our lives. We need to get down and find somewhere to rest where there aren't any rats."

Emily looked away, out through a grimy window onto the motorway. The sun was low, lighting up the horizon with a tinge of red.

She looked back again. "All right."

And then she was down, in amongst the rats, kicking and screaming and running.

She didn't have a chance. The rats were all over her, their claws snagging at her trousers, swarming up her little girl's body. Screaming, she staggered towards the stairs, beating at the rats, plucking them from her clothes and flinging them with all her strength as far as she could.

Daniel leaned forward, almost pushing himself off the counter top. He wanted to help her, but the thought of dropping himself into that sea of teeth and claws held him back.

"Emily!" he screamed.

The terrified girl couldn't hear him. She twisted and turned, pounding the rats with her fists. There were so many of them covering her legs it was as though the rats had become part of her. An undulating, twisting, frenzied second skin.

Daniel willed himself to push off the counter top, to sink into the mass of biting, scratching vermin, and go help Emily.

But his body simply refused to move.

Emily's screams got louder, and this, finally, was the trigger for Daniel.

He jumped off the counter top.

Daniel staggered as he landed on top of the squirming bodies, and he heard bones crack and squeals of pain. He grabbed hold of the counter to keep from falling over as a white hot pain shot through his ankles.

Already the rats were scurrying over his feet and up his legs. What had he been thinking? There was no way he could help Emily, he couldn't even get to her. He had to get back on the top of the kitchen counter once more, before the rats had dragged him to the floor where they would eat him alive.

One of the rats managed to climb up his clothing and onto the top of the kitchen counter. Daniel yanked his hand away as it nipped at his fingers. The quick, jerky movement caused him to lose his balance and with a loud yell he fell into the moving carpet of vermin.

The rats had swarmed over him within moments.

130

The stink of their squirming bodies overpowered him and his vision blurred with tears as he struggled to fight the rats off. But no matter how hard and viciously he smashed at them with his fists, more and more of them climbed on top of him, their long tails whipping at his face.

The rats on Daniel's chest suddenly flew off him, as though they had been caught in a mini whirlwind. A blur of movement, somebody roaring with anger, and more rats went flying. Daniel's vision cleared, and he saw Renton, wielding a large shovel.

The American slammed the shovel onto the floor, smashing into the rats, breaking their backs, crushing their skulls. He scooped them away, bent down and reached a hand out to Daniel.

The teenager took his hand and was hauled upright. Renton plucked a rat off Daniel's chest and squeezed until its bones cracked and blood spilt from between his fingers.

"Emily!" Daniel gasped.

They both turned to look. Incredibly, Emily was still standing, still fighting off the rats.

But it was a battle she was losing.

Renton swept the large, broad shovel across the floor, scooping up rats and throwing them into the air. Clearing a space as he walked, Renton was able to create a path to the young girl. He began pulling the rats off her and threw each of them away. Some of them hit the windows overlooking the motorway, leaving behind dark splodges of red where they smacked into the glass.

Overcoming his fear and revulsion, Daniel joined Renton in pulling the remaining rats off Emily.

When there were no more rats left on her, the three of them made a break for the stairs. Renton used his shovel to make a path for them through the mass of vermin. It seemed to Daniel that the rats knew they were in the presence of a predator in the form of Renton, as they quickly fled from his approach.

Daniel ground his teeth together as they walked. The pain in his feet and ankles was excruciating and if it hadn't been for the rats, he would have sunk to the floor where he was and refused to move any further until someone offered to carry him.

By the time they got to the top of the steps leading down to the main eating and shopping area the sweat was running down Daniel's face and he was feeling faint.

"What's wrong with you?" Renton growled.

"My feet," gasped Daniel.

Renton looked down, saw Daniel's tattered trouser legs, his swollen ankles. The American picked the teenager up like he weighed nothing and flung him over his shoulder. He carried him down the steps, closely followed by Emily.

Renton ran through the service station and outside. The sun was setting, casting long shadows over the mangled, twisted shapes that had once been cars in the car park. There was a humming, almost a vibration in the air as the insect population came to life.

Renton didn't pause in his stride and took them around the rear of the service station. They passed a large skip overflowing with rubbish.

"Where are you taking us?" Emily shouted.

Renton stopped and lowered Daniel to the ground.

"Here," he said.

They were by a delivery van, 'Tesco' emblazoned across its side. Daniel leaned against the van.

"What happened to you?" Renton said, looking at Daniel's feet.

"The pterosaurs took me, grabbed me by the ankles," Daniel said.

Renton grunted. "You were lucky."

"We thought you were dead," Emily said.

Renton stared at her, his one eye weeping, and he wheezed a couple of times. "You mean you hoped I was dead."

Daniel realised the wheezing had actually been laughter.

"How did you survive?"

Renton indicated the skip full of rubbish. "One of those damn flying monsters knocked me off the edge of the roof, but I fell into that." He slapped his hand against the side of the Tesco van. "Then I climbed in here and found this."

Daniel's eyes widened at the sight of the ignition key Renton produced from a pocket.

"Does it work?"

Renton shook his head. "No, the battery's dead. But if we can give it a push and get it moving, we might be able to jump start it."

Daniel's mind refused to believe it was possible, that they might have a vehicle, that they could travel faster than their frustratingly slow walking pace. He looked down at the tyres, expecting them to be flat. They weren't, they were full of air.

"I pumped them up with a foot pump I found," Renton said.

"But, how can we drive it up the motorway? It's all blocked with cars, there's no way through."

"That's only the northbound carriageway," Renton said. "The southbound into the city is mostly empty."

Daniel still couldn't work it out. "But how do we get the van across the barrier and over to the southbound side?"

"Take a good look, kid," Renton said. "That's the side we're on."

133

Daniel realised the American was right. In all the panic and the confusion he hadn't noticed they had crossed the bridge over the motorway and escaped through the service station on the opposite side of the motorway to the one they had entered.

Renton pulled open the door of the van. "One of you is going to have to drive while I push." He stared at Daniel. "Think you can do it?"

Daniel looked at his throbbing feet. He doubted he had the strength in them to push the pedals.

"I'll try," he said.

He climbed slowly into the driver's seat, gripping the steering wheel as he gingerly positioned his feet in the footwell. There was an open bottle of water on the dashboard. Where had Renton found that? In the back of the Tesco van, perhaps. Daniel was just glad he wasn't thirsty right now. He really didn't relish the idea of sharing a bottle of water with the big guy.

"You driven a car before?" Renton said.

"Yeah, my dad let me have a go a few times in his car."

Renton stared at Daniel, as though he knew he was lying. Professor Martin Atherton hadn't been the type of man to take his son out for driving lessons, and Renton probably had an idea that was the case. The only driving lessons Daniel had ever had were self taught on the Xbox.

"Put it into first gear for me," Renton said.

Daniel placed his foot on the clutch pedal and pushed. Pain shot up through his foot and his ankle. Gritting his teeth he pushed harder. He managed to get the pedal halfway to the floor before he had to give up and release it.

"I can't do it," he gasped. "The pain, it's too much."

Renton swore. Turned to face Emily.

"What about you? Think you can do it?"

"I'm not leaving here, I'm waiting for my mother to come

134

back," she said.

Renton punched the metal side of the van, leaving a dent in the bodywork.

"Your mother's not coming back," he snarled. "If she was, she'd have been here by now. She's dead, you got that? Now, to get this bloody van moving one of us needs to be pushing it while the other one sits in the driver's seat and slips it into gear. Neither of you are big enough or strong enough to get this thing moving and he can't even push the clutch pedal which means it's down to you. Got that?"

Renton was towering over Emily, his face stretched tight with anger.

Emily stepped back. "All right, all right, just get out of my face, will you?"

Renton pointed at Daniel. "Swap places with him."

Emily and Daniel did as they were told.

Renton stood by Emily's side, scowling at her through the open door.

"You ever driven a car before?"

"No, but it can't be that difficult if adults can do it."

Emily and Renton eyeballed each other for a moment. The young girl seemed to have no fear in the presence of the big man and his wounds, that permanently weeping eye with no lids, the heat emanating off him. Didn't she realise that she needed to be careful around him? That she was in the presence of a killer?

Renton shoved the key into the ignition and turned it.

He pointed to the clutch.

"Put your foot on that and push it to the floor."

Emily had to perch right on the edge of the seat and lean her weight on the clutch pedal before it moved.

"All right, let go," Renton said. "You," he pointed at

135

Daniel, "will have to operate the gear stick. You need to put it into second gear. You know how to do that?"

Daniel nodded.

"Go on then."

The boy gripped the gear stick and waggled it from side to side. It was in neutral. He looked at Emily.

"You have to put the clutch out before I can put it into gear."

Emily shook her head, as though this was the most ridiculous thing she had ever had to do, and was everybody crazy apart from her? Gripping the steering wheel and leaning forward she put all her weight on the pedal and pushed.

Daniel put the gear stick into second.

"Now ease back slowly on the pedal," Renton said. "And when I'm pushing the van and we're doing this for real you need to push on the gas pedal at the same time."

"He means that one, the accelerator," Daniel said, pointing.

"Yeah, I know!" Emily said. Her foot slipped off the clutch pedal and it sprang back into place, knocking against her ankle. "Ouch!"

Renton shook his head. "Try again."

Emily pushed all her weight on the clutch pedal again, shoving it to the floor.

Renton watched her. "Now ease it back up again."

Emily let the pedal go a little, and it rose back into position jerkily. But she kept her foot on it this time.

"I guess that'll have to do," Renton said. "All right, let's do it."

Daniel had a sick feeling in the pit of his stomach. If they really could get the van started they could cover so much more distance than by walking. On the one hand that meant leaving his friends behind in Birmingham, but on the other hand it meant possibly getting to the Lake District, getting to his father and the *IntelliCorps* compound and safety. The throbbing in his ankles reminded him that he was hurt pretty bad, and if the wounds were infected, he would need a doctor, maybe some antibiotics.

Renton gripped the edge of the driver side door, ready to slam it shut. He paused, and leaned in close to Emily, his face only inches from hers.

"Young lady, let me tell you now, if we get this van going and you try driving off and leaving me here I will hunt you down and I will kill you without a second thought. You got that?"

Emily nodded and kept her mouth shut for once.

Renton slammed the door closed.

"He's crazy," Emily said, as Renton walked away and round behind the van.

"I know," Daniel muttered. He wasn't so sure about Emily, either, but he wasn't going to tell her that. "You think you can do this?" he said, instead.

Before she could answer, Renton shouted, "Okay, put it into second and let the handbrake off!"

"He never told me about the handbrake," Emily said.

"It's all right, I'll do that," Daniel said. "You just push on the clutch pedal."

Gripping the steering wheel again, Emily leaned her weight forward onto the pedal. Daniel shoved the gear stick into second and then got hold of the handbrake. He had to pull the handbrake up to release the catch and at first it refused to move.

"What's wrong?" Emily said.

"It's stiff."

"Are you ready yet?" Renton shouted.

137

"It's the handbrake, I can't release it," Daniel shouted.

Silence, and then Renton appeared at the passenger side window. He yanked open the door, leaned in and pulled hard at the handbrake, pushing the button to release it and then let it down.

He slammed the door shut and headed back around the van. Emily and Daniel looked at each other in silence.

The van started rolling forward.

Emily's eyes grew wide. "What do I do now?"

"Keep looking where we're going," Daniel said. "We don't want to crash into anything."

"Oh!" Emily gasped, and she gripped the steering wheel even harder.

"Put the clutch in!" Renton shouted.

They were picking up speed, heading down the service road towards the car park.

"Should I do it now?" Emily said.

Daniel gripped the dashboard. He had realised neither of them were wearing seat belts.

Emily's foot slipped off the clutch pedal and the van bucked and came to an abrupt halt. Both Emily and Daniel shot forward, Daniel hitting his head on the windscreen. There was a grunt from behind the van.

Daniel rubbed at his head.

"Ouch, that hurt," Emily said, rubbing at her chest where she had banged into the steering wheel.

The open bottle of water had fallen over on the dashboard and the clear water was spilling out. Daniel grabbed it and placed it upright.

"Let's try again!" Renton shouted from the back.

"Let's put our seat belts on first," Daniel said, reaching over his shoulder to grab the metal buckle.

They both fastened their seat belts. Emily gripped the steering wheel again as though it was a lifeline.

"You can do this," Daniel said. "It's already in gear, you just need to press the clutch pedal down again and then ease it back up once we're moving, and remember to press the accelerator down slowly."

Emily shook her head. "Why is driving a car so difficult?"

"What are you two waiting for?" Renton shouted.

Emily shoved the clutch pedal to the floor, and they started rolling forward again.

"Now?" Emily said.

Daniel was staring out of the window at a line of cars they were swiftly approaching. "Let it pick up speed just a little more."

He took the steering wheel and adjusted their course slightly.

"Now!" he said.

Emily eased back in her seat and pumped at the accelerator pedal. The engine caught, coughed and spewed out a plume of black smoke at the rear.

"You did it!" Daniel shouted, just as the van stalled again and jerked to a halt.

The teenager closed his eyes and sank back into his seat. They had been so close. At least the seat belts had caught them this time when they jerked forward.

Renton appeared at the passenger window, a cloud of black smoke drifting by him. "All right, we almost had it that time. Let's try again."

"We're going to have to change direction first, and get onto the slip road," Daniel said.

Renton grunted as he looked where Daniel pointed. He was wheezing and bright red in what remained of his face. How much was this taking out of him? Would he have the strength for many more attempts at starting the van?

"Okay, I'll push, you steer. Shout when we're straightened up and ready to go again."

"Why can't I steer?" Emily said. "I'm the one in the driver's seat."

Renton ignored the young girl and pointed at Daniel. "You steer."

Daniel nodded and swallowed. His dry throat clicked painfully. He hated to think how ugly Renton's mood might turn if they failed to get the engine started.

"We need to put the gearstick back into neutral," Daniel said.

Emily scowled at Daniel.

"Emily, please. We need to put the gears into neutral so that Renton can get us lined up in the right direction. Put your foot on the clutch pedal."

Emily scowled at Daniel some more.

"What's the hold up?" Renton shouted from the rear of the van.

Emily jabbed her foot on the clutch pedal and Daniel slipped the gearstick into neutral.

"Okay, push!" Daniel shouted.

The van started moving once more. From his position in the passenger seat, Daniel steered them around the bend towards the slip road. The steering wheel was stiff and sluggish without power and the teenager had difficulty in getting the van going where he wanted.

Emily sat with her arms crossed in the driver's seat, still scowling.

They passed parked cars and Daniel noticed one with a bike rack full of bicycles on it. His heart ached for a moment at the thought of his BMX, of a time when his days were much simpler, of when his mother was still alive.

When they were straightened up on the slip road with a clear run ahead of them, Daniel shouted, "Ok! We're ready!"

The van picked up speed.

"Try again," Daniel said.

Emily, still scowling, shook her head.

"Emily, please!"

Incredibly, the van was still picking up speed. They were almost on the motorway. Renton shouted something, but Daniel couldn't make out what it was. He looked in the side mirror. Renton was standing in the middle of the slip road, bent over, his one hand on his knee as he gasped for air.

They were slowing down. Renton had given it everything he had, this was their last chance.

"Emily, if we don't get this van started then Renton will kill us, I know he will. Please."

Without a word, Emily grabbed the steering wheel and shoved hard on the clutch pedal. Daniel slipped the gear stick into first, and then remembered that was the wrong, putting it into second instead.

"Okay, put your right foot on the accelerator pedal," he said, "and push down as you release the clutch."

The van was still moving, but slowing down all the time. Did they even have enough speed to make this work?

Emily stamped on the accelerator pedal and lifted her left foot. The van jerked, the engine coughed and growled, coughed again, more black smoke billowing past them. The van was almost at a stop now.

Daniel gripped the dashboard and screwed his eyes shut.

The engine coughed again and roared into life. The van began kangarooing down the slip road, but the engine continued running.

Daniel snapped his eyes open. "You did it! Shove the clutch pedal down, quick before we stall!"

Emily, grinning wildly, stamped on the clutch and Daniel shoved the gearstick into neutral.

The engine roared at high speed. Emily still had her foot on the accelerator.

"Take your feet off the pedals," Daniel said, and yanked on the handbrake, bringing them to an abrupt halt.

Emily was jumping up and down in her seat, still grinning, her eyes wide with excitement. "I can drive a car! I can drive a car!"

The engine was idling, but unevenly. Almost like it might cut out at any moment.

"Rev the engine a bit," Daniel said.

Emily looked at him.

"Just tap the accelerator pedal lightly."

The engine roared into life again as Emily pushed a little on the pedal.

Renton appeared at her window.

"Move over," he wheezed.

Emily shuffled onto the passenger seat with Daniel. She couldn't seem to move fast enough. And Daniel could understand why.

Renton's disfigured face was dripping with sweat, and bubbles of snot and pus popped from the holes in his face where his nose had once been. The effort of pushing the van had obviously been too much for him. Blood trickled down his cheek where he had opened up a wound.

Daniel looked away as Renton climbed into the van and slammed the door shut.

"Let's go," he growled.

The Tesco van broke down after only two miles of halting, slow progress along the motorway, and refused to start again. Renton swore and pounded the steering wheel whilst Daniel and Emily sat in silence. Daniel knew Renton's temper, knew what he was capable of when he was angry. Best just to keep quiet and as still as possible, and hope that he exhausted himself quickly.

The sky was growing dark, night falling upon them faster than Daniel had ever experienced before. Then, when the first few large drops of rain hit the filthy windscreen, he realised why. The sky had become thick with black, heavy clouds.

More of the heavy rain drops splattered across the glass and hit the van's roof. A moment later and the rain had turned into a deluge, pounding out a rhythm on the roof and obscuring their view out of the windscreen.

Renton, breathing heavily from the exertion of his furious pounding at the dashboard and steering wheel, turned to face Daniel and Emily.

"We'll stay here tonight," he said. "Start walking again in the morning, when it's dry."

Daniel swallowed and nodded.

The wind was picking up, rocking the van. The teenage boy didn't relish the prospect of spending a night cooped up with Renton and his festering, charred flesh again.

"I told you, we shouldn't have left," Emily said. She was sitting and staring straight ahead out of the van's windscreen, in between Renton and Daniel.

"What did you say?" Renton growled.

Please don't, Daniel thought. *Just keep your mouth shut, please!*

"We should have stayed where we were," Emily replied, still

not looking at Renton. "We were safe there, we had food and water."

"What about the rats?" Renton said.

"They would have gone, eventually. We should go back. I should go back."

"Do what you want," Renton growled. "It makes no difference to me."

Emily reached across Daniel's lap for the door handle. He grabbed her hand and stopped her.

"You can't go out in this," he said. "It's too dangerous and, and, you'll get soaked."

"I don't care," Emily said. "Let go of me."

Daniel held on for another second, unwilling to let go. Finally he loosened his grip and Emily twisted her wrist out of his hand.

She pulled at the door handle and the door swung open.

Emily screamed.

"Hey, Dave, come and look at what I found!" shouted the man standing outside the van, a dark rain slicker pulled over his head and running with water.

He was holding a gun, pointing it at the occupants of the van.

Dave walked into view, a torch in one hand and a pistol in the other.

"Sweet," he said.

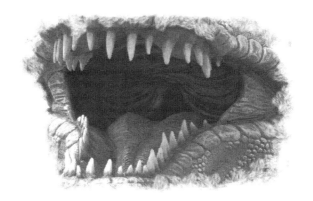

Chapter Fourteen

With the night came the rain. Not just rain but a deluge of water, a biblical torrent of rainfall. They had taken shelter inside a car, but by that time they were already soaked through. The windows quickly steamed up, increasing their sense of isolation and helplessness.

Lee was beginning to think they had made the wrong decision, that they should have fought their corner, stayed on at the compound. It would have been pretty unpleasant at first, maybe even for a long time, everyone blaming them for Matt Hooper's death. But surely that would have been preferable to this, outside where the dinosaurs roamed, nerves shredded at every little sight or sound of a possible threat, constantly on the lookout for water and food.

And yet, they couldn't have just left Daniel in Renton's hands. Yeah, the guy was intent on taking him back to the Lake District, back to his father, but how long before he changed his mind?

How long before he decided he wanted to kill Daniel, instead?

145

Lee shifted in her seat and wiped her hand across the window, clearing a space to peer through the misted up glass. It was no good, she couldn't see a thing.

The rain kept up a hard but regular beat on the roof of the car. It was too dark to properly see the others; they were just amorphous shapes in the gloom, and the thrumming of the rain just above their heads too loud to make conversation possible. Lee had no idea if Will and Helen were awake or asleep.

Lee shifted in her seat again. She couldn't get comfortable. She was in the back with Helen and Iggy. The dog had decided to sit at Lee's feet, which had been comforting at first. But now he was curled up between her legs and Lee could hardly move. She also had her rucksack on her lap, adding to her discomfort and a growing sense of claustrophobia.

On top of all that, she needed to go to the toilet.

This, it seemed to Lee, was the most ridiculous element of the situation they were in. None of the action movies that she had loved so much before the world turned upside down, none of the superhero adventures, addressed this problem of the hero needing the toilet at some point.

The need for a pee had been building for a while, pretty much since they had climbed into the abandoned car. Lee had done her best to ignore the call of nature, and for a while it had been okay. But, as the night wore on and the rain showed no sign of easing off, the pressure in Lee's bladder grew and grew.

Along with the sense of urgency to relieve it.

Lee wiped at the window again, desperate to see outside. There was no way she could relieve herself inside the car. She had nothing to pee into and even if she had, did she really want to be pulling her pants down in front of the others?

Okay, considering the situation they were in, and the fact that it was dark, she could do that. But with nothing to pee into and with the cramped conditions inside the car, she would just end up going all over Iggy.

Lee would just have to wait until the rain had stopped. Wait until morning, when there was enough light to see by, enough light to see any waiting dangers.

But she didn't think she could hang on that long.

Lee wriggled in her seat, trying to find a more comfortable position where the pressure on her bladder was less intense. She felt Iggy move against her legs and then shake his head.

"Are you all right?" Helen whispered.

"I need to pee," Lee whispered back.

"So do I," Helen whispered. "I've been holding on for ages, but I don't think I can much longer."

Lee felt a little better, relieved even, that she wasn't the only one in this predicament. "Same here," she said.

"Um, I need the toilet as well," Will said.

Lee giggled, nervously. "I thought you were both asleep, but we've all been sat here wide awake needing the toilet!"

"Hey, Iggy, do you need the toilet too?" Helen said.

Lee giggled again. "Don't make me laugh, I might pee in my pants!"

"I'm kind of really, really desperate to be honest," Will said.

Lee shifted in her seat. He wasn't the only one. It was weird, talking to the other two in the dark, the rain pounding on the car's roof. It was like a dream.

"To be honest, Will, you've got it easy, easier than us girls," she said. "All you need to do is open the window a crack and aim outside. Me and Helen are going to have to open the doors and hang our butts out into the dark."

Helen was snorting with laughter. "But if he points his willy out of the window something might come along and bite it off!"

147

"Willy? Is that what you English guys call it?" That was it, Lee was off, helpless with laughter. The two girls, both in the back seat of the car, managed to find each other and hold hands as they cried laughing. The car rocked beneath their movement which made them both laugh even more.

"Stop it!" Helen gasped. "I think I just wet myself a little!"

Lee had to concentrate hard to calm down and stop laughing.

"I've got an idea," she said. "Why don't we take turns at climbing over the back seat into the trunk and just pee in there?"

"Me first," Helen said, and scrambled over the seat.

"Hey, careful!" Lee said, when Helen banged into her shoulder. In the dark Lee couldn't tell what had hit her. Had it been Helen's knee? Her foot?

"Oh, that feels so much better," Helen said, a few moments later.

The rain continued pounding down on the car roof, obscuring all other noises.

"Hurry up, I need to go," Lee said.

"Almost done," Helen replied.

Lee did her best to concentrate, to think about anything other than her urgent need for the toilet.

"Lee?" Will said.

"Yeah?"

"I can't go to the toilet in the back of the car."

"Don't be stupid, where else are you going to go? It's dark, we won't be able to see your weenie."

Will didn't say anything.

"Come on, Will, you're not serious are you?"

"I don't just need a wee," Will said, finally. "I need to poo as well."

148

"Oh. You're right, you can't do that in the back of the car."

Helen bumped into Lee again as she climbed back into the rear seat.

"Watch out, will you?" Lee said.

"Sorry."

Lee took her turn climbing into the back of the car. She pulled down her pants and squatted, leaning a hand against the rear window to balance herself. Her hand slipped against the wet glass. Despite her urgent need to relieve herself, she couldn't let go at first. She tried not to think about what she was doing, about where she was and the situation they were in. The questions crowded in to her mind, the doubts.

What did they think they were doing, travelling to God knew where in a half-assed attempt at finding Daniel? Was it too late to turn around and head back to the Botanical Gardens? If they returned with Helen, then surely that would be in their favour? That Lee and Will would be let back inside, into the relative safety of the compound?

Lee realised she had let go and breathed a quiet sigh of relief as her entire body relaxed. The stream of urine seemed to last forever but finally she finished and pulled her pants back up. She climbed back into the rear seat, careful not to step on Iggy.

"Your turn, Will," Helen said.

"I can't," Will said.

"I know it's embarrassing, but honestly you'll be all right," Helen said.

"I need a poo," Will said.

"Oh."

The three teenagers were silent as they thought about this.

"Do you think you can hang on?" Lee said.

"I don't know," Will replied. Just as he finished speaking,

149

the silence was broken by a long, loud fart.

"Will! Was that you?" Helen said, and burst into giggles.

"Yeah." In the dark he sounded embarrassed.

Lee rubbed at the car window again, desperate for a glimmer of light to signal the approaching day.

Nothing.

"That stinks!" Helen gasped.

"Sorry," Will mumbled. "I've been constipated, I haven't been for a few days now."

"How long?" Lee said, pulling her top over her nose in anticipation of the smell.

Will mumbled something.

"What did you say?"

"I said, the last time I went was before we got here."

"What do you mean, got here?" Lee said.

"You know, the future, this place in the future, since we met at the museum."

"But Will, that's been like, a week!" Lee hissed.

"I know," Will said.

"Oh, man," Lee moaned. "Look, you're just gonna have to go in the back of the car."

"I can't do that," Will said.

"What else are you going to do?" Lee said. "You just gonna sit there and crap in your pants?"

Will was silent for a few seconds, and then finally he said, "I'm going to open the door, just a bit. I'm going to open the door and poo outside."

"Yeah? And what about when some gnarly monster comes up and bites you on the ass? What are you gonna do then?"

"It won't," Will said.

"Okay, okay, just do it then, will you?"

Lee waited. Will made no move to open the car door. The

150

rain thrummed heavily against the roof.

Finally, Will moved. He pulled at the door handle and opened it just a slither. The sound of the rainfall changed. Lee could hear the rain hitting the wet ground, sounded like they were sitting in the middle of a lake. She wondered if any newcomers had arrived, carried by the wormhole into a nightmarish future.

She felt sorry for them.

Will was shuffling about in his seat, getting himself into position.

Lee closed her eyes and waited.

* * *

Daylight came slowly, grey and wet and dirty looking. The rain finally stopped, but the thick cloud cover remained, threatening to spill its contents over them once more. Slowly and gingerly, stiff from the night, they climbed out of the car. They made sure to get out the opposite side from where Will had been to the toilet. When asked, Will told them the operation had been successful.

Lee really didn't want to know any more.

They stretched and shivered in the cold morning breeze. Lee knew the day would heat up pretty quick, but at this moment that didn't seem possible.

"Do you really think we can find Daniel?" Helen said, shrugging on her backpack.

"No idea," Lee snapped. "Why? Have you got other plans for today?"

Helen turned away, said nothing. Lee felt bad for snapping at Helen, but she didn't apologise.

Lee gazed down the long stretch of motorway ahead of

them, at the cars dripping with rainwater, abandoned bumper to bumper and disappearing into the grey dawn light. She thought about their dwindling supplies of food and water, of how the day was going to heat up, of the monsters they were likely to encounter as they travelled.

Do you really think we can find Daniel?

It was a good question.

Lee pushed the question to the back of her mind, buried the doubt out of sight. If they weren't going to look for Daniel, what else were they going to do?

The three of them shouldered their backpacks on and began walking along the motorway again, trudging through broad puddles of water. Who knew how far Daniel and Renton were ahead of them, or even if they had come this way? But the only way to find out was to keep walking.

Away from Birmingham.

North.

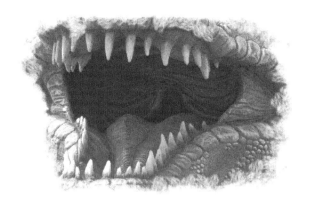

Chapter Fifteen

Slowly, very very slowly, Nuo twisted her hand inside the bracelet of the handcuff. She was at the point now where the bones in her hand were squashed painfully together, and she was also at the point of no return. If she gave up now and pushed her hand back through so that the metal bracelet was back around her wrist, all that effort and pain to get to this point would have been for nothing.

Nuo breathed deeply and calmly. She blocked out the sounds of screams, the rustling in the undergrowth. Twisted and turned that hand, her fingers and thumb all squashed together. It helped that she was slender, and flexible. And the man had been careless when he snapped the cuffs around her wrist and hadn't checked how tight the metal bracelet was.

Another scream in the grey morning light, followed by a gurgle and chomping, ripping, tearing noises.

Nuo closed her eyes, took a deep, shaky breath.

Twisted. Turned. Flexed her fingers, squishing them even closer together.

The metal bracelet was down to the knuckles and Nuo

knew that once she was past those bony protrusions, the handcuffs would fall off her hand and she would be free. But those knuckles seemed so impossibly prominent, so large. Nuo, the girl always described as delicate, slender, waif-like.

And now she felt so big and awkward.

She twisted and turned that hand, not thinking about the things with teeth and claws, about the men who had dragged her here and handcuffed her to the wrecked car, not thinking about the mangled skeleton in the back seat, its bones fractured, its cracked skull grinning up at her whenever she looked at it.

Twisted and turned and pulled, her fingers turning purple, the pain building and building. Nuo had long fingers, piano playing fingers her music teacher had told her. Would she be able to use this hand again if she even managed to pull it through that metal bracelet? Better to have a ruined hand and still be alive though.

Nuo ground her teeth together and screwed her eyes shut. Leaned back, pulling against the cuffs attached to the car door frame. Braced her feet against the side of the footwell and pulled.

The metal bracelet bit into her hand, clamped down on the thin, delicate bones. Ignoring the pain, thinking of her brothers and sisters, of sunshine and sunflowers, of days spent by the river and —

The handcuffs clattered against the car's metal frame and Nuo fell on her back. For a split second her mind couldn't grasp what had happened. Her hand, free of its metal bracelet, floated in front of her as though it was detached from her arm and filled with helium.

Another scream dragged her back into reality. Nuo pulled herself upright and looked out of the car's shattered windscreen. The morning was growing lighter, but the fog was still an impenetrable whiteness hiding the monstrosities that lay out there. For a moment it seemed safer to stay inside the car. After all, wandering around blindly in the fog was a surefire way to bump into a hungry creature, bearing its teeth and claws.

But the car was no protection against those teeth and claws. If she stayed here, she would die.

Nuo climbed out of the car.

Her hand throbbed from pulling it through the handcuffs, but she was able to flex her fingers fine. Her cheek hurt where the man called Dave had slapped her. Nuo remembered the boy watching as Dave manacled her to the car. She wondered briefly if he was still alive and then pushed him from her mind.

She had to look after herself.

Nuo took a couple of tentative steps into the fog. She glanced back at the illusion of safety that was the wrecked shell of a car. The temptation to climb back inside and curl up on the back seat with the mangled skeleton was strong.

Nuo turned her back on the car and took another step forward, and another.

A large, looming shadow materialised out of the grey, became a hedgerow grown wild and shaggy with no one to trim it. Its branches and leaves dripped with moisture. Nuo looked down at her feet. She was on the cracked, broken pavement.

Which way now? In the fog she had lost all sense of direction. Was the school where they had been kept prisoner off to her right or her left?

Voices, in the fog. Drawing closer.

Nuo shrank back against the overgrown hedge, disturbing it, the branches showering her with droplets of water.

"We were too late this morning getting out here, we need to start getting out earlier than this or we're gonna be eaten too."

"Are you blaming me? Like it's my fault?"

"Shuddup!" hissed the first man. "Did you hear that?"

Nuo could see the vague shadows of their forms now. From what she'd heard she recognised the second speaker as the man called Dave, the fat one, the one who had hit her and cuffed her to the car.

She knew she should run, get away from these two before they discovered her and took her back to the school to keep her captive until the next day when they would stake her out for dinosaur food again. But, lost in the fog, aware of the multiple dangers all around, Nuo was unable to move, frozen in place.

The man called Dave was the first to materialise, like a ghost, from the wall of swirling, grey fog.

His eyes widened, his mouth fell open. He looked like a caricature of a surprised person. The other man appeared alongside him. Finally freed from her paralysis, Nuo darted to one side, attempting to make a break past the two men.

She was too late. Dave already had one meaty hand around her wrist, the wrist that had just recently been handcuffed to the car. She screamed, but her scream was cut short as Dave pulled her to him and slapped his other hand across her mouth.

"Shush now, we don't want to be attracting attention to ourselves now, do we?" he whispered

"How the hell did she get free?" the other man said.

"I don't bloody know, do I?"

"You didn't cuff her tight enough to the car, did you?"

"Course I did!" Dave pulled Nuo even closer, his foul, meaty breath washing over her face. "She's a wily one, she is. Crafty, ain't you?"

"What are we gonna do with her?"

"Cuff her to the car again," Dave said. He pulled a bunch of keys from his belt and shook them in front of her face. "But

156

this time I'll make sure those cuffs bite nice and tight, I will."

Dave still had his hand clamped over Nuo's mouth, but his grip had relaxed enough that Nuo was able to work her mouth open slightly. She bit down on a finger, gouging her teeth into his soft flesh.

Dave screamed and swore, letting Nuo go for a moment.

But that moment was too small, too short. Before she had a chance to move, to dart to freedom, Dave had grabbed her again, this time by her upper arm. His fat lips were curled back in a snarl, his other hand, clutching the keys and tightened into a fist, was raised and ready to smash into Nuo's face.

"Hit her, Dave! Slap her right—"

The man, whatever his name might have been, never finished his sentence. A monstrous shadow loomed out of the fog and descended upon him, almost seeming to swallow him whole. There was a brief flurry of movement, a sense of limbs being torn apart, the muffled sound of liquid splattering across the ground.

Followed by the sounds of chewing and snuffling, of grunts and wet ripping sounds.

Nuo pulled free of Dave's grip and ran.

She blundered into the hedge. Branches scraped at her face, her arms, showered her with more water. Dave was screaming, something had latched itself onto him. Whatever it was, it was growling, shaking Dave around like it was a dog with its favourite toy.

Nuo pressed herself against the hedge, shrinking from the violence in the fog just in front of her. She couldn't move, paralysed by the carnage happening only a few feet away. Her mind tumbled over and over with panicked thoughts. What if there were other things out there, just feet away? If she turned and ran she would blunder right into them. Into open jaws,

157

teeth fastening around her arms and legs, claws ripping at her flesh.

Dave screamed again. Something flew from the fog at Nuo, landing at her feet. It was an arm, ripped from its owner at the elbow, a scarlet pool of blood expanding across the ground.

Dave's arm, his hand still tightened around that bunch of keys.

Nuo ran.

She tripped and fell, scraping her knees.

She picked herself up and ran again.

She didn't know where she was going, she didn't care, she just ran.

The fog was too thick, visibility too low for her to keep running. Her hair was plastered to her head, her face dripping with cold moisture. Monstrous, hulking shapes appeared and disappeared in the fog. Abandoned, rusting cars, sitting on flat tyres, windows smashed in.

But she only saw them, only recognised them for what they were, when she got up close. Until that moment those shapes materialising out of the grey fog were monsters, ready to snatch her up between bloody teeth and crunch her into a raw, fleshy pulp.

Nuo stopped running, panting with fear. She had hardly gone any distance at all. There were muffled sounds in the fog. Animal like sounds.

Nuo was standing by the wreck of another car and she put her hand against the cold metal, resting for a moment.

"Hey! Help me!"

Nuo's heart felt like it had juddered to a halt for a split second at the sound of that voice. She snatched her hand away from the car like it had suddenly grown searingly hot.

"Don't leave me! Please!"

Nuo bent down and looked inside the car, through the shattered rear windscreen. The boy she had seen earlier, the one who watched her being manacled to the car, he was in there. Wide eyed, staring back at her, handcuffed to the car door frame.

"Can you get these cuffs off me?" he whispered.

Nuo shook her head, her wet hair slapping against her face.

"But I saw them cuff you to the car!" the boy hissed. "You got free, tell me how you did it!"

Nuo couldn't speak. Her tongue seemed glued to the roof of her mouth, her lips frozen into place by the cold.

The boy tried pulling himself closer to her, his arm straining against the cuffs.

"There are things out there," he whispered. "You've got to help me."

"I slipped my hand out of the handcuffs," Nuo whispered.

The boy tugged at the metal bracelet circling his wrist.

"I can't do that, they're too tight," he said.

Gathering more courage as the seconds passed, Nuo crept around the car until she was next to his cuffed hand. The man called Dave had made sure this boy wasn't going anywhere. He had locked the metal cuff down tight around the boy's wrist. There was no way he could pull his hand free like Nuo had done.

The boy leaned forward, got right in Nuo's face.

"Help me," he said.

Nuo bit her lip, and then said, "I can't, they're too tight."

Someone screamed.

". . . ohgodnopleasegodnogodnonono . . ."

Nuo thought of Dave, of him being eaten by a monster in the fog. Thought of his arm landing in front of her, severed at the elbow. Of his fist, still clutching the bunch of keys.

159

She took a deep, shaky breath.

"Okay, I think I can get the keys. I can get you out."

Nuo glanced over her shoulder, at the wall of fog behind her, where she had just come from. Why was she doing this?

"Please, hurry!" the boy said.

Trying to not think about what she was doing, Nuo turned away from the boy in the car and entered the grey mass of fog. How could she even find her way back to where Dave had caught her? The fog was too thick, the surrounding sounds too disorienting.

Why was she even risking her life for someone she did not know?

Because she needed help too. Because she needed companionship in this terrifying new world she had been thrown into. So far she had been all alone.

The rusted, abandoned cars helped her guide her way back. She had only been aware of them as monstrous shapes rising from the fog as she fled, but she knew she hadn't come far. Nuo hoped that whatever had eaten the man called Dave wasn't still there. And that it hadn't taken the arm with it.

Nuo stopped, peering at the ground. Had she gone too far? It was so difficult to tell where she was.

Something shifted in the fog. Animal like eating sounds, crunching of bones, snuffling and grunting.

Nuo was standing with her back to a car, against the cold, damp shell.

This didn't feel right. Was she in the wrong place? Had she followed the wrong line of cars?

Nuo lifted a foot and slowly, quietly, took a single step closer to the sounds of eating.

The large hedge that she had stumbled into appeared out of the fog.

160

And there on the ground was the chewed up, severed arm.

The fist still clutched the bunch of keys.

How was that possible?

Again, purposefully not thinking about what she was doing, Nuo crouched down and edged closer to the keys. On her hands and knees she reached out. Careful to avoid touching the dead man's fingers, she closed her hand around the keys and pulled.

The fist refused to let go.

Nuo pulled again, desperate to not have to touch the dead man's fingers. The keys wouldn't come out of his fist. Somehow, the hand on the end of the severed arm was keeping tight hold of the bunch of keys.

Nuo crawled on her hands and knees closer to the arm. She froze as she heard movement in the fog again. A rustling, more chomping and ripping noises. The sound of something wet hitting the ground.

Gritting her teeth, Nuo picked at the fingers, closed tightly into a fist. Already the flesh felt cold to her touch. She prised the fingers open, and the keys dropped to the ground with a soft clink.

Nuo froze. Had the thing, whatever it was, heard? Would it come bearing down upon her from the fog, mouth open to reveal razor-sharp teeth?

The sounds of feeding continued, and no heavy, dark shapes materialised from the fog.

Nuo picked up the keys and began crawling backwards, back towards the hedge and the nearest car.

She was shivering and had to hold the keys tight to stop them rattling and giving her away.

Once she felt she was far enough away from the thing in the fog, Nuo slowly stood up on shaky legs and followed the line of cars back to the boy. He stared wide eyed at her as she approached him.

Nuo held up the keys.

"I got them," she said.

The boy snatched them from her and began trying out each key on the handcuffs. After only a few tries the cuffs suddenly fell free, clanging against the side of the car. His head shot up, eyes darting around, searching the fog for encroaching danger.

"Let's get out of here," Nuo said.

The boy shook his head. "We can't, not yet. There's a girl, in the school, Emily. We have to help her, set her free."

Nuo shook her head. "Uh uh, no way. If we go back into that school the men will catch us and we'll just end up being staked out as tasty treats for dinosaurs again."

The boy was rubbing his wrist, his head turning this way and that all the time.

"We've got to help her, I can't leave her there." He looked at Nuo. "You need to help us too."

Nuo folded her arms and stared at the boy. "Why should I?"

"How long have you been here?"

Nuo's bravado faltered a little, and she lowered her head. "I'm not sure. A couple of days maybe. I'm still not sure what happened. Do you know?"

"I've got a pretty good idea, yeah. Listen, I've been here longer than you, I know what it's like out here. I've got friends here too. We can help you."

Nuo lifted her head and looked at the boy again. "What's your name?"

"Daniel."

"Nuo." She took a deep breath. "Okay, I'll help you. But I am not getting caught by those crazy men again. If we even

162

look like we're about to get into trouble I am running, and you can come with me or not, I don't care. Okay?"

"Fair enough," Daniel said.

He climbed out of the car, through the window.

"This way," he said, and limped into the fog.

Yeah, I know where it is, Nuo thought. *I can't believe I'm doing this. I only hope this Emily girl is worth it.*

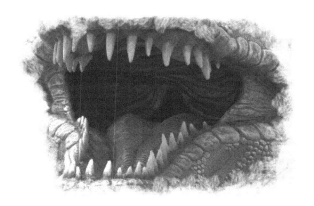

Chapter Sixteen

Will stared at the Tesco van like it was an alien creature. It bothered him, but he couldn't pin down why. Lee and Helen watched him, while Iggy padded around their feet.

"Come on, we should keep moving," Lee said.

"The key is in the ignition," Will said. He could see it, through the open driver's door. The passenger door was open too, and he could see all the way through the van's cab to the central reservation and the other carriageway.

"So?" Lee said. "You think you can get it going?"

Will shook his head. He kept looking at the Tesco van. It wasn't the whole van that bothered him, he realised that now. It was something to do with the cab.

"So what's the problem?" Lee said. "We need to hustle, we need to move."

"Did you search the back of the van?"

"Yeah, I told you already, we got water, we got some tins, we can't carry any more." Lee stared at Will, the frustration plain on her face. "Let's go."

"You got water," Will said, and there it was, the thing that

164

had been bothering him all this time.

He climbed in the cab and picked up the water bottle from the dashboard. Getting back out of the cab he held the water bottle out in front of him, like a talisman.

"Look, it's got water in it," he said.

"Yeah, and so have all the bottles we collected from the back." Lee glanced at Helen and then back at Will. "But ours are full, and that's half empty."

Will tipped the bottle until it was horizontal and clear water began pouring from the neck.

"But this is open," he said. "There was no cap on it."

Lee opened her mouth to reply and then snapped it shut again.

"That's right, someone's been here, recently," Will said, and turned the bottle upright again. "If this bottle had been sat on the dashboard, in the driver's window, the water would have evaporated in only a few days, never mind years."

"Do you think it was Daniel?" Helen said.

"And don't forget Renton," Lee said.

"Maybe," Will said, and dropped the bottle on the ground.

"Well, whatever," Lee said. "It looks like maybe they were driving this thing and then it gave up on them and so they started walking again."

"But why did they leave all the food and the water in the back?"

"Maybe they didn't. Maybe they picked up as much as they could carry and this is what was left."

"Maybe," Will said again.

"Come on, Will!" Lee said. "If they were here recently, we need to get a move on, try to catch up with them. For all we know they could be close."

"Okay, okay," Will said, turning his back on the Tesco van.

Lee pointed at his bulging backpack sitting on the pitted tarmac. "Me and Helen filled it up for you while you were in your trance staring at the van."

Will picked it up, grunted at the weight of it. He swung it around and over his shoulder, onto his back. He fastened the strap around his waist. Hard, angular shapes jutted into his back.

"Thanks," he said.

The three teenagers started walking again, along the motorway. Helen had put Iggy on a leash and she kept him close. Nobody knew what was hiding in the undergrowth on either side of the motorway. Back a couple of miles they had come across a service station. They had approached it, hoping to find food and drink. But then they had seen the rats inside the main building, a brown carpet of them flowing down the stairs, their mass undulating as they scuttled through the eating areas and the cafes.

They had soon backed off and kept on walking.

Now they walked along the motorway, constantly on alert for danger lurking in the bushes. Seemed like the whole world had become a forest, trees everywhere of all shapes and sizes. Made Will feel claustrophobic. He hadn't realised that trees could grow so fast if just left alone, that they could take over the landscape so quickly.

And with the trees had come the wildlife, the insects and the birds. Sometimes it seemed like the world was noisier now with fewer people on the planet than it had been before the dinosaurs arrived and started eating everybody.

Take humanity out of the equation and it seemed the world could not only look after itself, but flourish.

Made Will feel even worse than he had been. That humanity was nothing more than a pest, and that they should be

166

exterminated for the sake of planet earth. After all, they were the ones causing the problems. Wars, climate change, pollution, plastic.

Without people the pollution problem had disappeared, that was for sure. Will had never breathed air that smelled so fresh and clean before. And surely that meant the planet's climate was fixing itself.

But plastic. He still saw plastic everywhere. Mainly empty water bottles, scattered across the pathways and roads. That made him think of all the plastic in landfill, accumulated over the decades, and all the plastic in the ocean.

How long would it take the planet to recover from that?

Trapped in his own thoughts like this, his mood spiralled ever downward. Adding to his belief that they could never survive out here. Even if they found Daniel alive and unharmed, which was near impossible given the fact that not only were they in danger of being eaten by a dinosaur every single moment of every single day but Daniel was also travelling with a psychopathic killer, how would that change anything? How would it increase their odds of survival?

Lee would say that they were stronger in numbers, that they were better off together.

And that might be true.

But being a group of four instead of three didn't seem to be much of an increase to Will.

They were going to die.

It was only a matter of how soon.

Something clattered against an abandoned car wreck as Will walked past it, the noise jolting him from his thoughts.

"What was that?" Lee said, spinning around on the spot.

Helen grabbed Iggy's collar.

"I don't know," Will said, staring at the car, every nerve

ending in his body screaming at him to turn and run.

The car sat there, nothing moving within or around it.

Will felt something whoosh past his head, missing him by only an inch or two. It clattered against the car, making the same sound they had just heard.

And then Will saw it, lying on the ground with its companion.

An arrow.

"Nobody move, or we'll shoot you through the eyes."

Will slowly lifted his gaze to see a line of five teenagers standing on wrecked car roofs on the opposite carriageway. Each one had a bow and arrow trained on Will and Lee and Helen. There were two boys and three girls. One of the girls was taller than the other four teenagers, and looked older, and harder.

She was the one who had spoken.

"Drop the kit bags and empty your pockets," she said. "If any of you try anything, you will all die."

Will slipped the rucksack off his back and let it drop to the ground. Lee and Helen did the same. Will could hardly take his eyes off these five warriors with bows and arrows, but he managed a swift glance at Lee.

She was scowling so hard, Will was scared she might lose her self-control any moment and charge, screaming her head off and fists flailing, straight at the five teenagers.

"Now put your hands in the air," the girl said. "All of you, do it now."

Will raised his hands. So did Lee.

Helen was still holding on to Iggy's collar. The dog had bared his teeth, and he was growling at the newcomers.

"Put up your hands," the girl said, pointing the bow and arrow directly at Helen.

"I can't," Helen said. "If I let go of Iggy, he'll attack you."

The girl thought about this for a moment. "All right, keep hold of him. But do anything stupid and I will kill you and your dog. Okay?"

Helen nodded, tightening her grip on Iggy.

At a signal from the girl, all five teens jumped off the cars and climbed over the rusted barrier separating the north and south carriageways. They never wavered once with their bows and arrows.

Will studied them as they drew closer. The tall girl, their leader, she was strikingly beautiful, and she knew it. Long, tousled golden hair, a ring through her nose, and dark, piercing eyes. She wore skin-tight, black trousers and a tank top which showed off the muscular definition on her arms. A black belt buckled around her waist was studded with bright, shiny metal.

The other two girls looked like they were trying to emulate their leader's appearance but, possibly out of deference to her, they looked shabbier and less striking. The two boys both looked hostile, their eyes narrowed into hard stares.

They quickly surrounded Will, Lee and Helen. They kept their bows and arrows pointed at the three teens.

"Your weapons, show them to us, lay them on the ground," the leader said. "Carefully and slowly."

Lee slowly pulled the rifle off her back and over her head and laid it on the ground. Will and Helen placed their knives down. Helen still held onto Iggy.

"Are there any more of you?" the girl said.

"No," Lee replied. "It's just us."

"Don't lie to me!" the girl snapped. "We heard you talking about others. Where are they?"

"They're on ahead, maybe a couple of days' worth," Lee said. "We've been following them, trying to catch up."

169

The girl looked at the others.

One of the boys said, "They got taken by the others."

"Others? Which others?" Lee said.

"A group of adults, over in the village," the girl replied.

"They're bad news," one of the other two girls said. She looked to be the youngest in the group.

The other boy, the one who hadn't spoken yet, snorted and said, "Yeah? So are we."

"Are you sure it was our friends?" Lee said. "What did they look like?"

"There was a man," the first boy said. "He only had one hand."

"That's Renton," Lee said. "Talk about bad news? He's terrible news."

"And there was a boy and girl with him," the lad said.

Will and Lee looked at each other.

"All right, that's enough talk," the leader said. "Pick up your kit bags and let's get moving."

Will bent down to pick up his rucksack and paused when he saw Lee hadn't moved.

"Where are you taking us?" Lee said.

"Back to the Towers," the leader said. "Nemesis is going to want to meet you."

Still Lee didn't move. "What if we say no?"

Still holding the bow and arrow pointed at Lee, their leader didn't hesitate. "We'll kill you."

Lee held her ground a moment longer. Will picked up his rucksack, slowly hauled it onto his back.

Come on Lee! Don't be so stubborn!

Lee finally dropped her stare and picked up her rucksack, slinging it casually over her shoulder. Helen still had hers on her back.

"Move over there," the leader said, indicating a spot a little further away from the line of cars.

Once the three teens had walked away far enough, the two lads slung their bows across their backs and put their arrows away and picked up the weapons lying on the ground.

"Get moving," the leader said, and pointed at a gap in the trees beside the motorway.

They had to climb over the bent and rusted barrier, but once in amongst the trees Will found the going easier than he had expected. They had to walk in single file. Lee took up the front, adjusting her direction only when ordered to by the leader of the group, and then Helen and Iggy came next followed by Will.

And the whole time they walked, a spot between Will's shoulder blades tingled with anticipation of an arrow piercing his flesh.

* * *

They walked for a couple of hours, only leaving the forest briefly when they had to cross a country lane or a main road. Even then the trees were doing their best to reclaim the areas of ground covered in tarmac and concrete. The roads were cracked and bulging with roots, and long swathes of grass had grown between the gaps almost completely hiding the roads in some instances. They passed houses just visible between the closely packed trees, and the once former homes now looked deserted and reclaimed by nature.

But after those first couple of hours of walking, the forest opened out slightly and they began following a much wider trail. Will soon realised that this was because they were following a proper road again. At first he thought it had once been a motorway, but threw that idea away when he realised there was no central reservation, no barrier.

Besides which, it just didn't feel like a motorway. It didn't feel like any kind of regular road, and Will wondered what it had been.

The trees began thinning out and soon the group started walking through more open spaces, although they were still surrounded by forest. Will couldn't work it out. The landscape had become odd, a combination of wild, unruly nature and yet displaying signs of order, even design. It was the clear spaces they kept walking through. The trees lined these spaces like walls and Will had the idea that if he could get high in the sky and look down he would see a geometric pattern of large gaps in the forest.

Car parks! That had to be it. They were walking through a series of interlinked car parks. Although the tarmac was ruptured with roots, and plenty of vegetation was growing through the cracks, the forest hadn't fully been able to reclaim these areas.

But why so many car parks situated in one area?

Where were they being taken?

Ten minutes later and Will had his answer. The forest had opened out again to reveal another wide, unclaimed space. But this space had a series of barriers blocking the teens' progress. Barriers comprised of turnstiles and ticket booths.

A massive, twisted length of iron, looked like a helix or a computer representation of a chain of cells, was mounted in the middle of this space. It was this that Will recognised first.

A section of track from an old theme park ride.

The Corkscrew.

They were at Alton Towers theme park.

"You lot get yourselves ready for eating, we've got work to

172

do this afternoon remember," the leader said to her group. "I'm taking these three to Nemesis."

Will immediately thought of the roller coaster ride, called Nemesis. Riders were seated underneath the track hanging from the rails and were plunged through narrow canyons and twisted through loops at high speed. Why was this girl taking them to the roller coaster?

And then he remembered her saying that Nemesis would want to meet them. So, Nemesis had to be the leader of this group.

Following on from that thought came another one.

Why would anyone name themselves after a roller coaster ride?

The three teens' captors had long since packed their bows and arrows away, no longer seeing them as a threat. Especially now they were back at their base. The two boys and two girls headed off together. The group leader stared at Will, Lee and Helen.

"You two don't say much," she said, pointing at Will and Helen.

Will looked down at the ground. Ridiculously he could feel his cheeks growing warm as he began to blush. He didn't need to wonder why. This girl, this tall, striking teenage woman, she was just the kind of girl that Will had been terrified of at school. Terrified of, and yet insanely attracted to at the same time. Just the knowledge that she was even looking at him had his heart hammering and his face glowing bright red.

"There's not a lot to say when you're being held captive," Lee said, speaking up for all of them. As usual.

"Come with me," the leader said. "I'm taking you to Nemesis."

A silence followed, and no one moved.

Will looked up.

173

The girl, that strikingly beautiful young woman, hadn't moved. She was standing perfectly still, gazing at the three teenagers.

Then she shook her head softly, and said, "I don't know what she's going to make of you three. Just keep quiet, and only speak when you're spoken to, all right? That way she might decide to let you live. Maybe."

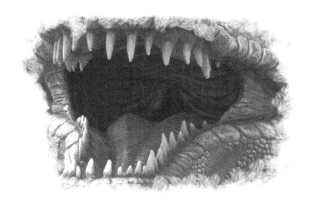

Chapter Seventeen

All the adults were out, apart from one man guarding the prisoners. He stood at the entrance to the sports hall, a rifle clutched in both hands. Nuo had told Daniel how she had escaped, and how the two men had almost caught her before being eaten by the monsters in the fog. It was obvious that nothing had gone to plan this morning, and it looked like maybe the others were out searching for their missing mates.

Daniel wasn't convinced that this solitary guard was the only person left at the school. So far Daniel had only seen the men called Dave and Nige, and the muscular man who seemed to be the leader. According to Nuo, Dave was dead along with his companion. Had that been Nige?

That still left the guard standing here and their leader, at the very least. Daniel knew there had to be more, and that wasn't even taking into account any women and children there might be. From what little he had seen in the fog, Daniel suspected the school had been a large one which meant it could now be housing a number of survivors.

Daniel knew if they were going to rescue Emily they had to

do it quietly.

But that was going to be difficult even if they managed to incapacitate the man standing guard. Once they got inside, there would be a riot as everyone made a bid for freedom. There was no hope of keeping everyone quiet.

"What do we do now?" Nuo said.

"I don't know," Daniel muttered.

"We should leave, before the others come back and find us."

Daniel shook his head. "I'm not leaving without Emily."

"In that case, I'm going," Nuo said.

"No!" Daniel hissed. "Just give me a minute, let me think."

From their position around the corner of the sports hall, Daniel stared at the man with the rifle. The fog was lifting, he realised. He could see much better than he had been able to. Was that a bad thing? The fog had been a hindrance, but at least it had hidden them.

Someone screamed, someone outside of the school grounds. The man looked in the direction of the scream. Daniel got his first good look at his face. He was chewing his bottom lip, his were like wide, round saucers.

Another scream, turning into loud sobs and cries for help.

The man took a step away from the sports hall. It was obvious he wasn't sure what to do. Perhaps he already knew about Dave and Nige being eaten, and now he didn't know if he should stay here, guarding their prisoners, or go and help the others.

Go on, go and help, go and find out what's going on!

As if obeying Daniel's mental command, the man set off running away from the sports hall, in the direction of the screams.

"This is our chance," Daniel whispered.

The two teenagers turned the corner and sprinted towards the doors.

Daniel pulled up short in front of them and his heart sank into the pit of his stomach. A thick, heavy chain had been looped through the door handles and secured with a padlock.

"No!" Daniel hissed. "No, no, no!"

He grabbed the chains, and they rattled in his hands.

Nuo took a step back, taking a long look at the front of the sports hall.

"It's okay," she said. "We can get in."

Daniel joined her, looking where she pointed. The large windows running along the front of the sports hall were all protected by black, metal grills. But one of them had been damaged, the lower right-hand corner bent back away from its housing in the wall.

"If we can bend that grill back some more, there'll be enough room for your friend to climb through."

"What about the glass?" Daniel said. "We need something to smash it with."

They both looked around at the ruined playground. Daniel's stomach churned painfully. Any moment now he expected the man with the rifle to return.

"There! That'll do," Nuo said, pointing to a chunk of masonry lying on the ground.

"Okay, let's do it, quickly," Daniel said.

They ran together to the window and wrapped their fingers around the cold, metal grill. Together they both pulled, leaning back to add weight to their strength. The metal grill bit into Daniel's palms, but he clenched his jaw tight and kept on pulling.

"That's enough!" Nuo gasped, letting go.

Faces had appeared at the window, peering through the

grime. When they realised what was happening the people inside started knocking on the window and shouting.

"Get back!" Daniel hissed. "You have to move back and stay quiet."

Nuo had run to get the chunk of masonry. Daniel was more convinced than ever that they were about to be discovered. That they would be caught and thrown back inside the sports hall, or maybe just shot where they stood to save their captors any more problems.

Nuo returned with the lump of masonry clutched in both hands. It looked heavy, but Nuo was stronger than her slender frame suggested. She hefted it up, over her shoulder.

"Get out of the way!" she yelled and hurled the rock at the window.

The glass in the bottom corner shattered as the masonry chunk hit it, and then a moment later the rest of the windowpane dropped from its frame and exploded on the ground.

The gap between the window frame and the corner of the protective grill that had been bent back was suddenly filled with bodies scrambling to get through.

"Oh no!" Daniel groaned. "We're never going to get to Emily now!"

The gap was too small to let many people through, but it gradually widened as more bodies pushed against the metal, bending it further. With a sudden grinding the grill popped off the wall and fell on the ground. More bodies immediately filled the larger gap.

"Emily!" Daniel shouted, leaping up and down in an attempt to see her over the people filling the open window.

He ran against the tide of escapees, fighting his way through. He'd almost reached the windowsill when he was shoved to the ground. Suddenly he was nothing more than an object to be scrambled over or to be kicked out of the way. Daniel threw his arms over his head, curling himself up in an attempt to protect himself.

A gunshot, followed by a scream. The horde of people scrambling over Daniel stopped, frozen in their tracks.

"Get back inside!" a voice shouted.

No one moved.

Daniel turned his head, looked between the legs of the adults all standing around him. It was the man who had been standing guard, but he looked as though he was on his own. He also looked terrified. He was holding the gun up, pointing it at the sky.

The crowd of adults shifted uneasily. They weren't going back inside that sports hall easily.

The man lowered the rifle and pointed it at the mass of men and women.

"Get back inside, now!" he screamed, his voice high-pitched and wavering.

The adults suddenly surged forward with a combined roar of anger. The man managed to fire off one shot before they were all over him. Daniel looked away as they started punching and kicking the man, but he could still hear the man's screams.

Nuo joined Daniel by the window as he climbed to his feet.

"Where's your friend?" she said.

Daniel scanned the inside of the sports hall.

It was empty.

No, wait. There she was, crouched in a far corner.

"Hey, Emily!" Daniel shouted. "We're getting out of here!"

Emily stood up.

Glared at Daniel.

"Well, it's about time," she hissed. "I knew I shouldn't have come with you."

They helped Emily through the window and then ran. The fog was clearing quickly now and Daniel felt exposed, visible to all. And with the clearer view came confirmation of what he had suspected. The main school building was occupied by more survivors. He saw children's faces pressed against the dirty windows, and he saw some women too. Watching Daniel, Emily and Nuo as they made their escape.

They left the school grounds and ran down the street, avoiding looking at the bloody, ripped shapes still hanging from the mangled cars. Something roared, something hidden by the row of houses and trees on their left. From the same direction came the sound of branches snapping and something big and heavy lumbering through the undergrowth.

"This way!" Daniel hissed, cutting right, down along the side of the school.

They kept running, jumping over erupted tarmac and thick roots bursting through the pavement. At times they had to fight their way through thick patches of forest, and then they were back out in the open again. They paused to catch their breath. Daniel leaned against the side of a car. Tendrils of some sort of vine had grown up through the ground and covered the car, its limbs snaking through the smashed windows and over the dashboard and steering wheel, over the seats and the gear stick.

"Now what?" Nuo said. "Any ideas what we do next?"

"We should go back to the service station," Emily said. "We were safe there, and my mother might be back by now."

"No, Emily, we weren't safe there," Daniel said. "What about all those rats?"

Emily snorted, making plain how stupid she thought Daniel was being. "Those rats will have long gone by now, you idiot! We should have waited them out, instead of running away."

"Was it safe there? Seriously?" Nuo said.

"Yeah, duh," Emily said. "We had food and water and shelter and everything. We should go back, it's not far."

"Maybe she's right," Nuo said, looking at Daniel. "Maybe we should go back. Unless you've got a better idea."

A better idea, Daniel thought. *If only I had any ideas.*

It seemed the only idea he had, the only thought in his mind, was to get back to the nuclear power plant in the Lake District and find out if his father was still alive.

Find out if there was any way of fixing this mess. Of sending the dinosaurs back to prehistory, where they belonged. And of sending him and Lee and Will back to their own time, twenty years ago.

"Look, Nuo, I know what Emily is saying might seem to make sense," Daniel said. "But we—"

Nuo held up her hand and silenced Daniel. She was looking over the top of the car's roof, at something further away.

"What is it?" Daniel said. "A dinosaur?"

Emily peered around the edge of the car. She turned back around and said, "No, it's worse than a dinosaur. It's *him*."

Daniel peeked over the top of the car.

Renton. Further down the street. And he was manacled to a car wreck.

Daniel turned back and let himself slide down the side of the car to a sitting position.

"What's wrong?" Nuo said.

"He's a maniac," Emily said. "He's, like, got one hand and he hasn't got a nose and he's a monster, he's horrible. We should just leave him here."

Nuo looked at Daniel.

He took a deep breath and slowly blew air out from his lips, his cheeks bulging. "She's right, he murdered a friend of mine

181

and kidnapped me."

"So we leave him there then, right?" Nuo said.

"Absogodamnlutely," Emily said.

Daniel didn't reply.

Nuo squatted down in front of him. "What?"

Daniel put his hands over his face.

"What? Tell me."

He took another deep breath. This was hard.

"I'm not sure I can leave him behind," he said. "I left him behind once before, left him to die. His hand was trapped, we'd just survived a plane crash, but the plane was on fire and Renton, his hand was trapped in the wreckage and he was begging me to set him free. But I didn't. I ran and left him to die."

"And that's why he's only got one hand?" Emily said. "Did he like, saw his hand off or something? Cool!"

"You can't blame yourself for that," Nuo said. "Sounds to me like you had no choice."

"Yeah, I know," Daniel replied. "Thing is, this time I do have a choice."

He held up the keys for the handcuffs.

"Oh," Nuo said

Renton shouted something. It was indistinct, not like any word that Daniel recognised. More of a guttural roar.

Daniel slowly lifted his head above the car roof. Renton was tugging at the handcuffs, pulling away as far as he could from where he was locked to the car door. Something was approaching him. It looked like a giant chicken with a long neck and a sparse covering of feathers. Its head swayed from side to side as it watched its prey.

"You gonna fight that thing to rescue this man who you say murdered your friend?" Nuo said.

"No," Daniel replied. "But one of us could distract it while I free him from the handcuffs."

Nuo shook her head. "You are one strange boy, did you know that?"

"Yeah," Daniel said, and paused for a moment in silence. "Maybe that's because I've been here longer than you. You'll be strange soon, too."

"Are you seriously thinking of setting him free?" Emily said.

Daniel ignored her. "Grab some branches or rocks, whatever you can find, and throw them at that car over there. If you can distract that thing, get its attention focused over there, I can unlock Renton's handcuffs and get him back here."

Emily huffed loudly and sat down. "I'm not doing anything to help him out."

"You should creep up a bit closer first," Nuo said. "I'm going to count to sixty, and then I'll start throwing stuff, like you said."

"Thank you," Daniel replied.

With one last look at Nuo and Emily, he squatted down and made a dash for the next car. He peered around from behind that one and saw Renton still leaning as far away as he could from the approaching dinosaur. Daniel could see Renton's hand had turned purple from the pressure on the metal cuff.

He darted to the next car along, keeping low. Slowly inched along to the car's bonnet and peered around it. He was closer now, close enough he could hear Renton's tortured breathing. Again, Daniel couldn't help but wonder how the American had survived for so long in the state he was in.

A sudden clattering from behind the dinosaur made Daniel jump. The dinosaur twisted its long neck, and it took a moment to look at the wreck of the car from where the sudden sound had come. Bored it turned its head back to Renton. Another clatter, closely followed by a third, had the dinosaur switching its attention back again. This time it turned its whole body, but it didn't run to the wrecked car. Just stayed where it was, its attention fixed on the tangled metal wreathed in green and brown vines.

Go on, Daniel thought. *Go closer, go and investigate what's making all that noise.*

Another crash from the car wreckage, louder than before, and this time accompanied by the tinkling of broken glass.

That was it, the dinosaur was intrigued enough by now to run towards the wreck, its long legs covering the ground quickly.

Daniel sprinted towards Renton, who grunted in surprise when he saw the teenager.

Almost gagging at the stink of Renton's putrefying flesh, Daniel fumbled the key into the lock.

"How did you—?" Renton said.

"No time," Daniel replied as the cuffs fell off Renton's wrist. "Come on, we need to run."

Daniel darted back towards the last car he had been hiding behind. As he reached the car he turned. Renton was shuffling along, having covered only half the distance that the teenager had. His breathing was hard and laboured, and his face was a mask of agony.

He's dying, Daniel thought. *He's actually dying.*

Renton finally got to the safety of the car and sat down heavily next to Daniel. Snot and pus bubbled from the holes in his face where his nose had once been. Daniel had to look away as his stomach was rolling so much he thought he might throw up.

184

Emily ran up to them. "We need to go! That thing knows it's been tricked, it's looking for us!"

Nuo was close behind Emily. "Let's go now!"

Something crashed about in the trees in front of them. Leaves fell off the branches as they swayed violently.

"What was that?" Emily said, wide-eyed.

"I don't know and I don't care, we need to get out of here," Nuo said.

Daniel climbed to his feet. He grabbed Renton by the arm and helped him up.

"This way," Nuo said, pointing.

There was a clear path leading back towards the school. Away from Emily's sanctuary at the motorway service station.

The monster hidden amongst the trees thrashed around again. A branch snapped, the loud crack like a gunshot.

"Back to the school?" Daniel said.

"It's the only clear path," Nuo hissed. "We'll cut straight through and out the other side."

And with that final statement she was off, sprinting for safety.

"Hey, wait for me!" Emily hissed, and ran after her.

Daniel looked at Renton.

"Come on then kid," Renton grunted. "Let's get moving, don't worry about me."

He staggered after Emily and Nuo, wheezing asthmatically.

Emily and Nuo were both out of sight by this time. Daniel kept pace with Renton and just hoped that the two girls would wait for them when they found a safer place. As they half-walked, half-ran past the school gates again, Daniel saw some survivors milling around aimlessly on the playground. They had been set free, but now they had no idea where to go, how to survive in their new world.

185

Daniel felt for them, but he couldn't do anything to help. He was having enough problems looking after himself.

Suddenly Nuo and Emily appeared in front of Daniel, running back towards him.

"We've got to hide, quick!" Nuo gasped. "There's a whole herd of hungry looking monsters back there, and they're heading this way."

"The school," Renton wheezed, pointing.

"Are you serious? We just escaped from there," Emily said.

"No, he's right," Daniel said. "But not back in the sports hall, we need to get into the main school building, upstairs."

Renton was already shuffling across the tarmac playground. Daniel looked at Emily and Nuo, feeling utterly helpless.

"All right, let's do it," Nuo said.

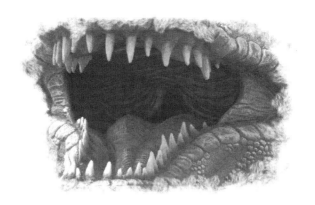

Chapter Eighteen

The teenager led Lee, Will and Helen through the park past the abandoned theme park rides. They walked past the Smiler, thick green tendrils wrapped around its tracks, strange, white flowers hanging from the vines that Lee had never seen before. Through the tangle of growth the Smiler logo still grinned at them.

The girl took them to a restaurant, leading them between tables which were surprisingly clean and neatly laid out. Two younger children were setting cutlery out and Lee was reminded of the efficiency of the commune in the Botanical Gardens. She glanced at Helen, wondering if she was thinking the same, and if maybe she was feeling homesick. But Helen was staring straight ahead as she walked, Iggy by her side, and betrayed no emotion.

The restaurant was laid out in an L shape, with the serving counter and the kitchen behind it in the inside corner of the L. It was only when they had rounded the corner that they saw Nemesis.

Lee almost stopped walking with surprise. She had been

expecting another child, another teenager. This whole setup so far felt like something out of The Lord of the Flies. Kids having claimed a theme park for themselves, run riot and then become tribal.

But no, Nemesis was an adult.

Her skin was a deep ebony, so black it almost seemed to be an absence of light in the room. She was wearing a faded Wickerman T-shirt, baggy camouflage trousers and a Smiler cap. An armchair had been dragged in here and placed on a set of four tables pushed together. Nemesis sat in the armchair looking down on these new intruders. The expression on Nemesis's face told Lee exactly who was in charge.

Surrounding Nemesis were things from the shop on the park, set up in a display.

"Who are these three sorry looking travellers?" she said.

Lee clenched her teeth together, biting back a sarcastic reply. She'd been advised to keep quiet, and for once she felt it might be best to take that advice.

"Found them on the highway, just where we've been having all that trouble," the girl said.

Highway? Lee thought. *That's something I would say. Don't they call them something else here?*

Nemesis leaned forward in her chair and rested her forearms across her knees. She was tall and gangly, looked to be maybe in her early twenties. If that was true she'd been a little girl when the dinosaurs came, which meant she had been amazingly fortunate to survive all this time. Of course she could have been a recent arrival, but Lee didn't think so. New arrivals were always scared, disoriented, powerless.

Nemesis was in charge here, that much was obvious.

"Blade, bring that one closer," Nemesis said, holding out a long arm and pointing at Lee.

188

The teenage girl, Blade, took Lee by the arm to pull her closer to Nemesis. Lee pulled her arm out of Blade's grip.

"Hands off," she said. "I can walk all by myself."

Blade stared at Lee, narrowing her eyes slightly. Lee couldn't tell if Blade was squaring up to her or if there was a hint of a warning in that look.

Lee approached Nemesis, looking up at the young woman in the armchair.

"What's your name?" Nemesis said.

"Lee."

Nemesis curled her lip in disgust. "That's a rubbish name. I'm going to give you a better name than that."

"I don't want another name," Lee said. "I like the one I've got."

Nemesis ignored Lee and looked over her head. "What are they called?"

"Why don't you ask them yourself?" Lee said. "They can talk, just like anybody else."

"I ain't talking to them, I'm talking to you," Nemesis said. "Now tell me, what are their names?!"

Lee sighed. This was nothing but a display of power, Nemesis showing Lee who was top dog around here. Lee had seen it plenty of times at school. And it got boring very quickly.

"Will and Helen, and the dog's called Iggy. Say hello to Nemesis, Iggy."

"I don't like dogs," Nemesis said. "Maybe we could eat him."

"No!" Helen shouted.

"Somebody else already suggested that," Lee said. "It didn't turn out too well."

Nemesis lifted her chin slightly, gazing down at Lee once more. "How long you been here?"

189

"I'm not sure, it's getting difficult to tell. A week, maybe two."

"You tough, to survive this long. There just the three of you?"

"There is now," Lee said. "We had a friend who was taken by this man. We've been following them, trying to rescue him. We were catching up too, and then you guys came along and ruined it."

Nemesis smiled. "You don't take no shit from no one, do you?"

"I try not to," Lee said. "Especially not off bullies."

The smile disappeared from Nemesis's face. "You saying I'm a bully? Is that what you're saying?"

Lee shrugged, looked away.

"I ain't no bully, I've been looking after these children for years now, once the adults all left. Alton Towers, this is a place of refuge for children, like it always was and always will be. This is a place of safety, and you should thank the Wicker that you were picked up and brought back here for safekeeping."

"Safekeeping?" Lee yelled. "We were marched here as captives against our will. We didn't want safety here, we wanted to find our friend."

Nemesis leaned back in her armchair and waved her hand languidly at Lee.

Blade took Lee's arm. "You need to go now."

Again, Lee pulled her arm free.

"You need to stop touching me without my permission, or I might get angry," Lee hissed.

"Lee, leave it," Will said.

Lee turned around to face her friends. Helen was squatting by Iggy, holding on to him and whispering in his ear. Will was staring at Lee, his eyes round and wide with fear.

190

"We should go!" he hissed. "Before you make her angry."

Lee unclenched her fists by her sides.

"All right," she said. "Okay."

They walked back out of the cafeteria with Blade.

"What is her problem?" Lee said when they were outside, rounding on Blade.

"She's our leader, we do what she says," Blade replied.

"Yeah? And what does she say you're going to do about us?"

"I'm going to lock you up, until Nemesis has decided what we should do with you," Blade said.

"You can forget all about that," Lee said. "Come on guys, we're leaving right now."

Before any of them had moved, three teenage girls stepped out of the shadows. They were armed with bows and the arrows were pointed directly at Lee and Will and Helen.

Iggy growled.

"Shush, Iggy," Helen whispered, ruffling his fur.

"No, you're not going anywhere," Blade said. "Nemesis will keep you here until she has decided what she is going to do with you. She doesn't like the unknown, including visitors."

Lee was clenching and unclenching her fists again. She knew she had to stay calm, that she couldn't fly off the handle and wade into Nemesis with her fists flying. But it was hard. Her instinct was to fight, to go down fighting if need be. That was how she had always conducted herself at school, never giving an inch, never allowing herself to be labelled as weak, as a pushover.

But this was different. Back then, before the dinosaurs, Lee risked a beating and little more. That could be pretty bad sometimes, painful, humiliating even. But here, now, she risked more than a beating if she let her temper get the better of her.

She risked death.

Lee took a deep breath, let it out nice and slow. Blade seemed to sense that Lee had come to a decision, that she had come to the right decision, and she nodded at the archers to relax, stand down.

"Hand over your rucksacks," Blade said.

Lee looked at Will. Again the urge to say no, to fight, began bubbling up within her chest.

Will shook his head.

Lee knew exactly what that meant.

Don't resist, don't fight. Just do as you're told.

Lee shrugged the backpack off her shoulders and let it drop to the ground. Helen and Will both did the same.

"You'll get them back when Nemesis has made her decision about you," Blade said.

Lee said nothing, just stared at Blade, dead-eyed.

Blade walked them through the park, overgrown now with trees and climbing vines. They followed a footpath, pitted and bulging with large roots bursting through the tarmac. After about five minutes the forest suddenly opened up and Lee saw the towers, the ruined stately home that was the centre piece of the park.

"You'll be spending the night in here," Blade said as she took them inside and began climbing up a spiral, stone stairway.

The stone steps were worn away from hundreds of years of use, a depression in each one like the bottom of a bowl. As they climbed the tower they passed holes in the wall where there had once been windows. As they climbed higher and higher, Lee was able to see more of the jungle stretched out into the distance.

She hadn't seen much of England before the dinosaurs arrived and she was picked up and thrown twenty years into the future, but she was sure it hadn't looked like this. Again, there was that feeling that something was accelerating the climate, the change in the environment.

They reached the top of the tower and stepped out onto a stone landing. With no lights inside the old building, the landing was gloomy, and they had to watch where they put their feet as they walked along the uneven floor. There were flaming torches placed along the walls, the fire giving off a greasy, stinking smoke which made the teenagers cough. Lee started feeling sick.

"In here," Blade said, pushing open a wooden door.

The empty chamber had no torches on the walls, but it didn't need any. Not during the day anyway. There was no roof, and daylight streamed into the stone built room. The walls and floor were bare, and puddles had gathered on the floor along with piles of rotting leaves and branches.

"You're expecting us to stay here?" Lee said.

"Only for a few hours," Blade replied. "Until Nemesis has made her decision."

Lee looked at the others for support. Will looked utterly miserable, with his head bent and his body sagging in apparent defeat. Helen was focusing all her attention on Iggy, as though if she looked after him she could look after her herself, keep some semblance of control in her life.

Lee thought about shoving Blade out of the way, making a dash for the tower steps and down to the park. She dismissed the thought. There were too many kids around, too much in the way of obstacles.

"I'll be back for you later," Blade said. She stood in the doorway, her hand on the huge iron ring ready to close the door on them. "I'm sorry."

And with that she closed the door and slammed the bolt

into place.

"Dammit!" Lee hissed.

"They're going to kill us, aren't they?" Will said.

Lee rounded on him. "Don't start with that crap! We're going to find a way out of here, okay?"

"Oh yeah?" Will shouted back. "How the hell are we going to do that? We're at the top of a tower in a locked room surrounded by crazies with bows and arrows! And let's not forget about all the dinosaurs wandering around out there looking to gobble us up!"

"We're just going to give up then, is that it?" Lee yelled back. "Just wait for Blade to come back and tell us that Nemesis has decided we're for the chop? You're a waste of space, Will! You're a coward!"

Will suddenly ran at Lee and began pounding his fists against her torso and arms. Lee grabbed him and they both fell on the hard floor, kicking and punching at each other.

"Stop it!" Helen screamed.

Iggy started barking and ran over to the two teenagers.

"Iggy! Here!" Helen shouted.

Lee pulled herself away from Will. With the fight paused, Iggy returned to Helen's side. But he kept staring at the two teens, and he was growling quietly.

Lee and Will stood up, panting heavily.

"If you start fighting again, Iggy will attack you," Helen said, squatting by Iggy and stroking him. "If you're fighting, he sees you both as a threat to me."

Will wiped dirt off his face. He looked like he was crying.

"I'm sorry I called you a coward," Lee said. "You're not a coward."

"Yes, I am," Will said, and wiped his shirt sleeve across his face.

194

Lee didn't respond, she knew it was pointless. She looked up at the grey sky and then at the walls imprisoning them. The towers had been built with stone, and over the decades since it had been left to fall apart, since the roof had fallen in, the weather had beaten at the walls and carved foot and hand holes into them.

"I'm going to climb up to the top and take a look outside," Lee said, approaching a wall that looked like it might be the easiest one to climb. She was only partly interested in what she might be able to see. Secretly, Lee just wanted to find somewhere she could be on her own, even if only for a minute or two.

"And then what?" Will said, his voice quiet, subdued.

"I don't know," Lee replied, grabbing hold of her first hand hold. "I'll let you know when I get up there."

She took the wall slowly and carefully. The stone was gritty which made it hard for her fingers to get purchase sometimes. But there were plenty of hand holds, and places for her feet. Despite having to go slow, she still made it to the top in good time. Hoisting herself up on the edge, Lee sat on the top of the wall and took a good long look from her high view point.

The theme park had mainly been taken over by nature. The forest was a dense canopy below her, preventing her from seeing much at all. The wide footpath that Blade had walked them along was still visible, and Lee saw figures running backward and forward. In the distance she noticed movement and saw a long necked dinosaur raise its head from the covering of the forest. What were they called? They were herbivores, she was pretty sure of that.

Dotted around this new, young forest were the theme park rides, their metal, curved structures rising from the green like monuments to once modern gods. Gods who had abandoned

195

their servants, left them to fend for themselves in a hostile world.

"What can you see?" Helen said.

"Lots of trees," Lee replied.

She shifted position on the wall to look down at Helen and Will, and stopped. And stared.

"Guys?" Lee said. "I think I've found us an escape route."

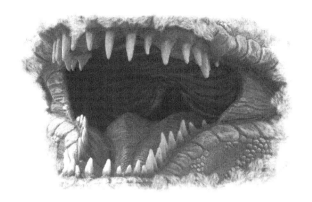

Chapter Nineteen

Daniel had seen faces at the school windows, he knew he had. Children mainly, their faces pressed against the glass, but some adult women too. He'd had the impression that the school was full of women and children. But now they were inside, standing in the school reception, it seemed as though the school was empty. Abandoned long ago and left to fall into disrepair.

Renton was leaning against the reception counter, breathing heavily. Sweat poured down his face, and his cheeks were scarlet with the effort he had made to get across the playground and into the building. He looked like he might just fall down at any moment.

"We have to hide," Nuo said.

"Why?" Emily said. "We're inside now, we're safe from the dinosaurs."

"It's not the dinosaurs I'm thinking about," Nuo said. "Those men who kept us prisoner, who were feeding us to the dinosaurs, they live here, I'm sure of it."

"I saw faces at the windows earlier," Daniel whispered. "Children, women."

197

"I suppose it's too much to hope that one of you guys went to this school and know your way around?" Nuo said.

Daniel and Emily shook their heads.

"I thought so," Nuo said, softly.

"Let's go do some exploring," Daniel said. "If we stay on the ground floor, we should be able to get out easily if we get into trouble."

"Yeah, we can't stay here, that's for sure."

"What about him?" Emily said, pointing at Renton.

"What about me, kid?" Renton growled. "I ain't finished yet, if that's what you're thinking."

"Come on, let's go," Nuo said.

Nuo took the lead, and they followed her down an empty corridor. Faded posters and signs hung in tatters from the walls, noticeboards that had once been packed with school notices now dirty and torn. The corridor was dark and gloomy as it didn't have any direct lighting and so they walked with their hands running down one wall to guide them.

They got to a door and Nuo pushed it open, its bottom edge scraping against years of dirt and grime. Once through the doorway they found themselves in another corridor, but this one had classrooms leading off either side. They walked in silence down the school hall, Renton's grunts and snuffles echoing off the walls and ceiling.

The classrooms looked like they'd had a gale force wind blow through them, picking up tables and chairs and throwing them everywhere. In one classroom there were sprays of blood against a wall.

They kept walking, Daniel's every nerve ending alert for the slightest movement or sound. He was about ready to jump out of his skin, he was so uptight. As he followed Nuo, watching her slender frame lead the way, it suddenly occurred to him that she had seemingly taken charge without anyone having said a word. But then, if that's how she wanted it Daniel wasn't going to complain. The dynamics had changed now, and Daniel no longer felt like he was being held captive by Renton. The teenager knew that he could simply run now, if he wanted to.

But not yet. Not now that he had been joined by Emily and Nuo.

They were approaching a junction in the corridor when Nuo froze and held up her hand, indicating that the others should stop walking.

Daniel heard voices, getting louder as the speakers drew closer. Two men, it sounded like, walking down the corridor from the left, that joined the one the teenagers were standing in. Nuo turned and looked behind Daniel.

"We'll never make it back down the hall," she whispered

Daniel pointed at the nearest classroom. The door was ajar.

As quietly as they could, Daniel and Nuo darted inside the classroom. Emily followed them, with Renton shuffling behind, wheezing and snorting.

"Can't he be quiet?" Emily hissed. "He sounds like a broken down steam train."

"Get down," Daniel whispered.

They all squatted behind the classroom wall, beneath the windows that looked into it from the hallway.

The voices grew louder.

"What the hell's been going on, Mick?"

"I dunno, it's that big ape if you ask me, the one with no nose and only one hand. He got free somehow, came back and let all the others go."

The two men stopped outside the classroom. Daniel stayed completely still and held his breath. Stared at Nuo, who stared round eyed right back at him.

199

"You sure about that? The big guy looked like he was about ready to fall down, you ask me."

"Yeah, but I've seen his type before, they just keep going long after you think they should be done for."

"Maybe. We need to round up the ones we can still find and get them back in the sports hall. We need to have food on the table for those dinosaurs when they come back tomorrow morning."

Daniel heard a zip being pulled.

"What are you doing?"

"I need a piss."

"You can't go out here, what do you think this is, a toilet?"

The two men laughed.

Daniel's body temperature dropped several degrees as he saw one of the men enter the classroom. He was standing side on to them, all he had to do was turn his head and he would be looking right at them.

Instead he turned his back on them. A few seconds later and Daniel heard the splatter of urine against a wall.

The other man joined him in the classroom, standing with his back to Daniel and the others and began urinating against the wall. Daniel hadn't thought he could grow any more terrified than he already was, but he did. This was the leader of the group, the tall, muscular one with the braided hair. It seemed impossible to Daniel that the two men would not see them now. Surely when they had finished relieving themselves and they turned to go they would see the group hiding behind them?

Daniel's thighs had begun to burn with pain. He was squatting, rather than sitting, on the floor and his muscles were starting to protest. The two men seemed to be taking forever to relieve themselves and Daniel wasn't sure how much longer he could stay still in this position. But the slightest movement might betray them.

"You think we should go and help Mick out there?" the man who had first come into the classroom said.

"Nah, it's about time the lazy bastard did some work."

They both chuckled.

"Besides," the leader continued, "the number of people we've been getting chucked at us recently is crazy. I don't think we need to worry, there'll probably be another storm tonight and we'll get some more."

They both finished relieving themselves. Daniel winced as he heard the two men zip up. The sound was like a death knell. Now they would both turn around and see Daniel and Emily and Nuo and Renton.

And that would be the end of them.

The two men stepped back from the wall, turning slightly to face each other. The leader pulled a battered packet of cigarettes out of his camouflage trouser pockets and offered one to the other man, saying, "Here, enjoy it, we haven't got many left."

The leader struck a match, cupped his hands around the flame as the two men both leaned in to light the ends of the cigarettes.

Daniel held his breath.

"Come on, let's get out there and see what's going on," the leader said.

They stepped out of the classroom. Daniel continued holding his breath as he listened to their footsteps receding.

Then he let his breath out in a whoosh of air.

"I thought we were done for," Nuo said, almost laughing with relief.

Renton was snorting and snuffling again.

201

He must have been holding his breath too, Daniel thought.

"We should get moving," Daniel said. "We've got to find somewhere to hide until it's safe to go outside again."

"Are you crazy?" Emily said. "We can't hide in here?"

"Where else are we going to hide then?" Daniel snapped. "As soon as those two see all the dinosaurs outside they'll be coming back in here, but we can't exactly go out there at the moment, can we?"

"Hey," Nuo said, placing a hand on Daniel's arm. "Chill, all right? She's just a kid."

Daniel shrugged Nuo's hand off his arm and poked his head out of the classroom door. The hall was clear.

"Follow me, quick!" he whispered.

They ran down the hall and took the left turn at the end. They were faced with another long corridor, classrooms leading off it.

"How big is this school?" Nuo said.

They ran down the hall, slowing as they came to windows looking into classrooms to check they were empty before running past them.

They stopped as they heard a high-pitched scream of terror.

A moment later a child appeared at the opposite end of the hall, sprinting towards them and screaming again.

Behind the child appeared a two-legged dinosaur, covered in feathers. Its clawed feet scrabbled on the floor as it changed direction to chase the child. It looked to be about waist high to an adult which made it taller than the child it was chasing. It also looked to have vicious claws and teeth.

"Oh no," Daniel muttered.

Nuo grabbed the child, a little girl of about three or four years old, as she tried to run past them and clasped her tight.

"Up the stairs!" she shouted.

Daniel hadn't noticed them before because they were still a few feet away. The problem was they were further down the hall towards the oncoming dinosaur.

We'll never make it, he thought. *And that thing will rip us to pieces.*

Something large and bulky hit Daniel in the side, almost pushing him over. It was Renton, letting out a guttural roar as he charged at the reptilian monster skittering towards them. He held a plastic school chair out in front of him and jabbed at the dinosaur's mouth, pushing it back.

Nuo was already taking advantage of the distraction and running up the stairs with the young girl in her arms. Emily was right behind her. With one last look at Renton, Daniel followed them.

They dashed up a couple of flights before Nuo had to stop, gasping with the exertion. The little girl was still screaming and beating her fists against Nuo's chest and shoulders. Nuo let go of her and she dashed off, through an open doorway.

"You're welcome," she gasped. "It was my pleasure saving your life, no need to thank me."

"We need to keep moving," Daniel said.

"You think those things can climb stairs?" Nuo said.

Daniel glanced back down the stairwell, and thought of the raptors learning how to climb the escalators. "I don't know. But I've seen raptors do it."

"I think he's right, we should keep moving," Emily said.

"Yeah, but which way?" Nuo said. "Do we go up another flight or do we follow that kid?"

Emily was already running up the next flight of steps.

"I guess we follow her," Daniel said.

They ran up the stairs behind Emily until they got to the top floor. Another corridor met them, but this one had windows to the outside world running down one wall. The three children gathered at the windows and looked down onto the school playground. It was filled with dinosaurs picking off the adults who had escaped from the sports hall but then hesitated, not knowing what to do next.

Daniel wanted to look away, to tear his eyes from the grisly spectacle, but he couldn't. The prehistoric monsters were ripping their victims apart in sprays of blood and flesh. There were too many dinosaurs for anyone to escape, and some of the creatures were fighting over scraps.

Emily cried out and threw her hands over her eyes. Nuo placed an arm around her shoulders.

Movement at the top of the stairs startled them. Daniel tensed, ready for another attack from a dinosaur.

Renton appeared through the doorway, breathing heavily. His flesh looked yellow and shiny, and his breathing seemed more tortured than ever.

"You need to go," he said, his voice little more than a raspy wheeze. "Those two men we saw earlier, they're on their way up here. They saw me fighting that thing downstairs."

Daniel's stomach plummeted to the floor once more. It felt like they were never going to get a break, a chance to get to safety.

"That thing's attacking them at the moment but it won't be long before they finish it off," Renton said. "And then they'll be after you. I'll hold them off as long as I can, but you need to run."

Nuo and Emily started backing up.

"Come on, quick!" Nuo hissed.

Daniel couldn't move. He kept staring at Renton.

"They'll kill you," he said.

Renton laughed, a wet, gurgling sound. "I'm already dying,

204

haven't you noticed? Get back to your father, kid. He's the only one can fix all this."

"We don't even know if he's still alive."

"He's alive," Renton said. "I know he is. Now get your ass out of here."

Daniel turned and ran.

Nuo and Emily had already reached the opposite end of the corridor. On their right was another set of stairs going down, and on their left two steps up to a closed door.

"Which way?" Nuo said.

"This way," said Emily, climbing the two steps and opening the door.

They stepped into a darkened, musty smelling room. When Nuo closed the door behind her, the room grew even darker. But there was some light coming from somewhere. Daniel realised there was a window set into one wall, but a blind had been pulled down and light was leaking around its edges.

Emily had already spotted the blind, and she was walking over to it.

"Wait!" Daniel hissed. "Just leave it down for now, we need to stay quiet."

Nuo slid to the floor with her back to the door. Emily stood in front of the blind, peering through the narrow gap between the blind and the wall.

Daniel stayed where he was, too scared to move. Part of him wanted Emily to lift the blind and shed light on the room. If there was someone, or something, else in there with them they would have no idea until it was on top of them. On the other hand they needed to make as little noise as possible, for fear of being discovered.

Footsteps, outside.

"That bastard bit me," a voice said.

205

"You should get the doc to look at that, you might have rabies now," another voice said.

"Yeah? And what's she going to do? Kiss it better? She's bloody useless, she is."

"All right, deal with that later, right? We've got to find those kids first."

The sound of the voices grew quieter as the two men headed down the stairs.

Nuo tipped her head back and let out a sigh of relief.

Emily opened the blind.

Light flooded the room, hurting Daniel's eyes and forcing him to squint.

The room was full of children.

All huddled at the far end, staring wide-eyed at the newcomers. They ranged in age from primary school to teens. They were all gaunt, their faces sharp with prominent cheek bones and round, sunken eyes. They had their knees drawn up to their chests, arms wrapped around their legs. And they were silent, totally and absolutely silent.

Nuo climbed to her feet. "Hey, we're sorry, we just needed to…"

She looked at Daniel, lost for words.

"The dinosaurs have gone," Emily said.

Daniel joined her at the window and looked down at the playground. Bodies, ripped and bleeding, lay scattered across the black tarmac, but Emily was right. The dinosaurs had obviously had their fill and left.

"I think we should leave," Nuo said. "Like, now."

The mass of huddled children were still staring silently at the three intruders, but it seemed to Daniel that Nuo was right. They needed to leave now, because it seemed to him that there was a growing atmosphere of hostility in the room. And that at

206

any moment that mass of silent children might suddenly come to life.

Daniel grabbed Emily's hand. "Come on, let's go."

Emily didn't protest.

They slipped out of the door and headed back along the corridor they way they had come in, ignoring the stairs directly outside the room. They slowed as they approached the figure lying on the floor, a dark pool of blood spreading around him.

As they stepped past the body, Daniel couldn't bear to look at Renton. He felt utterly conflicted right now, knowing the things Renton had done, and yet today he had sacrificed himself for Daniel and the others.

They ran down the stairs, pausing at the corners to make sure there was nobody coming up. At the bottom they took the hall back to the main reception, running as fast as they could past the empty classrooms. If they were discovered now, they would have to fight their way out.

And Daniel didn't fancy their chances.

They got to reception and the open school doors. A torn, bloody body lay in the doorway, one hand outstretched over the threshold as though still seeking sanctuary from the monster that had ripped it to pieces.

"You ready?" Nuo said.

Daniel nodded.

Emily simply sprinted for the open doorway.

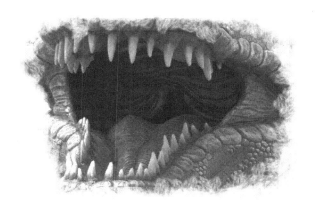

Chapter Twenty

Will wasn't sure, he wasn't sure at all, but then it seemed like he was sure about nothing these days. He'd thought the world was bad enough before he got thrown twenty years into a dinosaur dominated future. But now, looking back on those days when all he had to worry about was climate change and avoiding the school bullies, it seemed like a lazy stroll in the park.

Living now, in this time, in this moment, was the hard part. Trying to keep from getting eaten was bad enough, but then having to deal with other people, other children, who were intent on killing him, was much worse.

Will's neck was beginning to hurt, having to keep his head craned back to look at Lee. She was sat on the top of the wall still, looking down at Will and Helen and waiting for their answer.

"Come on, guys, we can do this," she said.

"I don't know," Will replied, and immediately hating himself for saying it.

"What else are we going to do? Wait for Blade and her pals to come back and kill us? You heard what she said, that

Nemesis woman is going to decide what to do with us, and I don't think she's going to want to keep us hanging around."

Will hung his head, tired of looking up all the time. He knew Lee was right. But the thought of climbing up that wall, then leaving the wall and climbing onto the branch of the huge tree next to the towers before inching along that to the main trunk and then getting onto the rope walkway that formed part of the high-ropes experience, left him giddy with nerves. Even that wouldn't be the end of it as they would have to make their way along the footpaths along the treetops until they could find their way down somewhere close to an escape route out of the park.

It was all right for Lee. She was the physical one, the Tomboy. What about Helen? Will had no idea if she was able to do something like this.

And at that moment, looking at Helen crouched on the floor with her arms around Iggy, Will realised Helen wouldn't come with them anyway.

He craned his head to look at Lee once more. "What about Iggy? He can't climb up the wall, or crawl along tree branches. He's not a cat."

Will heard Lee say something, but didn't catch what it was. He was pretty sure he hadn't wanted to hear it, either.

"Okay, okay," Lee said. "I'll get out this way and then I'll come back up for you."

"They'll catch you again," Will said. "You don't have a chance."

"Wait there," Lee said, and disappeared from view.

Will kept looking up, his neck aching as he kept his head craned back. After a few moments he saw the leaves and the branches rustling. Lee was on the tree.

"Will she really come back?" Helen said.

"Yeah," Will replied. "She'll be back."

* * *

The sweat poured down Lee's face, stinging her eyes. This was harder than she had thought it would be. The branches swayed beneath her and her feet kept slipping off the smooth bark. At all times she kept one hand gripped firmly onto a branch while the other hand sought out the next hold. The branches up here were dense with leaves. On the one hand that was good, as she was unlikely to be seen from the ground. But on the other hand they were too dense, and she had to fight her way through, every inch of the way.

Lee wiped at her face. How far was she from the trunk? It was hard to see, having to keep blinking her eyes free of sweat. She couldn't be too far, surely? Gripping a branch with both hands, Lee hauled herself further along. The leaves shook and made rustling noises and Lee heard something snap.

She paused.

Slow down, she thought. *If they discover you up here, they'll probably just shoot you down instead of trying to catch you again.*

Lee took a deep breath and exhaled slowly.

Edged along the thick branch once more. She could see the massive trunk now, and the ropes and metal clamps bolted into it that formed part of the high-ropes experience. About ten feet beneath that she could see the wooden platform.

Not far now.

Lee had to bend down to get beneath a thick, gnarly branch that crossed her path. She gripped it tight as she bent double, her foot slipping and twisting on the branch below. The leaves made those rustling sounds again, surely giving her away to anyone who happened to be nearby. Once she had managed to straighten up again on the other side of the branch, Lee paused and listened.

Nothing. No shouts of alarm, no running feet, no arrows flying at her.

Lee continued inching her way along the branch. It was growing much thicker now as she drew nearer to the trunk. She was able to move a little faster.

When she reached the tree's massive trunk, she wrapped her arms around it, hugging it like a dear friend. The bark was rough against her skin, against her cheek, but she didn't care. For the first time since leaving the safety of the tower wall, Lee looked down. The ground was a terrifying distance away. She saw movement down there, between the branches, kids walking to and fro.

Further out, in the distance, she could see some of the park's rides. She recognised the Smiler, its bright black and yellow swirling designs now looking faded and dirty. Beyond that she saw the car parks, and queues of cars waiting to leave. Lee could almost hear horns being pressed, the long wails sounding a note of impatience and frustration.

What must it have been like, that day? A sunny day, full of screams and laughter suddenly dampened with the arrival of the storm. And then the screams would have started up again, but not the laughter.

Lee looked away, trying hard not to imagine the scene. She looked down at the platform beneath her, circling the thick tree trunk. It seemed an awful long way off. It was thick with a layer of mouldy leaves and twigs. And there seemed to be what looked like pale mushrooms growing through the composting vegetation. The only way Lee could see of getting down there was by dropping onto the platform from where she was. But she didn't know how strong the platform was after all these years. When she dropped onto it, she might just crash straight through and continue plummeting to the ground.

Lee looked around for another branch she could climb onto, one that was lower down the trunk, nearer to the platform. There was nothing. All the branches had been sawn off to enable people to stand on the platform before they continued their trek across the treetops on the ropes. There weren't even any hand or foot holds along the trunk for Lee to use to climb down.

The only way down was by falling.

Lee swallowed.

She would have to hang from the branch she was standing on to reduce the distance she fell.

Or, she could go back the way she had come, back to the tower. Back to Will and Helen and Iggy.

Lee shook her head. "No, I'm not going back. Come on, you can do this. It's easy."

She looked down at the platform again.

Yep, as easy as falling off a log. Or in this case, a branch high up in a tree, and possibly falling to your death.

Lee lowered herself down until she was squatting on the branch. Holding tight onto whatever she could grab hold of she pulled her feet out from beneath her and swung her legs out into thin air so that she was sitting on the branch.

Sweat had popped out on her forehead again and ran down her face. She wiped angrily at her eyes and forehead.

Next she turned herself around, so that she was hunched over the branch on her stomach. Holding on tight, Lee slowly let herself go, the bark scraping against her arms and chest.

Finally she was hanging from the branch by her hands, her body swaying gently.

And now she didn't want to let go.

This had been a stupid idea. Stupid and dangerous. What the hell had she been thinking?

Lee tried pulling herself back up, but she was too tired, too weak. The muscles in her arms started burning. Her fingers were slipping on the branch.

Just let go!

She fell.

For a moment she was free. The air rushing past her face, cooling her cheeks and drying the sweat, felt good. It was a moment of escape from responsibility, from being tied down, not just to the ground but the others.

And then she smashed into the wooden platform. The mouldy leaves and twigs, the composted mulch that had gathered there over the decades, shot into the air beneath the impact and she was covered in it. Her booted feet crashed through the rotten boards and her legs swung freely. Lee had fallen through the wooden slats up to her stomach before she had stopped her fall by grabbing at the edges of the platform. She hung on tight, her feet kicking the tree trunk as her legs flailed helplessly.

"Did you hear that?" she heard someone say, someone on the ground.

Lee willed herself to stay still. She bit down on her tongue, mentally commanding her legs to stop their wild kicking.

"Look at all this," she heard someone else say.

They were right beneath her. If they looked up, when they looked up, would they see her? Would they see her feet and her legs?

"It's part of the high-ropes platform. It must be rotten."

"Can you see it?"

"No, the leaves are too thick, I can't see anything."

Lee kept biting her tongue. She could taste blood. She

213

didn't care.

"Do you think we should tell Nemesis?"

"No way. She's crazy, I just keep away from her as much as possible."

"We'd better get moving, we're going to be late."

Lee listened as the two speakers began walking away, their voices growing fainter. Late for what?

The teenager pushed that thought out of her head as she concentrated on hauling herself up through the hole she had made. She moved slowly, trying hard not to cause any more damage or make any more noises that might give her away. Once she was back up on the wooden platform, she sat with her back against the tree trunk and breathed heavily, letting her heart rate settle down into a regular rhythm.

The smell of rotting leaves was thick in her throat. The platform ran all the way around the trunk, and a little further to her left Lee could just see what she had thought were pale mushrooms. Getting on her hands and knees she shuffled a little closer for a better look.

And froze.

Those weren't mushrooms.

They were eggs. Huge, pale eggs covered in a fine tracery of zigzagging lines.

Lee glanced up, fearful of seeing some monstrous bird descending upon her, claws out and ready to shred her to pieces. If the mother of these things came back now, she would assume Lee was there to steal the eggs and would attack her. It was time to get off the platform and onto the rope bridge across to the next tree.

Lee shuffled over to the rope bridge. It didn't look damaged or worn at all, which was the good news. The bad news was that Lee would be fully exposed to view as she crossed it. The rope bridge ran across one of the main thoroughfares between the rides. Anyone looking up would see her.

Except, if she stayed down low and crawled across. The base of the bridge was like a cargo net made of thick ropes. Someone lying flat out across it would only be seen from below by people actively looking. But a quick glance up would reveal nothing.

Lee got down on her front and began inching her way onto the thick lengths of rope entwined around one another and creating diamond shaped gaps. With every movement she made the bridge swung slightly. Lee paused for a moment. Instead of using her whole body, including her legs, to shift herself along, she had to think of some other way.

Stretching her arms out in front, Lee laced her fingers through the gaps in the ropes and dragged herself forward.

The bridge swayed slightly, but much less than before.

Using this technique, Lee continued her journey across the rope bridge towards the next platform bolted to a tree.

Fortunately the park was quiet. Lee wondered if maybe everyone was at a meeting, and that was what one of the speakers beneath her had meant when he had said they were late. But if that was the case, what were they meeting about?

Lee and Will and Helen, obviously.

Lee suspected this might be their best chance to escape, maybe even their only chance. She had to get down on the ground so that she could run to the towers and rescue Will and Helen. That meant finding a platform on a tree that had access to the ground.

Lee paused.

Surely they all had safe access to the ground? They would need to, in case someone needed bringing down.

215

Lee swore. She should have stayed where she was, looked for a ladder or some other method of getting safely down.

Too late now, she was over halfway along the rope bridge. She just had to keep going. But her fingers were growing tired and sore, and her shoulders were aching from the constant tension of dragging herself along. Shoving all thoughts of tiredness and pain aside, Lee dug deep and continued dragging herself towards the next tree.

When she finally got there, she clambered onto the platform and sank down to the wooden boarding on her back, grateful for a moment's respite. There wasn't time to be lying around feeling sorry for herself though. If every one of the kids who lived here were in a meeting with Nemesis right now, then Lee had to capitalise on that and get herself and the others out.

Dragging herself upright, Lee looked for a way of getting down from the tree. There was nothing obvious, until she leaned out, over the platform edge, and looked down. There, running alongside the tree trunk was a ladder. But it was underneath the platform, so how could she get to it?

Like the other platform this one was covered with mouldy debris from the branches overhead. Lee sifted her hands through it about where she thought the ladder was and revealed a trap door. She pulled it open.

With one swift glance out across the park to make sure there was no one around, Lee lowered herself through the square hole, her feet finding the ladder almost immediately, and began climbing down.

Once on the ground she began running towards the towers. Even though every one else might be in a meeting with Nemesis, Lee realised there would probably be a couple of guards keeping an eye on their prisoners.

She was right. There were two of them, both holding bows,

216

standing at the top of the wide, stone steps leading to the entrance. They looked bored. Lee stood and watched them from her hiding place behind one of the many trees. Not that she needed to try too hard at keeping out of sight. The two boys who had been given guard duty weren't exactly trying their best to keep a look out. And, of course, they wouldn't expect to be watching for someone on the outside, they were guarding their prisoners inside the towers.

Lee decided to take a look around, see if she could find another way inside. Keeping low she was able to run around to the side of the old building whilst remaining hidden by the long grass. There was a broad walkway running up beside the towers which had access to a large courtyard. From the courtyard was an open doorway into a massive, empty hall. The inside was almost like a church, with stained glass windows and a decorated, vaulted ceiling. Amazingly the stained glass windows were intact.

On the other side of the hall was a small door. Lee grasped the iron rung and tried pulling at it. The door refused to budge. She tried pushing, and the door ground open.

Lee froze, scared that the noise might attract the two boys at the front of the building. Then, realising she was stupid for just standing there, waiting to be discovered, she pushed herself through the gap between the door and the old, rotting frame and into the cool darkness.

Lee left the door open slightly, not wanting to risk making any more noise but also needing the little bit of light the gap gave her. Walking quickly through the gloom, running a hand along the rough stonework of the wall beside her, Lee tried to get her bearings.

It was no good. Between her escape route from the top of the towers and through the trees to her unorthodox entry back inside, she had no idea how to get back to her friends. But the building was mostly a ruin, which at least cut down her choices. And the first thing she had to do was simply find a way to get upstairs.

Creeping through the ruin, alternating between gloomy passageways and empty rooms filled with light from large windows, Lee began to worry she would never find her way back to Will and Helen. At one point she found herself back outside again, in what looked like it might have once been a garden area alongside a long greenhouse. All the glass had had been shattered, and her boots crunched over the broken glass as she walked.

Lee doubled back and finally found herself at the bottom of the narrow stone steps she had been taken up with Will and Helen. The boys guarding the entrance were close by, Lee could hear the murmur of their voices as they talked, although she couldn't make out what they were saying.

Quietly, Lee took the worn steps two at a time. Once at the top she found herself back in the gloomy corridor, lit only by the flaming torches shoved into ragged gaps in the walls. The door to the makeshift prison had been bolted shut, but there was no lock on the bolt.

Lee pulled it back and opened the door.

Will and Helen were standing in the middle of the chamber, Iggy by Helen's side.

Will actually smiled.

"I told you she'd be back," he said.

"Let's get out of here," Lee said.

She told them about the two boys guarding the entrance.

"I don't know why they're bothering though," she whispered. "There are more ways out of here than I can count."

Lee took them back down to the area that had once been a

218

garden and greenhouse, at the back of the ruined building. It seemed to Lee that the light wasn't as good as it had been when she was here earlier. She looked up at the sky, filled with clouds.

Will looked up too. "Do you think there's going to be another storm?"

"I don't know," Lee said. "Maybe."

Iggy whined and Helen ruffled the fur on the back of his neck.

"Let's get moving," Lee said. "It looks like everyone's in a meeting with Nemesis right now. We're not going to have a better chance of escaping."

The three teens ran through the long grass until they got to the outer wall of the gardened area. A section of the wall had collapsed and led out onto one of the main thoroughfares. Lee took a quick look outside and then began running, signalling the others to follow her. They crossed the pitted, cracked tarmac path and disappeared into the long grass where there had once been immaculately kept lawns.

"I think we need to get back to the main entrance, unless anyone knows of another way out?" Lee said.

Will and Helen both shook their heads.

They kept moving. Lee wasn't sure she was heading in the right direction, but she knew she had to keep moving. Anything was better than standing still, doing nothing. The grass made a soft swishing noise as they pushed their way through it.

Suddenly they were back outside in open space again. A massive structure rose up in front of them, curved lengths of metal twisting and contorted, rising and falling in a concrete pit.

"It's the Smiler," Will whispered.

A giant, black and yellow face grinned maniacally at them. Perched on top of the Smiler sign was a big, black crow. With a single caw it lifted into the air and flew away.

219

"Which way to the exit, do you know?" Lee said.

Will shook his head.

"We'll never find our way out of this place, it's like a maze!" Helen said.

Lee looked back up at the house, just visible still between the trees and the long grass.

"Maybe we should head in the direction the ruin is facing," Will said, looking at the house too.

"Yeah, that's just what I was thinking," Lee replied.

They had run away from the towers to its left, but if they headed in the direction, it faced they might well find themselves at the exit. It would make sense that the house faced the entrance and exit to the park.

They scurried along the perimeter fence to the Smiler ride, past the entrance. Before they had got very far they stopped, frozen in their tracks by the sound of voices drawing closer.

Lee stared wide eyed at Will. They were stuck out in the open with nowhere to hide. Any second now the two teenagers who were talking would round the corner and see the fugitives.

"In here!" Helen hissed.

Lee and Will turned to see Helen and Iggy disappearing through the gate to the Smiler. They followed her and ran down the long passageway between the chain-link fences until they reached an underground passageway.

With one last glance behind at the darkening sky and the two figures who appeared on the thoroughfare beside the Smiler, Lee stepped into the gloom of the tunnel.

She hoped they were doing the right thing.

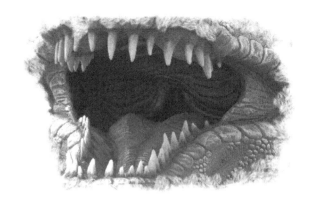

Chapter Twenty-One

They ran.

They simply kept their heads down and ran, sprinting for safety.

Like animals, they weren't running for something or to somewhere they were just running away from the school. From the horrors of what they had seen, of what waited for them if they were caught again and taken back.

Despite being the youngest and the smallest, Emily kept up with Daniel and Nuo. They dashed between houses and through overgrown gardens thick with strange plants and chirruping insects. They bolted down streets littered with wrecks of cars and more strange vegetation fighting its way through the erupted tarmac. The sweat began pouring off Daniel's face and his chest began to hurt, but still they ran.

Finally, in a back garden overgrown with thick-stemmed plants that towered over the children, they halted and took refuge in a broken down shed. Although there wasn't much of the construction left, there was enough that, together with the unusual plants, they were hidden from casual view.

221

The three youngsters collapsed on a tarpaulin-covered mound, unable to speak while they struggled to get their breathing under control once more.

Emily was the first to speak. "What do we do now?"

Nuo shrugged, still panting heavily.

"I think we should keep heading north," Daniel said.

"What for?" Emily said.

"My father, he lives up there, he might be able to help us."

Emily stared at Daniel, her face streaked with sweat. "Yeah? Well my mum will be back at the motorway station now, which you took me away from, and she will definitely be able to help us."

Daniel closed his eyes. He didn't want to have this argument. He wasn't even sure if Emily's mother was real or just some kind of wish fulfilment on her part. But one thing he was sure of, his father was more likely to be able to help them than this mythical mother figure of Emily's could, even if she turned out to be real.

"What about you, Nuo?" he said, his eyes still closed. "What do you want to do?"

"I want food and water," Nuo said. "I want to go back home and crawl in my bed and fall asleep, and then I want to wake up tomorrow and realise this has just been a terrible nightmare."

Daniel opened his eyes and looked over at Nuo. "Yeah, I know."

They sat in silence for a while, gazing at the overgrown garden, listening to the wildlife hidden deep inside the undergrowth. It wasn't just the chirruping and the ticking noises, but the sounds of movement, of things shifting and stirring.

"We can't stay here," Daniel said, at last. "They might come looking for us."

"Have we agreed what we're going to do?" Nuo said, looking at Emily.

The young girl turned her head away and said nothing.

Daniel sighed. "Let's head a bit further out, away from the school, and then maybe we can break into a house, spend the night indoors at least while we think about what we're going to do next."

And we need to find food and water, Daniel thought. He doubted it had occurred to the other two yet, but they were now without any supplies at all. They needed to find something to eat and drink soon. The utter futility of it swept over Daniel and almost sent him into a tailspin of despair. This was his life now, desperately searching for something to drink, something to eat, whilst trying to avoid being eaten himself.

"Why don't we just stay here?" Nuo said, pointing at the house that backed onto the garden they were sitting in. They could just see it over the tops of the huge, swaying flowers.

"No, I don't like it here, we're too close to the school, to those people," Daniel said.

"We should go back to the motorway," Emily said, turning to face the others. "At least then we'll know which direction to walk. We might be able to get another car."

"That's a good idea," Daniel said. "And the motorway takes us north—"

"Or back the way we came," Emily said.

Daniel snapped his mouth shut, before he started arguing with the girl. What was it to him if she wanted to go back? Why should he try to stop her? But he knew he couldn't just leave her on her own. As resourceful and tough as she was, she wouldn't last long by herself. Daniel decided to say nothing for the time being. At least while they were walking back towards the M6 they had time to think, to delay making any decisions.

It was only once they reached the motorway they would have to choose.

Daniel stood up. "Let's get going, before it grows dark."

Nuo joined him, stretching. "I would so love to just find a nice, clean bed I could sink into. I haven't slept properly in days."

Daniel looked at the wall of the thick stemmed, strange flowers in front of them. He hadn't paid much attention to them when they had pushed their way through to the back of the garden, seeking shelter, somewhere to hide. But now he had a chance to examine them he realised they unsettled him. Their thick stems shooting straight up, like sunflowers. But these were shiny, like they were coated in some sort of oily substance. Large, wide leaves hung from the stems, their green surfaces shiny with the same greasy film. And the flowering heads at the top of the stems, they sort of did look like sunflowers except they were purple. Something shifted inside the teenager, looking at those flowers. Something unnerved him.

Mostly though, Daniel didn't like they way they seemed to crowd in on the teenagers. It was almost as if they were closer now than they had been when he first got here. Which was stupid.

Wasn't it?

The other thing that unsettled him was the sounds of movement from within the mass of flowers. Nothing poked its head out at them yet, baring its teeth in a nasty, hungry smile. But there was so much movement going on in there, and Daniel could see the flowers swaying as the things, whatever they were, scurried and darted here and there, that the teenager had begun to wonder why they hadn't seen anything.

Why nothing had tried to eat them yet.

"What's wrong?" Nuo said.

Daniel hesitated. If he asked Nuo if she thought those flowers had drawn closer in on them while they had been sitting here, what would she think? That he had gone crazy, that's what. And yet . . .

"It's those flowers, isn't it?" Nuo said. "Have you noticed it too?"

"You mean, how they seem to have a life of their own?" Daniel said, and cringed inside, still half-expecting Nuo to laugh at him.

"Yeah, exactly," Nuo replied. "All those sounds we can hear of things shuffling around in there, I don't think there is anything. I think it's the plants making all that noise."

"But how?" Daniel said. "There's no wind—"

Emily screamed. A long, thick tendril had wrapped itself around the young girl's ankle and it was wrapping itself around her lower leg.

"Get it off me! Get it off me!"

Before Daniel had chance to react, he gasped as a slimy vine curled itself around his neck and began squeezing.

Daniel grabbed the thick stem and pulled at it as it began to tighten its grip on his throat. Already his breathing was constricted, he was choking and spluttering. Emily screamed again, but Daniel was too busy fighting off the thing trying to strangle him to see what was happening. More things wrapped themselves around his legs and his arms. The strange flowers seemed to be right on top of him now, their purple heads blocking out the daylight as they loomed over him.

The things dragged him to the ground. More roots and vines, smelling of damp earth and compost, squirmed over him, cocooning him in their grip.

Panic had seized him and he thrashed about as much as he

could and tried to scream, but managed little more than a strangled gurgle.

All of a sudden a scream did fill his ears. A scream of anger and defiance.

Nuo! With what sounded like a war cry, Nuo swung a garden spade over her head and then brought it down with a sickening snap. The tendrils around Daniel's neck went limp. Nuo swung the spade again, slamming it edge down into the ground. Another of the tendrils, this time around his left arm, went limp and fell off him.

When Daniel sat up he saw that Nuo was slicing the roots, the vines or whatever they were, in half with the sharp edge of the spade.

Emily screamed again as more thick, snake-like plant tendrils unfurled towards her. Daniel grabbed a garden rake and began slashing at the things attached to Emily. The rake wasn't as effective as the spade, and Daniel had to keep chopping at the roots until they let go of Emily.

Another curled around Nuo's wrist and she screamed and dropped the spade. Daniel threw the rake to the ground and picked up the spade, hacking at the long, thick, writhing roots.

Emily had shrunk into the shadows at the back of the shed. Daniel pulled Nuo free and dragged her deeper into the shed too.

The tall flowers swayed in front of them, their stems glistening, their roots squirming out of the soil like pale, thick worms.

Daniel looked up. There was a large hole in the shed's wooden roof. It was the only way out, the monstrous purple flowers had blocked any other route to freedom.

Nuo and Emily both had the same idea. Working together, Daniel and Nuo gave Emily a leg up so that she could climb through the hole in the roof. The two teens were showered with slivers of rotten wood and bugs as Emily climbed out. As soon as she was on the roof she jumped down, behind the shed.

"You next," Daniel said to Nuo.

The teenage girl nodded and put her foot in Daniel's cupped hands. He gave her a boost as she reached up and pulled herself out. More of the shed's rotten roof gave way and Nuo almost fell, before wriggling her way up and out on her stomach.

Daniel yelled as a root curled around his ankle and tightened its grip. This one felt like it had tiny teeth or claws, it was so painful. The root squeezed at his bruised ankle, and Daniel screwed his eyes shut as tears ran down his cheeks.

Nuo reached down.

"Grab my hand!" she yelled.

Another tentacle whipped around Daniel's other ankle.

He looked up at Nuo, wide eyed. "I'm caught, they've got me!"

"Use the spade!" Nuo shouted.

Daniel had forgotten about the spade. He grabbed it off the ground and attacked the squirming roots with its sharp edges. As the spade's blade cut through the sinuous roots, it seemed to Daniel that he could hear a high-pitched scream of pain, just on the edge of his hearing. He kept hacking at them until his legs were free.

Dropping the spade, Daniel reached up and Nuo grabbed his hands and pulled. Daniel's legs kicked, and he swung as Nuo hauled him up.

"You've got to help me!" she screamed. "I can't hold on any longer."

The boy's foot found purchase on a shelf just as his one hand slipped out of Nuo's. He managed to grab hold of the edge of the shed's roof, but the rotten wood crumbled beneath his fingers. Nuo still had hold of his other hand and continued pulling him up, but both of their hands were slippery with sweat and Daniel could feel her grip on him loosening.

Using his one foot on the shelf to push up and kicking out with his free leg, the teenager managed to thrust himself a little higher and got his arm out of the hole and onto the shed roof. With Nuo's help he hauled himself out, even as more of the rotten wood crumbled beneath him.

"Let's get off here before the whole thing collapses," Nuo gasped.

Daniel didn't need telling twice. The two teens jumped off the roof and landed in a lane between the houses. Daniel cried out as the impact drove a hot spike of pain through his ankles.

Emily was waiting for them.

"Which way?" she said.

Daniel panted, struggling to get his breathing under control. "I don't know, give me a minute."

"Err, no," Emily said, her voice mocking. "We don't have a minute."

Daniel looked up. The plant tendrils were slithering out of the shed roof and down the back wall towards them. Now and then they paused to weave from side to side, as though using whatever senses they might have had to detect their prey.

The three children began running down the lane.

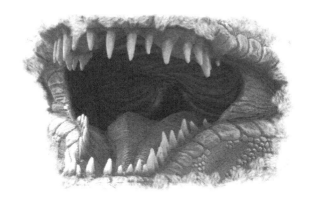

Chapter Twenty-Two

Hiding down in the concrete pit in the bowels of the Smiler ride, Will could hear them. The kids who lived in the theme park, out of their meeting now, were running around screaming and whooping. Sounded like they were glad to be out. Will couldn't imagine that sitting in a meeting chaired by Nemesis would be much fun.

The question was though, what had the meeting been about? Presumably they had been discussing their captives, and what to do about them. Will had the feeling that the meeting would have been less of a discussion and more of a decision taken by Nemesis, and Nemesis alone. She didn't come across as the touchy-feely type who loved listening to others' points of view.

Will, Lee, Helen and Iggy were all hiding in the basin where the cars would have come to a stop for riders to get on and off. There was a Smiler car stationary at the point where the cars entered the boarding station and a second frozen in the act of travelling around the bend and on its way to its first incline.

There were no remains of riders in either of the cars.

The teenagers were crouching under the track where there was just enough space for them to hide.

"How are we going to get out of this place now?" Will said.

"We're going to have to wait until it goes dark," Lee said. "When everyone's asleep we can sneak out."

Iggy growled, a low, ominous sound in the back of his throat.

"You've got to keep him quiet," Lee said.

"I know, I know," Helen replied, stroking Iggy along his back. "It's just that he's scared, he thinks we're in danger."

"Well he's right," Will said. "We are in danger."

"Just keep him quiet," Lee said. "If he starts barking and making a racket, he'll give us away and we'll be caught again."

Helen bent down over Iggy and hushed him, whispering soothingly to him.

"How long till it goes dark?" Will said.

Lee and Will both looked up at the sky, visible between the rails of the track looping overhead. "I don't know, not long I don't think."

"Thing is, if anybody goes to the towers to check on us and finds we're not there, how long do you think we can hide from them?"

Lee blew out a long breath in frustration. "We've just got to do our best. Unless you've got a better idea."

"No," Will said, and lowered his head to look at the concrete floor.

He snapped his head back up again at the shrill sound of the whistle. Three long blasts and then silence.

Complete silence.

"That's about us," Lee whispered. "They've discovered we're gone."

"What are we going to do?" Helen whispered. "We can't

hide down here, they'll find us."

"We'll just have to keep moving," Lee replied.

Iggy started growling again, louder this time. Helen stroked him and tried soothing him.

"Look, there's a door down there," Will said. "It looks like an access point of some kind, for the workers. Maybe we can hide in there."

The three teens shuffled along the concrete basin beneath the track until they reached the metal door that Will had seen. Lee pushed it and it opened inwards. The interior was dark and smelt of rust and something else, a rotting, decomposing smell.

The teens looked at each other.

Above them they could hear distant shouts. It sounded like the children were being organised into search parties.

"I think it's our best chance," Lee said.

Without another word they climbed through the doorway one by one. Lee was last and once she had pushed the door shut behind her, the darkness became complete. Will blinked, trying to focus on something, to make something out in the gloom. Slowly, shapes became discernible. Light was leaking in from somewhere, although where from Will couldn't tell.

"We'll have to go carefully," Lee whispered.

"Do you think there is another exit?" Will said.

"I don't know, but it might be worth exploring."

They shuffled forward, painfully slowly, being careful not to bump their heads into the thick, metal framework that ran diagonally through the space and up through the roof. Will stepped in something wet and squishy. Whatever it was released a hideous stink and Will threw his hands over his face to try to stop the smell.

"Ouch!" Helen gasped.

"What's wrong?" Lee whispered.

"I banged my head."

"This is stupid," Will hissed. "Even if those psycho kids don't catch us we're going to have an accident down here and probably die."

"Just walk carefully," Lee said. "We can do this."

Will clenched his teeth, telling himself not to reply with a sarcastic comment. Lee was always so gung-ho, so typically American, it annoyed the hell out of him. Sometimes all Will wanted to do was lie down and give up, but Lee had to keep him moving, keep him trying. It was like she enjoyed suffering or something.

But Will knew that if he made a comment, then they would just argue. And Will was tired of arguing, tired of talking and running and hiding.

The teens all threw their arms in front of their eyes as light exploded around them.

This is it, Will thought. *They've caught us.*

"Sorry bout that, sorry, sorry, sorry bout that."

The light moved, became less harsh. A man, holding a torch. He was wearing neon yellow work clothes and a yellow hard hat, but they hung off him like rags on a scarecrow.

"Follow, follow, follow," he paused and screwed his face up. "Follow Smiler."

With that he turned and walked away, the bright torchlight illuminating his path. The teens followed him, ducking beneath the girders and low sections. Iggy was growling again, but Helen had hold of him by his collar.

"Do you think he's safe to be with?" Will whispered. "Can we trust him?"

"We don't have much choice," Lee whispered back.

They didn't go far before the man stopped and abruptly sat down on a striped deckchair. He shook his head and started

232

laughing, and the hardhat swiveled around on his skull because it was too big for him.

"It's been a long, it's been, it's been a long time since Smiler had company," he said. "Company? A long time. Company."

The teens glanced at each other.

"Who are you?" Will said.

The man looked up at Will, and his expression was a blank, as though the question made no sense to him.

"What's your name?" Lee said.

The man's eyes widened as he realised what was being asked of him. He stretched his mouth into a wide, crazy grin, showing off his brown, rotten teeth.

"Smiler," he said, through gritted teeth.

"I don't like this," Helen whispered.

Will didn't like it much either, but at least the man seemed friendly enough.

The man had led them into what could only be described as a den of sorts, a tiny space in a corner of the basement surrounded by boxes and pallets piled high like walls. Everything the man had collected was merchandise from the shops on the Alton Towers site. There were T-shirts and hoodies bearing the Alton Towers logo, the Smiler, Nemesis, Oblivion, the Wicker Man, there were plastic water bottles, pink, blue, red, lunch boxes, caps, board games, phone covers, miniature statues, and sweets, so many brightly coloured sweets.

Will jumped when he heard the whistle again above ground. The teens looked up as they heard movement above them.

Smiler started shaking his head, stilling grinning that loony smile.

"Not down, not down, down here, no not down here, they don't, down, not down here they don't come," he said, and his voice trailed off as he continued muttering the words.

Lee squatted down in front of Smiler. "How long have you lived down here?"

"Oh, oh, oh!" He dropped his torch on the concrete floor and put his face in his hands.

"He's crazy," Will said. "He's freaking me out."

"I know," Lee said. "He's freaking me out too, but he might know a way out of the theme park, a secret way out."

Smiler was rocking back and forth, sounded like he was crying into his hands.

"It's all right," Lee said, reaching out a hand to comfort him. "I didn't mean to upset you."

When her hand touched his shoulder the man leapt to his feet and backed away, his tear-stained eyes wide with fear.

Lee held her hands up, palm out. "I'm sorry, I scared you, I'm sorry."

"Children bad," Smiler said. "Children bad, bad, Smiler not like children."

"Which children are bad?" Will said.

"Children upstairs, children on rides, on rides, children bad."

"Why are the children bad?" Lee said.

"Hurt Smiler, hurt Smiler lots."

The door clanged open and light spilled through the darkness.

"Hey, Smiler, are you down here?"

Smiler stood up and pointed into the darkness, away from the direction of the door.

"That way, that way," he hissed. "Go that, go that way."

Lee grabbed the torch from where Smiler had dropped it on the floor and the three teenagers plunged into the darkness.

"They're down here!"

Lee kept her head low as she stumbled between pipes and

234

cables and past machinery in cages. She didn't dare turn her head to check the others were with her in case she collided into a pillar or a wall. She could hear the kids streaming through the doorway, whooping and yelling. To Lee they sounded like they were a baying pack of rabid dogs.

Why had Smiler sent them this way? Did he even know where they would end up?

And then Lee saw the set of concrete steps, going up. Finally pausing to glance back, she saw Helen and Will right behind her.

Without a word, Lee sprang up the steps and pushed open the door at the top. The others quickly followed her through.

Sunlight streamed through large windows caked with dirt, illuminating the rows of shelves and hangers. Notebooks, pencil cases, lunch boxes, toys, key rings, T-shirts, hoodies, all bearing the Smiler logo, were displayed neatly and cleanly. It was as though the shop would open up at any moment and welcome in visitors to Alton Towers.

Lee ran up to the nearest window and peered through the dirt. Despite the sunshine the park was falling into darkness. Thick, black clouds hung low over the theme park, but the setting sun had managed to find a space in the clouds to cast a deep orange glow over everything before it disappeared behind the horizon.

But the theme park was empty.

Down below them the noise of their pursuers echoed up the stairway and into the shop.

Lee pushed open the shop door and Iggy ran past her. She stepped outside. A single drop of rain touched her cheek.

This was their best chance to escape. But they had to run, and fast.

"Wait!" Helen shouted.

Lee turned. "Whatever it is, there's no time! We have to run!"

Helen was standing in the open doorway to the Smiler shop. "It's Will. He's not coming."

Lee could just see him, behind Helen, sitting on the floor of the shop. He'd pulled a hoodie off its hanger and he was cuddling it like it was a favourite teddy bear.

Pushing past Helen, Lee ran back into the shop and grabbed Will by the arm, hauling him to his feet.

"Don't you dare give up now!" she screamed in his face.

Will pulled himself free.

"Leave me alone," he said. "It's my decision, you can't make me change my mind."

He sat down on the floor again.

The first of the theme park kids chasing the teens erupted into the shop, streaming through the doorway and down between the shelves and the hangers. So many of them, filling this space. Their faces crazed, hungry for violence. Within seconds they were streaming around Will, yelling and screaming at him. Will kept on looking at Lee, until he disappeared behind the mass of bodies surrounding him.

Lee turned and ran.

With Helen and Iggy she sprinted through the park, between walls of long grass. They sprinted over a wooden bridge and past a pirate ship built beside a large lake. The surface of the lake's water looked green and stagnant. Without talking they continued running up the hill towards the block of buildings that Lee suspected were part of the main entrance. Lee's lungs ached with each breath she took in and she could feel her legs turning to jelly. How much longer could she do this?

Slowing to a halt, Lee turned and looked back down

towards the Smiler ride. Helen paused too.

No one was following them. Why? Were they satisfied with capturing Will? And what would they do with him?

The shop wasn't visible from where they were standing, but Lee didn't need to see it. The image of Will as he was surrounded by the feral, theme park kids had been burnt into her mind's eye.

"We have to go back and get him," she said.

"We can't do that," Helen said. "There's too many of them, they'll kill us."

"And if we don't do anything they're going to kill Will!" Lee snapped, turning on Helen.

Iggy barked and started growling at Lee.

"I know he's your friend," Helen said, her face twisted with misery and anxiety, "but we can't go back, we just can't."

Lee knew she was right, but still she couldn't move, couldn't command her body to turn and run for the exit, for freedom.

"Please, we should go now, before we're spotted," Helen said.

Lee lowered her head, bit her bottom lip, chewed at it.

"All right," she muttered.

But when they turned to leave, they saw a figure standing by the exit, watching them.

Blade.

The young woman stood with her feet planted apart and holding her bow, relaxed by her side and in her left hand. She didn't appear to be a threat.

"What are we going to do?" Helen whispered.

"We're going to escape, like we planned on doing," Lee replied.

They walked the rest of the way towards Blade and the

237

exits. Blade stood and watched them approach. She made no move to lift her bow or to take an arrow from the quiver slung across her back.

As they drew closer, Lee said, "You can't stop us."

"Where is the other one?" Blade said. "The boy."

"Your friends caught him," Lee said.

Blade said nothing, simply looked at Lee, her face impassive.

"What will they do with him?" Helen said.

"Kill him," Blade said, her voice flat, emotionless.

Lee's stomach dropped at those two words. It wasn't a surprise, she'd known this would be their plan all along. But still, hearing the words said out loud hurt.

"Are you going to kill us too?" Lee said.

Blade continued looking at Lee in silence. Seemed like she was never going to speak, but finally she did.

"No. You should go, run, before you're discovered."

"You're letting us go?" Helen said.

"Yes," Blade said. "Is it that difficult to understand? Now get out of here before the others find you."

Still Lee and Helen didn't move.

"Why?" Lee said. "Why are you doing this?"

"Because not all of us are the same, not all of us agree with . . . Nemesis. Some of us want change, for the better."

Blade lifted her right arm high and then let it drop. From the shadows of the buildings around the exit, the shops and the cafes and the ticket offices, figures emerged. More young people, a mixture of boys and girls but all around the same age as Blade.

"Now go on, get out of here," Blade said. "I'm not going to tell you again."

"We can't leave without Will," Lee said.

238

Blade shook her head.

"You could help us rescue him," Lee said.

Blade shook her head again.

"Why not? Why can't you help us?"

"There are too many of them, too few of us," Blade said. "Besides, we have to live here. It's not perfect, but it's safer than being outside."

"So you're just going to let them murder him?" Lee said. "That makes you a murderer too."

Lee spun around on her heel, turning her back on Blade, and looked back down the path they had just run up. The park was empty still. If Lee and Helen wanted, they could run now.

Get away.

Escape.

"I'm going back," Lee said. "I can't leave him."

"Wait," Blade said.

Lee turned back to face her.

"Maybe we can help," Blade said. "Maybe. I need to talk to the others, we all have to agree."

"There's no time for that!" Lee hissed. "They could be killing him right now!"

"No they won't," Blade said. "Nemesis wants a sacrifice, tonight, when it is dark. She wants to put you all in the Wicker Man and set fire to it. She wants to burn you to death."

"Oh no," Helen whispered.

"Which means they won't hurt your friend yet," Blade said. "We have time."

"All right," Lee said. "Well, go and have your stupid vote. And then we can start planning our next move."

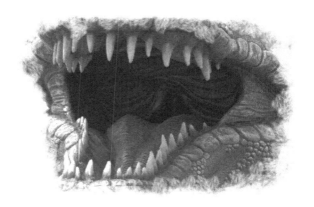

Chapter Twenty-Three

They broke into a house. It didn't take much; the windows were already smashed and the lock on the front door had been busted off. The interior smelt of damp and disuse. Of an accumulation of emptiness.

They decided they would be better off hiding upstairs. That way they wouldn't be taken by surprise if someone entered the house, and they could keep a lookout from the upstairs windows. Daniel offered to keep watch first.

Emily climbed on the double bed, still made as though ready for someone to have a good night's sleep on it, and fell immediately into a deep slumber. Nuo sat by the window with Daniel for a while, looking out across the night enclosed streets. With no streetlights or windows glowing with lamps and televisions, the town took on a different feel. Nuo's eyes were constantly drawn up to a patch of clear sky visible between the thick clouds and filled with stars. It seemed like she'd never seen stars properly before.

"What are we going to do tomorrow?" Nuo said.

Daniel said nothing for a few moments and when he finally

spoke he was looking up at the stars too. "We need to find water and food."

"And then what?"

"I'm sticking with my plan and keep heading north."

"To find your father?"

Daniel nodded.

"But why? How do you know he's alive still?"

"He's alive," Daniel said. "He's too clever to die."

Nuo shook her head. "What does that mean?"

Daniel finally lowered his gaze and looked Nuo in the eye. "There's a lot you don't know, and I'm too tired to try and explain to you right now. But my father might just be the one man who can correct all of this. He might be able to put things right again. But I need to find him, let him know what happened to me. That I'm alive."

"Will that make a difference?" Nuo said.

"Maybe not," Daniel replied. "But Renton was so obsessed with returning me to my father, oh, I don't know." He paused. "It just feels like maybe some of Renton's craziness has passed onto me. Whether I find my father or not, it won't make any difference to him. He's either going to find a way to fix all this, or he isn't. But still, I need to find him. Besides, what else am I going to do?"

Nuo looked over her shoulder at Emily, curled up into a ball in the middle of the bed. "And what about Emily? She wants to go back to her mother. Doesn't she have the right to do that?"

"Emily's mother doesn't exist," Daniel said. "She's just a figment of Emily's imagination."

"Really?"

"Yeah, really. I think she invented her just so she could cope with what had happened, and now she's as real as you and

241

I, but only in her head."

"So what are you going to do?"

"Take her with us."

"Us?"

"Yeah, us. We're sticking together, right?"

Nuo arched an eyebrow. "You're assuming a lot. Did someone put you in charge?"

"No, but. . ." Daniel faltered.

"You say that your father is somehow part of all this madness, that maybe he can fix it, but how can I believe you? Why should I believe you, but not believe Emily about her mother?"

"Because it's the truth," Daniel said.

"According to you."

Daniel looked up at the stars again, as though seeking help from a higher being. The clouds were closing in, the gap becoming smaller. "Are you saying you're not coming with us?"

Nuo placed a hand on Daniel's. He flinched, as though he had been shocked by static electricity.

"No, I'm not saying that. Well, maybe. I just need to think about this some more. I don't know what to believe."

"You mean you don't know who to believe."

Daniel took his hand away from Nuo's and folded his arms.

"Daniel, it's not like that."

"You can do what you want," the teenage boy said. "Go with Emily to find her imaginary mother. I'm heading north. I know where my father is, I've been there before. Even if he can't fix everything, I'll be safe up there."

Nuo sighed. She wanted to punch Daniel, slap some sense into him. "How are you going to get up there all by yourself? We need to stay together."

"I'll be all right. I've survived so far."

242

Nuo turned away. "I'm going to get some sleep."

She climbed on the bed next to Emily and placed her arm gently over the young girl's body.

Daniel continued sitting at the window, gazing up at the stars until the thick rain clouds finally closed in and buried them from view.

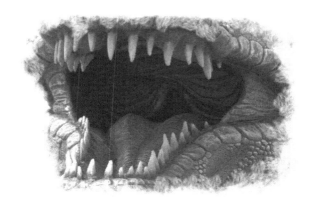

Chapter Twenty-Four

Helen had her hands clapped over her ears, and even Iggy was lying on the floor with his head between his paws, and his ears flattened down along his head. The drum beat, if you could call it that, had begun about half an hour ago and slowly built in intensity from then on. There was no discernible rhythm to the beat and Lee thought the kids had to be using whatever they could lay their hands on to create that awful noise, but if its intent was to unsettle Lee and the others then it was working.

Poor Will, in the middle of all that noise, had to be losing his mind.

Lee wondered how long it would be before Helen lost it too and became even more of a liability than she already was. Helen might have grown up in this world of flesh-eating dinosaurs, tribal groups intent on destroying each other and none of the resources available to Lee in her own time, but she was soft. Hooper had done his job of protecting her too well. Helen was used to living within the confines of a secure compound, milking dinosaur cows and preparing food for the menfolk. Now that she thought about it, Lee realised that the

244

group living at the old Botanical Gardens had reverted to old-fashioned male to female power roles. The men had been the ones with the guns, the ones who ventured outside of the compound's walls, who hunted and explored and rescued the newcomers. The women had to stay inside where it was safe, and cook and clean.

Once they got away from this madhouse, Lee was going to start teaching Helen a few things. Maybe try toughening her up. Her and Will both. It seemed like Lee was having to do everything, to be the alpha leader, and it was exhausting.

Blade and her group of rebels had voted to rescue Will. There seemed to be something else going on too, a decision to mutiny and take control of the theme park for themselves. But Blade wasn't saying anything and Lee was fine with that.

All she wanted was to save Will, and then they could leave.

Blade's group numbered fifteen teenagers, all of them thankfully at the upper age limit and all of them looking reasonably battle hardened. They were split pretty evenly between boys and girls. There were two of the girls in particular who looked tougher than all the boys. They were both lean and hard looking and neither of them spoke much, mainly just muttered comments to each other. One of them wielded a machete, spinning it around in a complicated series of loops and swings. The other, her sister from the look of them, had a crossbow.

Lee was impressed.

"We're going now," Blade said, her face grim. "You stay here and wait for us. We will bring your friend back as soon as we can."

Lee shook her head. "No way, we're coming with you."

Blade glanced over Lee's shoulder at Helen, still sitting on the floor with her hands over her ears. "I would be happy for

245

you to come with us, you look like you can take care of yourself, but what about her?"

"I'll take care of Helen," Lee said.

"No, she'll slow us down, she'll cause problems, we can't risk it. You come with us, but her and the dog stay here."

"No," Lee said. "That ain't happening. We have to stick together. I'm already looking for one friend I've lost, I don't want to be looking for another. We stick together, which means Helen and Iggy are coming with us."

Blade stared at Lee, a muscle twitching in her jaw. Finally she spoke. "All right, do what you want. But if you get into trouble because of her, the rest of us won't be there to rescue you."

"Yeah. Whatever."

Blade turned to face her group. "This is it! The day has come. Maybe it's arrived a little sooner than we thought it would, but we knew it was on its way. Nemesis can't be allowed to carry on like she has, spreading fear and hate and distrust. Today we are going to take back control of the Towers."

Blade's group of teenagers raised their hands and began yelling and whooping.

When the battle cries had died down, Lee said, "And rescue Will."

Blade looked at Lee. "Yes, and rescue your friend."

"Don't forget that bit, will you?"

"We won't forget," Blade replied, and smiled.

Somehow, Lee couldn't take much comfort from that smile.

"Are you ready?" Blade shouted.

"We're ready!" her soldiers shouted back.

"Then let's go."

Will had been pushed and pulled along a maze of paths until he was completely disoriented. Not that he could see much anyway over the heads of the group of children surrounding him. As they walked, they kicked and punched him and tripped him up. Every time he fell down he was hauled back to his feet and slapped and punched again.

And the kids laughed every time he fell over.

Their leader, Nemesis, strode on at the front of the group, leading them through the theme park and past rides almost hidden by the tangle of vines and greenery covering them. The way she held herself, the way she walked, it was as though she believed she was a queen, maybe even a god. And from what Will had seen and heard on this parade to wherever they were taking him, all the kids agreed with her.

Will was shocked at how young some of these children were. Some of them were feral, screaming and hooting unintelligible noises, their bodies and faces covered in dirt and bruises, their clothes ripped and dirty. Nemesis had them under her control but she wasn't caring for them, she wasn't a benevolent leader.

Will tried to not look anyone in the eyes, tried to keep from provoking anyone. It was bad enough that they kept slapping and tripping him, but if they really took it into their heads to hurt him he dreaded to think what they would do.

Onward they moved, deeper into the theme park.

Will's chest tightened as the kids cheered, and he saw the wooden structure appear above the treetops.

It had two faces, one on the front and the other on the back. It looked pagan in its design.

Will glimpsed a signpost as he was shoved closer to the

247

structure.

The Wickerman.

Of course.

He recognised it now.

And his stomach shrivelled into a tiny knot at the thought of what might be happening next.

Will had never been to Alton Towers before. It wasn't the kind of place his parents approved of. But he had read about the Wickerman when the ride had first been built. How Alton Towers had claimed that it was not based on the film of the same name, and yet the ride involved the participants being offered as a sacrifice to the Wickerman and the roller coaster cars shot through an opening in the huge, wooden structure as fake flames licked at its sides.

In the film the lead character had similarly been imprisoned in a huge wooden effigy which was then set on fire, while the pagan revellers danced around it.

Was this what Nemesis and her followers had in mind for Will?

As they entered the lane that organised the queues on busy days they had to order themselves into single file. The kids began banging sticks on the handrails as they walked, and the awful noise grew and grew as more of Nemesis's followers joined in.

Will twisted his head this way and that, looking for escape routes. But the lad behind Will was holding his arms tight as they walked and drew closer to the Wickerman.

They held their flaming torches high, flickering orange and yellow in the darkness, casting a hellish glow over the pagan symbols carved into wooden signs stationed along the path. Backwards and forwards the procession zigzagged along the lane. Because there was no queue they could have simply walked straight to the Wickerman, but this parading up and down in tight formation seemed part of the ceremony.

Nemesis stopped at the station where riders would have boarded the cars. The only way up to the Wickerman from here was by climbing the track up and down its loops. Nemesis lifted her arms, holding a flaming torch in each hand. The fire crackled and sparked, but none of that seemed to bother Nemesis.

The children gathered on the platform with her, as many as could fit on there. Will was dragged through the crowd and placed directly in front of Nemesis. The drumming and the laughter and shouting had stopped. Other than the sound of the burning torches, there was a heavy silence.

Everyone was waiting.

"Tonight," Nemesis shouted, her voice ringing out clear and bright, "we make a sacrifice to the Wickerman."

The children cheered, as though they had just been told that school had been cancelled for the week and they could go home and do as they please.

Will struggled to get free, but his captor's grip was too tight.

"No, please don't," he said, looking up at Nemesis.

The young woman ignored him, as though he was of no consequence to her except as an offering to her god.

At a signal from Nemesis two of her acolytes pulled Will to the floor and began tying him up. Will kicked and punched and struggled but he was quickly overcome. They were too strong. Once his hands and feet were bound, they threw him into a ride car parked at the station. The children had begun their drumming again, hitting any surface they could find with sticks and hammers and whatever they could lay their hands on. The beat was growing wilder all the time.

The boys jumped down onto the track and manoeuvred

Will onto the seat and then locked the safety bar in place over his thighs. They began pushing the cart up the slope towards the Wickerman effigy. The children on the platform had begun howling and hooting and stamping their feet.

They were celebrating.

Once the boys had pushed the ride car underneath the Wickerman structure, one of them locked it in place and they ran back down the track. Will squirmed in the seat, trying to push himself out. He could smell petrol fumes.

The crowd of children behind him suddenly fell silent. Will tried to turn in the seat, to see what was happening. He was pinned in too tight by the bar across his lap. And then there was a cheer, and the night sky lit up with the glow of yellow flame.

* * *

From her hiding place Lee saw Nemesis touch the two flaming torches to the wooden base of the track, igniting them. Bright orange flames carved a path up the roller coaster track towards the Wickerman effigy where Will was currently trapped.

Blade gave the signal.

Her band of followers sprang from their hiding places. Arrows sliced through the air, clattering against the wooden track and the onto the ride station's platform. Lee hung back for a moment, waiting to see how this was going to play out. She wasn't interested in the power struggles between Blade and Nemesis, or who was going to win this fight.

All she wanted was to get Will out of that wooden monstrosity currently blazing with fire

"Wait here," she said to Helen, squatting beside Lee and holding on to Iggy.

Lee ran out from their hiding place. Already some of the

250

kids who followed Nemesis were fleeing into the woodland surrounding the Wickerman ride, whilst the braver ones were charging out to meet their attackers. Lee spotted the twins in front. The one with the crossbow fired off an arrow, and it sank into a young lad's chest. He collapsed, clutching at the arrow protruding from his chest, gasping in pain.

The twin ran up to him, placed a booted foot on his torso, pinning him to the ground, and yanked the arrow from his chest.

Lee looked away, sickened.

This wasn't a playground scrap between a bunch of kids. They meant business.

Keeping her attention set on the wooden structure where Will was being held, Lee dodged between fighting kids. More of the roller coaster track had become engulfed in bright yellow and orange flames. Lee leapt at the fence separating her from the ride and scrambled over it, jumping to the ground on the opposite side. This next bit would be easy, climbing up the slats and beams holding the ride together. Once on the track she could approach the Wickerman from the opposite end where the fire hadn't reached yet.

But she knew she had to be quick. Already the Wickerman itself was alight, and greasy, grey smoke spiralled up along with sparks, bright against the night sky.

Lee ran up the curving slope. The heat from the flames scorched her face and all her instincts shouted at her to turn and run before she caught fire too.

But she could hear Will coughing. She pushed herself on, up the slope, towards the dark hole into the Wickerman.

Lee began coughing as she scrambled inside. Shadows danced around the interior as the flames licked at the slats.

Will retched and coughed and tears streamed down his face.

251

Lee climbed into the car with him and began pulling at the ropes. Her fingers fumbled at the knots. She could hardly see anything now, the smoke had grown so dense and her eyes were blurred with tears. Between his hacking coughs, Will was shouting something, but Lee couldn't make out what.

Deciding to forget about the ropes, Lee grabbed the safety bar pinning Will into the seat and yanked at it. The bar moved an inch at the most before hitting a lock.

Unless she found the release mechanism, there was no way she could pull that rigid bar open.

Will leaned in close to Lee and coughed in her ear. But she heard a single word too.

"Push!"

Not understanding, Lee pushed down on the safety bar, thinking maybe that was what released it.

Will screamed as the bar dug deeper into his lap and locked into place.

"Push . . ." he coughed, ". . . the . . ." he spluttered and coughed more, ". . . car!"

Suddenly Lee understood. She scrambled out of the roller coaster car and leant her weight into it, pushing it off the apex of the upward loop they were on. The car was heavy. Despite pushing with everything she had it only moved an inch or two. Lee sank to her knees, coughing and retching. The fire had grown in intensity since she got here. From above she heard a crack from the Wickerman as it began to fall apart.

Lee pulled herself upright. They had to get out of now or they were going to die.

Drawing on every last bit of mental strength and willpower she could, Lee pushed everything she had against that car. It moved again, and this time it kept on moving.

Lee scrambled inside, landing half on top of Will.

The car kept travelling forward.

They rolled into a wall of flame.

Searing heat, charring her clothes, her skin.

And then they were out, gathering speed as they rolled down the slope towards the next incline.

Lee gripped the sides of the car, holding herself in inside and partly on top of Will. Going through the flames had felt like she was being burnt alive, but she could see they were both fine. Both of them were still coughing, but the fresh air, even though it still smelt of smoke, felt good in her lungs. The car sped down the incline and then began its ascent up the next slope. Without power it soon came to a halt and rolled back down to the dip between the two loops.

Lee looked back at the Wickerman. Through eyes blurred with tears she saw it crashing in on itself in a shower of sparks and flames. The fire was spreading quickly, swallowing up the roller coaster ride in vibrant yellow and orange flames.

Lee pulled at the bar pinning Will into his seat but it refused to budge.

"There's a lever on the side," Will said between coughs. "It releases the safety bar."

Lee found the lever and released it. The bar swung up easily. Will sat up and Lee began working at the knots on the ropes. Down below the ride were the sounds of warrior-like yells and screams of pain as the battle continued.

"What's happening?" Will said, as the rope fell from his wrists.

Lee quickly filled him in on the rescue plan while she worked on the knots tying his ankles together.

"The thing is," she said, "I think Blade is as much of a psycho as Nemesis. We need to get out of here as fast as we can."

"No argument from me," Will said.

The two teenagers climbed down to the ground. Immediately they were engulfed by bodies, children fighting each other, hacking and slashing and punching and kicking each other. But Lee and Will seemed invisible as no one paid them any attention.

They pushed their way through the fight, Lee fending off punches thrown her way and bodies pushed in their path. They kept shoving until they were through the mass of bodies and into a clearer space. A coffee shop in front of them was ablaze and smaller fires were starting amongst the trees.

"This whole place is going to burn to the ground," Lee said. "Let's find Helen and Iggy and get out of here."

They ran around the back of the blazing coffee shop, making sure to give it a wide berth. When they got to the spot where Helen and Iggy had been hiding, Lee stopped and looked around in confusion.

They were nowhere to be seen.

"Over here!" Helen shouted, emerging from a covering of trees and holding Iggy by his collar.

The dog had his tail down between his legs and his ears laid flat against his head. He looked utterly miserable and afraid.

"Let's go," Lee said.

They ran back the way they had come, along paths of erupted tarmac, weeds whipping at their ankles and long fronds swaying in a breeze.

Soon they were at the entrance to the park, and this time there was no one there to stop them leaving. The three teens climbed over the barriers whilst Iggy squeezed his way through a gap, and they ran between abandoned cars on the car park. They had no torches, but they didn't need any as the night was bright with the flickering light of the huge fire in the park. Once they were out of the seemingly endless number of parking sections and back on a main road, they paused and looked back at Alton Towers.

The theme park resembled a massive bonfire, the biggest bonfire the world had ever seen. A cloud of bright yellow sparks hung over the raging fire. It seemed unreal, like something from a fantasy film.

"What now?" Helen said.

Lee was about to speak, but Will got there before her.

"We need to find some shelter, somewhere to stay the night." He paused and looked at Lee. All of a sudden there seemed to be a steely determination in Will's eyes that Lee hadn't seen before. Maybe it was the reflection of the fire in Will's glasses.

Or maybe it was something more.

"And then tomorrow we're going to find our friend," Will said.

Lee nodded and smiled.

"That's right," she said.

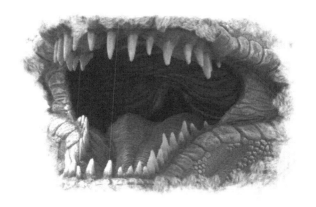

Chapter Twenty-Five

The morning dawned bright and cold. Daniel and Nuo searched the house and the neighbouring houses for food and drink, but every house they searched had already been cleared out. Daniel's thirst was building and his stomach was painful from hunger pangs. He knew the others were feeling the same.

When they had given up their search and returned to the house where they had spent the night, Emily announced her intention to return to the service station on the motorway. There was water and food back there.

And her mother would be waiting for her.

Daniel noticed the glance that Nuo threw his way.

He said to Emily, "That's a good idea, we'll come with you."

Daniel still didn't believe that Emily's mother existed. Somebody had set up the water catchers and the drainage system, but Daniel thought it was more likely that Emily had stumbled upon the place after whoever had set it up had been outside, hunting maybe or just exploring, and never come back. He agreed to return with Emily because it was a good idea.

There was food and water, and the van hadn't travelled that far before it broke down so Daniel reckoned they could be back at the service station well before nightfall. They just had to hope the rats had gone.

The other reason he decided to head back with Emily? He was tired of arguing. Tired of trying to make the decisions. Nuo was right, nobody had appointed him leader and so he needed to stop pretending to be one.

They followed the road signs to the M6 and then began the slow trudge south.

The blue sky looked set to stay with them all day, but there was a mass of dark clouds off in the distance.

"Hey," Nuo said after they had been walking in silence for a while, "did anyone see that huge fire last night?"

"Nah," Emily said.

"I saw it," Daniel replied. "It started not long before I turned in."

"It lit up the entire horizon, it was amazing," Nuo said.

Daniel turned and pointed to the shadow hovering in the distance. "I thought those were clouds, but maybe it's smoke."

"I think so too," Nuo said. "I hope the fire doesn't spread."

"Doesn't matter if it does," Emily said. "We're nowhere near it."

They kept walking, mostly in silence. Mostly looking out for creatures, listening for rustling in the long grass on the sides of the motorway, waiting for that moment when they would have to run.

But nothing pursued them, there were no prehistoric roars to ruin the beautiful day, the peace and the quiet. If he closed his eyes and paused for a moment he could almost convince himself he was out for a pleasant walk.

Almost.

257

It was mid-afternoon when Emily spotted the bridge over the motorway that linked the southbound and northbound services. They had made good time.

Although he was pleased to see the service station once more, and looking forward to drinking some of that water, his stomach still tightened up at the thought of the rats.

Please let them be gone!

"Are you sure there's water there?" Nuo whispered to Daniel as Emily strode ahead.

"Yeah, loads of it, and packet food too."

"Good, because I'm not sure how much longer I can keep doing this."

Despite their tiredness, despite their thirst and hunger, the three children picked up their pace.

As they walked up the slip road, Daniel slowed Emily down.

"We need to take care," he said. "The rats might still be there and even if they aren't, someone else might have turned up and not be happy about seeing us and having to share food and water."

"But it's my food and water," Emily said.

"I don't think that's how it works anymore," Daniel said. "Whoever has possession has ownership these days."

Emily didn't look happy with that answer, but she slowed down as Daniel requested.

Before they stepped inside, they had a good look around outside. Daniel was interested to see if he could spot something different, a sign that might warn them about intruders. But he wasn't really sure that he could see anything different at all and eventually gave in to Emily who kept prodding him let her go in.

They stepped through the shattered windows, glass shards

crunching beneath their shoes. It looked just as Daniel remembered, except there were no rats flooding down the steps that lead to the bridge, and then chasing them outside.

"I think all the rats have gone," Emily whispered.

"Why are you whispering?" Daniel whispered.

"I don't know, why are you whispering?" Emily whispered back.

Daniel rolled his eyes and Emily giggled. It wasn't much of a giggle, just a tiny one, but it lifted Daniel's heart for a moment.

"Let's look upstairs, shall we?" Nuo said.

They took the steps together, walking slowly in a line. With every step higher, Daniel's heart thudded as he waited for a rat to appear at the top of the stairs. It was only when they finally arrived at the top, looking along the covered bridge over the motorway, that Daniel truly began to believe that the rats really had gone.

Although they had left behind plenty of rat droppings.

"It stinks up here!" Nuo said.

"You should have been here when you couldn't see the floor for rats," Daniel said.

"Where's this water?"

"Follow me," Emily said, stepping carefully between the rat poo.

The water dispensers still worked and the water itself tasted sweeter than Daniel remembered. The three of them drank and then sat with their backs to the wall.

"I never thought water could be so lovely and tasty," Nuo said, wiping her lips and her chin. "Maybe we should just stay here from now on, we've got everything we need, right?"

Daniel shifted position a little. He didn't want to argue, but he had to say something.

"I can't do that," he said. "Tomorrow I'm going to head north again. I need to find him, find out what happened to my father."

"I don't believe it!" Nuo said. "Can't you just—"

The unmistakable sound of a gun being cocked silenced Nuo and had all three children looking up.

The woman stood with her feet planted apart and a shotgun in her hands pointing right at Daniel and Nuo. Her shaved scalp and the boots on her feet, the camouflage clothing and her stance gave her the appearance of a soldier.

"Emily," she said.

Emily jumped to her feet and ran to the woman and threw her arms around her.

"I knew you'd be here! I knew it!"

Emily's mother still had the shotgun trained on Daniel and Nuo.

"You two have got some explaining to do," she said. "And it had better be good."

Thank You

As usual, it is my pleasure to acknowledge the people who helped make this book what it is. If it wasn't for the following readers, writers, and friends, this story wouldn't be in the shape it is today.

First up, as always, I need to thank my friend and beta reader Carrie Rowlands for her first read-through, picking up of typos and continuity errors, and comments on the story.

The following generous and kind-hearted readers also contributed by reading and reviewing and generally encouraging me:

Julian White, Silvasurfa, Alan, Katherine Turner, Beverly Laude, Marjorie, Paul Willmott, Rick Bancroft, Tina C, and Shaz Richmond.

Thank you!

Books

Ken Preston

The Devil and Edward Teach

Caxton Tempest at the End of the World

Planet of the Dinosaurs Book One: Project Wormhole

Planet of the Dinosaurs Book Two: The Journey North

Visit me at

https://kenpreston.co.uk/books-for-young-adults/

47040434R00160

Printed in Poland
by Amazon Fulfillment
Poland Sp. z o.o., Wrocław